You Don't Have to Suffer

You Don't Have to Suffer

A Complete Guide to Relieving Cancer Pain
for Patients and Their Families

Susan S. Lang
Richard B. Patt, M.D.

New York   Oxford
OXFORD UNIVERSITY PRESS
1994

Oxford University Press

Oxford   New York   Toronto
Delhi   Bombay   Calcutta   Madras   Karachi
Kuala Lumpur   Singapore   Hong Kong   Tokyo
Nairobi   Dar es Salaam   Cape Town
Melbourne   Auckland   Madrid

and associated companies in
Berlin   Ibadan

Published by Oxford University Press, Inc.,
200 Madison Avenue, New York, New York 10016

Oxford is a registered trademark of Oxford University Press

Library of Congress Cataloging-in-Publication Data
Lang, Susan S. You Don't Have to Suffer /
Susan S. Lang, Richard B. Patt.
p. cm.   Includes bibliographical references and index.
ISBN 0-19-508418-7
1. Cancer pain.   I. Patt, Richard B.   II. Title.
RC262.L27   1994
362.1'96994—dc20   93-30173

Dose schedules are being continually revised and new side effects recognized.
Oxford University Press and the authors make no representation, express or
implied, that the drug dosages in this book are correct. For these reasons, readers are strongly urged to consult their physicians and the drug company's printed
instructions before taking any drugs.

1 3 5 7 9 8 6 4 2

Printed in the United States of America
on acid-free paper

In loving memory of my mother,
Beatrice Lang,
and my in-laws,
Jerry and Mickey Schneider,
all of whom taught me
lessons of life, love, and death.

S. S. L.

To yesterday's,
today's,
and tomorrow's cancer patients
who deserve the best.

R. B. P.

Preface

My father-in-law died in agony from lung cancer in 1980, the "dark ages" for modern cancer pain relief. When his wife fell ill with terminal brain cancer several years later, she begged us not to hospitalize her, thinking that it was her husband's hospitalization that caused him such misery. During a spell of strength, she flew up to visit us, but her first night, she collapsed. As she grew more ill, she stayed in our living room. Over the following six weeks or so, we cared for her as she declined. A dear and gifted physician, Bernard Friedman, M.D., helped us manage her pain, and she died a gentle death in 1984. By 1992, when my mom became gravely ill with a painful cancer (cancer of the septum that spread through the palate and mouth), I was so grateful that I already had some experience with knowing what we as family members could do in cooperation with a team of caring, well-informed, health-care professionals to work together to relieve the potentially intractable pain of cancer.

This book is the manual I wished I had from the beginning. It would have helped me understand how pain relievers work, what doctors need to know to do their job best, how other kinds of medications or treatments could contribute to comfort, how to relieve side effects and other distressing symptoms, including depression and anxiety, all of which can contribute to the suffering associated with cancer. We have tried to provide important background information about many aspects of cancer pain, so that when meeting with doctors, precious time may be used well, discussing the particular case in hand, instead of having to provide background information. We have also provided many comfort care tips so that the loved one caring for the patient can step in with confidence that he or she is well prepared.

This book is not, however, meant to be used in place of a physician's care. We mean to educate and offer tips for comfort care, but not to prescribe a treatment plan for any particular patient. Only a doctor who understands the patient's particular illness and condition can tailor the options to plan a well-thought-out treatment plan. Similarly, although we may refer to a medication or treatment as usually or often recommended for a particular condition, there are always exceptions, and physicians are best equipped to use that judgment. Nor do the listings of particular organizations or references necessarily mean we endorse them all, for they were too numerous to assess. This book is to be used as a tool to foster open communication between the health-care team and the patient and family, and to foster self-education—again, not as a recommendation or prescription for any particular treatments.

We hope that our use of gender pronouns and references to family members and loved ones will not offend anyone. Rather than using either or both male and female pronouns for physicians and patients, which seemed awkward, we have used masculine pronouns in places. There are, obviously, many female physicians and many female patients. Likewise, we often referred to family members as synonymous with caregivers. There are, of course, many nontraditional family units and loving primary caregivers who are not family members. Again, forgive us for not always including loving and primary caregivers who are not relatives. We made these language decisions only to keep the language simple and clear.

Ithaca, New York   Susan S. Lang

This book is among the most important accomplishments of my professional life, and the reason is because you are reading it. My day-to-day work involves working with cancer patients and their families to enhance comfort on a one-to-one basis. In an effort to widen that impact I teach groups of medical and nursing students, and even rooms full of trained health-care providers about how to better control pain and improve communication with their patients. Time though is limited, and since each day marks the needless suffering of countless patients, this book represents a special opportunity to communicate with those who need this information the most.

Both the practice of medicine and the experience of being a patient have become complicated and are changing rapidly. Cancer is a frightening, overwhelming experience—even to the treating doctor, and as a result, it is an experience around which our communication skills often falter. Consider the careful research and negotiation we engage in when buying a car or television, and then how something seems to strike us dumb when we sit in the same room with a doctor, especially when discussing serious or life-threatening illnesses. This book is intended to promote your role as informed partners to ensure your appropriate health care.

Pain is a very common problem in patients with cancer, and one that if allowed to persist not only degrades quality of life but interferes with cancer cure. Pain can almost always be managed effectively, but much too often, it isn't. We live in a drug-phobic society. We are so troubled about the specter of drug abuse that the beneficial effects of pain medications are too often ignored. They tell us "Just say no" when the postscript should read

". . . unless prescribed by your physician for a legitimate medical reason." Doctors are taught far too little in medical school about using pain medicines safely and effectively. Tragically, together we fail to distinguish between the drug addict who would break any law or trust to get a "high" from drugs and the relief that can come for the suffering cancer patient if just the right amount of the right drug were prescribed at the right time.

Important scientific advances have made some cancers easier to treat and have brought cure into sight for others. The point of this book is that having cancer is dehumanizing enough without the indignity of unrelieved pain. There is more and more attention being brought to bear on managing the suffering of today's patients while we continue to search for the cure for tomorrow's victims of cancer. These two priorities can and should exist together.

Managing today's pain is not about looking for a new technology or new painkiller, but about maintaining the same intensity of care for patients throughout the course of a cancer illness—whether that care is directed at shrinking the tumor or managing pain and distress. All of this gets easier when doctors act not out of treating a cancer, a tumor or a "case," but instead recognize that they are dealing with people who are ill. Similarly, health care works best when, as a patient, you are able to relate to your doctor as your partner in health care, engaged with you in a process that depends on communication and mutual respect, rather than as an impersonal, unapproachable authority figure. Relationships of this quality don't happen automatically, but are achievable. This book is also intended to help patients and doctors recognize how dependent they are on each other, and how the quality of their relationship can influence the outcome of health care. Armed with the information in this book, we believe that today's patients will be able to work more closely and confidently with their doctors to maintain the best quality of life available to them.

Austin, Texas   Richard B. Patt, M.D.

Acknowledgments

Thanks go to Dennis Meredith, for referring me to the Pain Management Information Center (PMIC) in the first place, to Jerry Nye of PMIC and Hospicare, Ithaca, whose choice of a co-author was right on target, to Susan Neiberg Terkel whose generous spirit opened yet another professional door for me, to Bob Silverstein, my agent.

For showing me how to actually put this information into practice and helping my family and me care for my mother dying of a painful cancer, my thanks go first to Linda Lerner, R.N., L.L.B., and Marvin Frankel, R.Ph., M.S., of HNS-New York, Inc. (part of Home Nutritional Services), whose constant support and expertise helped keep us steady, strong, and skilled. A special thanks to Peggy Kennedy, R.N., as the first "stranger" to come into our home when my mom was so sick and for throwing that first lifeline and convincing my dad, Solon Lang, to catch it and to accept help with home care. And thanks also go to Rose Rafanelli of HNS for her highly skilled nursing support and to Dr. Marc Citron of Long Island Jewish Hospital whose compassion and direction ensured that my mother need not suffer.

My final grateful words go to my husband, Tom Schneider, for his unflinching support, love, and perceptive insights that continue to nourish me and keep me on track, and to my daughter, Julia, who understood when some phone calls were important ones, and patiently waited for me to finish them.

S. S. L.

I am fortunate to work in a field populated by many compassionate health-care providers who have influenced me. My acknowledgment goes out to people like Russell Portenoy, Eduardo Bruera, Kathy Foley, and John Bonica who, by virtue of their work and their caring, have made my job easier. Special acknowledgments are due to my first teacher whose heart is as large as the population of India, Subhash Jain. I wish to thank my colleagues at the University of Rochester, where I started this book and was provided with the mortar and brick to build one of the most outstanding pain programs in the country. Special thanks go to my first chief, Ronald Gabel, for his vision, and to his predecessor, Denham Ward, Fred Perkins for his support, nurses Laura Hogan and Marie Flannery for their across-the-board quality, and Olga Welling and Eileen Smith, who provided the best administrative support ever. The gifts of my parents and all of those in my personal life who have shown me love are beyond thanking, but I shall do so anyway. Most of all, my patients and their families have always given me back more than I could possibly predict or imagine and are most directly responsible for my accomplishments. Special thanks go to the families of Hugh Cumming, Chuck Kayser, Karen Howe, Ray White, and Betty Jennison who, like others I have had the privilege to care for, will remain a part of me forever.

R. B. P.

And we'd both like to thank our editor Joan Bossert, whose enthusiasm for the project made it happen, as well as Neil Ellison, M.D., and Russell Portenoy, M.D., whose very helpful comments on the manuscript helped us improve it.

Contents

Death I understand very well, it is suffering I cannot understand.

Isaac B. Singer

Part I

CANCER AND ITS PAIN

1

Cancer Pain Undermines Cancer Treatment

Pain is a more terrible Lord of mankind than even death itself.
—Albert Schweitzer

To be struck with cancer, or have a loved one afflicted with cancer, is frightening. To endure the pain of cancer is overwhelming. To witness that anguish in a loved one is heartbreaking. To discover later, however, that the suffering might have been prevented is the worst of all.

The words of Albert Schweitzer, the legendary physician and humanitarian, still ring true today: pain is a more terrible lord than even death itself. Uppermost in the minds of many cancer victims are fears and anxiety about pain. Yet these fears may finally be put to rest. Today, we are equipped with a modern arsenal of drugs and techniques capable of eradicating cancer pain in most cases. Around the country, in doctors' offices, pain clinics, and leading medical colleges, patients, physicians, and pain specialists are working together to ensure that cancer pain is properly treated and quelled where possible.

Yet, tragically, many people still believe that unrelieved pain is inevitable with cancer. Anxiety about the agony of cancer has its roots in the haunting memories from earlier times when cancer pain could not be avoided. Loved ones suffered with quiet stoicism, or not so quiet rage, trying to bear the pain as best they could. Their physicians, having done all they could to treat the cancer, would shake their heads and apologize to the family that they could do no more. Families kept their vigil but despaired at their inability to ease the suffering.

Those "old days" were as recent as the early 1980s.

Today, new knowledge reveals that pain is not merely a side effect of cancer, but an integral part of the disease and a serious medical problem that needs to be confronted and treated as aggressively as the tumor itself. Pain is as much an enemy of the cancer patient as any virulent disease, because it robs a patient of the energy needed to fight the illness and to comply with demanding treatment regimens. Pain interferes with eating, sleeping, and the overall functioning of the body—all of which are vital in times of stress. Unrelieved, pain drains us of our emotional, psychological, and physical well-being, wearing down our natural abilities to fight disease. Some experts even suspect that pain can weaken the immune system, perhaps promoting the disease process.

Advances in pain management have also shown that pain is not a psychological problem. It is an experience that encompasses the whole body—the mind, the flesh, the soul, and the spirit. By not confronting cancer pain head on, we are not only denying our loved ones and ourselves the opportunity to live life to the fullest, and to value the life we have, but also to rally all the body's natural reserves and healing abilities against the disease.

CANCER PAIN IS NEEDLESS, YET UNDERTREATED

In most cases, cancer pain *can* be relieved, and yet we find it is too frequently left undermedicated. Despite great advances in biomedical knowledge and technological savvy in how to ease the pain of cancer, the majority of patients with cancer continue to suffer. The reason is because the readily available and relatively simple-to-use pain treatment methods, in general, are not being adequately used. This situation is changing every day, but unfortunately not quickly enough for some. Every day around the world, there is a silent yet deafening tragedy being played out—the tragedy of needless cancer pain.

To prevent needless cancer pain, patients, families, and friends must learn to put aside their fears about using narcotic medications, to abandon their stoicism in the face of pain, to ask for more help when the pain is unabated, and to learn how to help their doctors take full advantage of available resources to fight cancer pain. They should never give up and assume that there is little that can be done to ease the pain and suffering of cancer. If family members take an active role in helping the doctor and health-care professionals manage the pain of a loved one who has been stricken with cancer, they can be assured of the best possible quality of life for the patient even during the worst of times. By working with their doctor to achieve control of cancer pain and suffering, families can avoid the all-too-common and unnecessary agony associated with cancer.

At the same time, health-care professionals need to be vigilant about pain, assessing it properly and treating it aggressively. Communication between these professionals and patients and their caregivers must be open and responsive to the patient's changing needs. Together, the health-care professionals and caregivers must actively work to relieve the suffering of cancer;

that care requires nurturing and nourishing not only the body, but the mind and spirit as well.

Pain is fairly common with cancer, yet it is *not* inevitable—with proper care, the pain and suffering of cancer can be relieved.

MOST FAMILIES WILL BE AFFECTED

Despite millions of dollars of research spent in the quest for a cure, cancer is becoming more and more common. Every year, 1 million Americans and 6 million people more worldwide become victims of cancer. At any one time, some 14 million people around the world have active cancer. One in five of us will die from the disease: 500,000 die of cancer every year. This is one cancer death every minute all year long. Eventually, 53 million Americans alive today will be given a diagnosis of cancer, and three out of four families will confront this disease. Several exciting advances are taking place in research labs throughout the country, with much hope for the future, but what about today's patient and pain?

When a person is first diagnosed with cancer, the first two questions that typically come to mind are: "Am I going to die?" and "Will I be in pain?" The truth is and studies show that the public believes cancer pain is worse than it really is. Nevertheless, pain is among the most common symptoms of cancer—about one-third of those in the early stages of the disease and up to 80 percent of those in the late stages will have pain that is severe enough to warrant medication. Unfortunately, some 1.1 million Americans and 9 million people around the world suffer from cancer-related pain on any given day—and 3.5 million people every day around the world will not receive adequate treatment.

The situation is improving, but overall, cancer pain continues to be a major unresolved health problem that demands solution.

CANCER PAIN CAN BE RELIEVED

Although cancer pain can be agonizing if its symptoms are left untreated, relief can be achieved in 90 to 99 percent of patients. Relatively simple medical treatments can eliminate the suffering of about 85 percent of cancer patients; these include the use of analgesics (painkillers), such as morphine and other opioids, or other simple treatments that have been in use for quite some time and require only the doctor's prescription. For the remaining 15 percent who require more complex treatments, recent advances in cancer pain management—a burgeoning new medical subspecialty—can be applied to relieve pain in almost all cases.

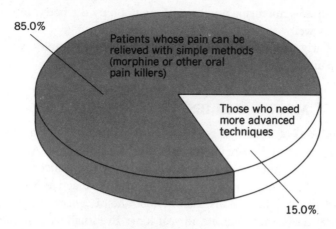

Figure 1.1. *Percentage of cancer patients requiring simple or advanced techniques of pain management. Pain can be controlled in most patients with simple methods.*

WHY DO SO MANY STILL SUFFER?

Studies of only a few years ago revealed that 50 to 80 percent of cancer patients in the industrialized "developed" world suffered unnecessarily. Although the situation is getting better, many cases of cancer pain are still undertreated. In developing countries, where medications are far more scarce and know-how severely limited, the situation is especially bad. (See Figure 1.2.)

What can explain the neglect of such a severe health problem? Why is our well-stocked arsenal of pain management tools underused? Unfortunately, myths, misinformation, and biases about narcotic (opioid) use abound among both the public and health-care professionals. On the one hand, patients fail to communicate the pain problems adequately to health-care providers. On the other hand, doctors and nurses need to take pain more seriously. Both sides harbor fears about narcotics. Moreover, addiction on the streets has led to laws and regulations that strongly discourage or inhibit doctors from prescribing appropriate doses of narcotics. How puzzling that U.S. scientists must fill out intricate forms describing how the comfort and pain relief of laboratory animals are being ensured, and yet no such guarantees are in place for humans.

CANCER PAIN EXPERTS SPEAK OUT

Around the world, an energetic and enthusiastic group of cancer pain experts are trying to underscore the unnecessary tragedy of cancer-related pain. And these experts assert that unrelieved cancer pain is a prevalent yet avoid-

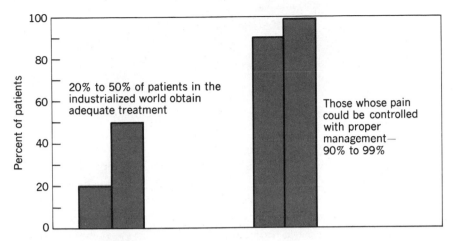

Figure 1.2. *The tragedy of needless pain. Cancer pain can be controlled in the majority of patients.*

able health problem in most countries, including the United States and other Western nations. In the words of Dr. Charles Schuster, former director of the National Institute on Drug Abuse: "The way we treat cancer pain borders on a national disgrace."[1] Another expert, one of America's leading cancer pain specialists and chief of Pain Service at New York's Memorial Sloan-Kettering Cancer Center, Kathleen Foley, M.D., adds: "Society has a strong anti-drug attitude, and cancer patients are caught in the middle. There is no excuse for a cancer patient to be suffering from pain."[2] And we hear a very similar message from an expert committee of the World Health Organization: "Freedom from pain should become the right of every cancer victim and access to pain therapy is a measure of respect for this right."[3]

And from the Wisconsin Cancer Pain Initiative, the country's leader in state efforts to relieve cancer pain: "Unrelieved pain destroys the quality of life for patients and family alike. Cancer is difficult enough to confront without the debilitating effects of uncontrolled pain. . . . Tragically, patients and the public do not know and are not being told that cancer pain can be managed."[4]

Finally, James R. Oleson, M.D., Ph.D., associate professor of radiation oncology at Duke University Medical Center and an advisory board member of the Pain Management Information Center, a national consulting service for physicians providing expert advice on controlling cancer pain (see Appendix) summed up his views and those of others we talked to: "Based on my experience, at least half the time cancer patients have inadequately managed pain. It's a distressing situation. With all of our modern medical technology, very simple approaches to cancer pain management are under-utilized. People need not suffer the kind of pain they frequently do suffer with cancer."[5]

THE FEAR OF NARCOTICS

Although the suffering from cancer calls for the legitimate and appropriate use of painkillers such as morphine, our entire society is programmed to "Just Say No." As a culture, we tend not to distinguish between legitimate and illegitimate use of narcotics, also called opiates or opioids, and as a result, many doctors are reluctant to prescribe these medications ade-quately. And even when prescribed, patients are reluctant to take them as part of their treatment.

As former director for the National Institute on Drug Abuse, Dr. Charles Schuster is all too familiar with our culture's view of drugs: "Unfortunately, in our culture, the phrase 'drug addiction' conjures up a mental image of street life with its hustling of drugs, its criminal entrepreneurs who exploit and victimize, its shooting galleries, disease, filth and desperation. *But this image of drug addiction has nothing whatsoever to do with treatment of cancer patients for pain.* . . . [T]here is simply no evidence that appropriate pre-scription of pharmacologic agents used to treat pain results in drug addic-tion."

In fact, clinical experience suggests that the actual risk of addiction is only about 1 in 10,000 for patients taking medications prescribed to control cancer pain. Dr. Charles Schuster continues: "The overriding ethic which must guide our use of the narcotic drugs for the treatment of severe cancer pain is that no patient should suffer needlessly, and no patient should wish for death, because of our failure to use properly our strongest weapons against pain."[6] Even though these same drugs destroy lives and families when they are abused, they restore lives and families of cancer patients when used properly, because they allow them to resume more active lives, to fight their disease, and to preserve an essential quality of life.

CONFUSION OVER ADDICTION, DEPENDENCY, AND TOLERANCE

Far too many people, including some health-care professionals, confuse sev-eral factors associated with the legitimate long-term use of painkillers. Un-fortunately, people often lump them together under the term *addiction*, a term that has been often misused, so much so that it has ceased to have a clear meaning. Outdated and unscientific ideas about opioids reinforce ir-rational fears about the safety of medication use among cancer patients.

Thus it is critical that the terms addiction, dependency, and tolerance are distinguished from each other and better understood so that unfounded fears will not interfere with the proper and appropriate care of cancer patients.

Addiction is a psychological craving for a drug. The need to obtain and use a drug completely overwhelms and controls the addict's life. Addiction involves the use of drugs for nonmedical purposes and is extremely rare among cancer patients.

Physical dependence, on the other hand, is a common and natural result of the body growing accustomed to a medication (including drugs other than opioids), so that physical problems and signs of withdrawal would occur if the drug were suddenly stopped. Physical dependence needn't and shouldn't interfere with good pain control. If physical dependence occurs and medication becomes unnecessary because the cancer improves, complete withdrawal without complications can be accomplished in a relatively short time by reducing the dose of the drug gradually.

Tolerance refers to a condition in which a patient will need larger doses over time to achieve the same relief. It, too, is also totally unrelated to addiction. It, too, needn't and shouldn't interfere with good pain control. There is no limit to tolerance—patients can continue to obtain relief from opioids—they may just need larger doses over time. As patients use and increase their doses of opioids, they may not only become tolerant to the analgesic (painkilling) effect, but also to the side effects of the opioid, so treatment remains safe.

Cancer pain experts agree on this matter: addiction should not be considered an issue for cancer patients or their doctors because it is very rare among them. In a review of almost 12,000 patients who received at least one dose of an opioid while hospitalized, only 4 patients (less than one-tenth of 1 percent) with no prior history of addiction developed this psychological dependency. In fact, studies have shown that addiction to sedatives, such as Valium, is far more common than it is to narcotic painkillers.

David Friedman, Ph.D., from the National Institute on Drug Abuse, finds that "the risk of addiction is greatly overestimated in part because many people do not understand the distinctions between drug abuse and drug addiction, on the one hand, and physical dependence and tolerance on the other." He continues: "Dependence and tolerance are virtually inevitable outcomes of long-term opioid use, but they are neither sufficient to cause addiction nor the equivalent of it." For Friedman, "We have become so afraid of opioid addiction that we have created a situation in which patients in pain—cancer patients [among others] . . .—are made to suffer because of the institutionalized barriers we have created to prevent addiction. One might justify this suffering if the medical use of opioids did indeed carry a significant risk of addiction. The evidence, however, indicates that it does not. We can only conclude that *the suffering caused by the under-use of opioids is in vain.*"

Pain is not just a side effect of cancer but is a legitimate health problem; treatment with medication is often required so the sufferer can resume a normal life, much like a diabetic or arthritis patient needs daily medication. Just as the diabetic and arthritis victim are not considered addicts, the cancer pain patient should not be thought of as addicted.

Yet, it is clear that some doctors and nurses still underprescribe because of unfounded fears of addiction. A 1990 survey in California revealed that almost one-third of 2,000 nurses believed that the chance of patients on opioids becoming addicted was 25 percent or greater. But leading cancer pain experts stress that the true odds are so minute that they are not a reason to let the vast majority suffer in unrelieved pain.

Fear of becoming addicted plagues patients and their loved ones as well. As a result, patients may be reluctant to comply with their doctor's instruc-

Table 1.1. *Differences Among Tolerance, Addiction, and Physical Dependence*

Developing Tolerance
Patient:
- Needs increasing doses to maintain same painkilling effect.
- Has a growing physiological (physical) need for larger doses that has nothing to do with desires or choices.
- Requires drug only to relieve pain, and does not necessarily get a "high" from medication use.
- May need larger doses over time.
- Has extremely low risk of developing a psychological dependence (addiction).

Developing Psychological Dependence or Addiction
Person:
- Has an obsession with getting and using a drug for nonmedical reasons.
- Desires for drug stems from psychological needs and choices; may have genetic predisposition.
- Wants drug to get "high," to boost mood.
- Has a psychological need to get drug that overwhelms all else, including economic, social, and physical well-being.
- Often develops tolerance, requiring larger doses to get original high, as well as physical dependence (see following discussion).

Developing Physical Dependence
Patient:
- May develop withdrawal symptoms (much like the flu) if medication is suddenly stopped.
- Would completely avoid withdrawal if medication were "tapered" or prescribed in gradually lowered doses.
- Wants drug only to relieve pain; does not seek a "high" from medical use of medication.
- Has extremely low risk of developing a psychological dependence (addiction).

Source: Adapted from J. A. Paice, The phenomenon of analgesic tolerance in cancer pain management. *Oncology Nursing Forum* 1988: (15) 455–460.

tions to take medications because they don't want to be viewed as being reliant on drugs, or families may indirectly or directly convey to the patient that he should abstain from the opioids as much as possible. Parents are especially concerned that children and teens who have cancer will grow up to be addicts if they take pain medication. "When we surveyed the parents of children dying with cancer, we asked them what their major concern was about their children receiving narcotics. It was that 'my child will grow up to be an addict,' " said Dr. Kathleen Foley of Memorial-Sloan Kettering. These children, however, were grappling with a life-threatening illness and suffering with pain which could have been avoided.

TOO MANY BELIEVE OPTIONS WILL RUN OUT

Many patients are reluctant to begin with opioids, fearing that active and aggressive treatment of their disease will no longer be pursued or that taking such drugs signals the "beginning of the end." The truth is that patients may need painkillers to resume a normal life during treatment. Another fear is that if they start taking narcotics too early, the drugs won't be as effective later when they are "really" needed. Yet pain can both be controlled early in the disease as well as later if it progresses. Nevertheless, it is estimated that these unfounded fears result in *half of patients not following their doctors' orders when it comes to taking pain medication.*

CULTURAL BARRIERS TO PAIN MANAGEMENT

Another reason that cancer pain is undertreated is that many people believe that the ability to endure pain is a virtue and reflects a strong character. Our culture depicts heroes as able to withstand pain without flinching or complaining. These images promote what could be called the "stiff upper lip syndrome"—the notion that not complaining and remaining stoical is somehow good for you. In fact, we talk of "no pain, no gain" in other contexts, and yet here it is grossly out of place. Some of us view people who complain about pain as being weak-willed or as having weak characters. People who feel this way, including some doctors and even families, regrettably may feel obligated to build the character of the "complainer" by withholding adequate pain relief.

Our culture also tends to compartmentalize the mind and body, and view pain in terms apart from the disease. These Western medical notions may interfere with treating the pain as an integral part of treating the disease. In this way, pain is viewed by some professionals as a "stepchild" of medicine—they may not focus on its problems unless forced to, failing to recognize how important pain management is to cancer treatment.

WHY PAIN IS HARMFUL TO HEALTH

It is hard to imagine any benefit that could result from enduring cancer pain. Pain relief is of utmost importance, not only for humanitarian reasons, but also for medical reasons—pain is harmful and debilitating. When patients are fighting pain, they cannot marshall their full strength to fight the disease. Pain also makes patients irritable, anxious, fearful, angry, depressed, and sometimes suicidal. In fact, those in pain are twice as likely to have a psychiatric problem in addition to their cancer compared to those without pain. Because they are fatigued, patients in pain may also be less likely to pursue treatment as aggressively as possible—treatments that could affect their outcome. Patients need to be at their best during these times— they can't afford to be compromised by pain.

Pain may also further debilitate a patient by disrupting lifestyle and well-being, interfering with work, social relationships, recreational interests, mobility, and perhaps even with the ability to take care of oneself, which in turn, affects self-esteem, body image, and feelings of competency.

Furthermore, patients in pain are ill equipped to fight their cancer. As discussed briefly on the first page of this chapter, pain may be harmful to the cancer patient's health. It can seriously affect a person's ability to get adequate rest and eat well and may even influence the growth of the tumor. Animal experiments have shown that the tumors of rats with pain who were not treated with morphine grew much faster than the tumors of those that received morphine. Some experts suspect that pain may even inhibit the normal functioning of our body's immune system, thereby increasing the risk of death. More studies are needed, but experts are convinced more than ever that inadequately relieved cancer pain may actually be hazardous to one's health.

Relieving pain is also economical. A Dartmouth University–Hitchcock Medical Center study showed, for example, that intensive-care patients whose pain was almost totally relieved spent three days less in the intensive care unit (ICU) and six days less in the hospital than those whose pain was not relieved—a savings of $9,200 per patient.

Moreover, patients with pain tend to receive lower grades on "performance status" (how well a patient is functioning and getting around) from medical staff. When doctors are selecting patients for experimental procedures or therapies, they often will bypass the patient who is in constant pain, unable to function and get around, in favor of another patient who is functioning well.

Cancer patients who try to keep a stiff upper lip and endure the pain related to their cancer without relief may also not realize that, while they are bearing the enormous physical and psychological burden of cancer pain, everyone around them bears that burden too. Cancer patients don't suffer in isolation—their family, friends, and other caregivers suffer along with them. And the suffering is in vain.

TRAINING OF DOCTORS AND NURSES

Although many patients are undermedicated for cancer-related pain, it is not because doctors are incompetent or uncaring. Pain medication is either improperly used or underused because medical training is primarily focused on disease and treatment of disease and not on relieving symptoms. Student doctors have been taught how to treat short-term or acute pain from surgery or trauma, but many have not learned how to properly use painkillers such as morphine, the cornerstone of cancer pain treatment, for chronic pain. Reviews of medical school curricula have found that few schools teach the basic principles of opioid use and other cancer pain treatments. "Medical schools and post-grad training programs devote little, if any, time to teaching physicians about . . . the chronic pain of cancer. Essentially, physicians have been taught only how to treat acute pain. Regrettably, undertreatment has become customary practice," says C. Stratton Hill, Jr., M.D., former Director of the Pain Service at the University of Texas System Cancer Center. Fortunately, more comprehensive pain education is now being added to medical school curricula, which bodes well for the future but doesn't improve today's situation.

Not even residents in oncology (the science and study of cancer) receive much training in cancer pain treatment, although this situation is improving as well. Among the enormous amount of teaching material about cancer, there is very little information about effective pain treatment. According to one review in the late 1980s of the eleven major textbooks on oncology published in the United States, totaling some 13,000 pages, only two books had a chapter on pain control. The other nine books combined had only 62 pages out of more than 10,000 pages on pain control.

"The situation is appalling, extraordinary, sad and distressing," says David Newman, medical director of the Pain Management Information Center, a consulting service for physicians in need of advice for treating a specific patient's cancer pain problems (see Appendix). "The good news is that physicians with a little background can teach themselves in two evenings what they need to know."

Yet many doctors are unaware of modern methods used to treat chronic cancer pain, and so they erroneously continue to apply the principles of acute pain management. For example, although all the current literature on cancer pain management strongly recommends that narcotics (opioids) be given on schedule around the clock (a-t-c) rather than as needed (known as prn from the Latin *pro re nata,* meaning as the occasion arises) when the pain comes on, more than two-thirds of the painkillers prescribed in cancer centers surveyed in the late 1980s in two studies were still being given as prn. This is only one example of how changing the behavior of doctors who treat cancer has been agonizingly slow when it comes to treating the pain. (More on prn versus "around-the-clock" dosing in Chapter 3.)

DOSES MAY VARY WIDELY

Another problem that contributes to inadequate treatment of cancer pain is that prescribing strong painkillers, while still a science, is often an inexact one. Determining the correct dose for a particular patient can be difficult and time consuming; it often requires well thought out trial and error until most of the pain is relieved with few side effects. One reason is because pain varies widely, even in patients with the same kind of cancer. Also, pain cannot really be measured objectively, so proper treatment requires a good relationship between patient and doctor. Patients must be willing to discuss their discomfort. At the same time, doctors must trust their patients' report of pain.

While an allergic reaction to narcotics is extremely rare, some patients do better (more relief and less side effects) with some medications than others. People also vary widely in their thresholds for pain (how much pain they can or want to tolerate) and their tolerance to painkillers (how much painkiller is needed), so what relieves the pain of one person may not relieve the pain of another. In addition, what relieves the pain today may not be adequate tomorrow as the disease progresses or the patient grows tolerant to a given dose of medication. Whereas one patient will stay on a constant dose for years, another may need adjustments hourly.

NARCOTIC DOSES AND TOLERANCE
HAVE NO UPPER LIMIT

Unfortunately, many health-care professionals fail to understand how tolerance to painkillers develops and how to respond to it, which may lead to undertreatment. The longer most patients use an opioid drug or the more severe the pain becomes, the more medication they may need to achieve the same relief.

In fact, there is no "ceiling effect" or upper limit for opioids such as morphine. Although "customary" or "standard" doses of narcotics are published in older medical texts, those doses are based on the needs of patients with acute pain (like labor pain or pain after surgery), not for the chronic pain of cancer. The truth is that some patients need much more medicine to get the same pain relief, either because their bodies grow used to it and they need more to get relief, or because their pain increases, or both. While a typical starting dose of morphine may be as little as 20 to 30 milligrams (mg) by mouth every four hours (or 8 to 10 mg intravenously), some patients have been reported to need the equivalent of up to 35,000 mg a day.

UNDERMEDICATION IS THE NORM

Since not all doctors are up-to-date on modern cancer pain management, many undermedicate cancer pain and then mistakenly teach young doctors to do the same. Since so many doctors undermedicate, other doctors feel pressured to stick to the norm of low "standard doses" set by their colleagues.

Yet, even when an adequate range of doses is prescribed, some studies of postoperative pain have shown that most patients still only receive as little as one-quarter of the prescribed amount—in hospitals, nurses usually dispense medications and many nurses have their own misconceptions about what are safe and proper doses. So despite good intentions, they tend to underdispense. Also, the drugs are often not administered or increased frequently enough to relieve or prevent pain.

MISINFORMATION ABOUT PAIN
AND BREATHING PROBLEMS

Although opioids can slow breathing (known as respiratory depression), even to a dangerous degree if not prescribed carefully, respiratory depression is not a serious risk when low starting doses are used. Since cancer patients rapidly grow tolerant to this side effect over time, it becomes less and less of a problem. Moreover, severe pain counteracts this side effect, even with seemingly large doses. Regardless of how large a dose may seem, its side effects will be minimized if the patient has been prescribed gradual increments in doses and it is the dose required to relieve the pain. In fact, the proper use of morphine is a recognized treatment for shortness of breath and can improve breathing problems in some patients, especially those with rapid or painful breathing. Unfortunately, exaggerated concerns about respiratory depression sometimes keep doctors from prescribing enough medication to soothe the pain.

UNDERUTILIZED OPTIONS

The frontiers of medical science are rapidly expanding, and keeping up with them is a challenge. Doctors who have mastered the use of simple painkillers (effective for most patients) may be unaware of different ways to administer morphine, of alternative drugs, and especially of effective drug combinations (some drugs that aren't normally considered painkillers can relieve certain pains very effectively when used properly, or can enhance the painkilling effect of opioids). Electrical stimulation, nerve stimulation, surgical procedures to cut nerve pathways, and nerve blocks (see Chapter 9) as well as nondrug approaches—such as relaxation training, biofeedback, hypnosis, acupuncture, and massage—may also help relieve pain in many cases, but are usually only prescribed by pain specialists.

LOW EXPECTATIONS AND LOW ENTHUSIASM ARE TOO COMMON

Many people, including some physicians and patients, often incorrectly believe that severe pain and cancer go together. This is a normal result of having seen other patients or family members undertreated. As a result of these false beliefs, some doctors undertreat the pain and patients accept their doctor's unfounded fears about addiction and about serious side effects, as well as their low confidence and low expectations of success. Cancer pain often does not completely go away, but in almost all cases, it can be controlled or, at least, kept to a low and tolerable level.

THE NEED TO DISCUSS PAIN

A busy doctor may not ask a patient about pain, assuming that if it's a problem, the patient will bring it up. *Patients should not wait for a doctor to ask about the pain.* Sometimes the doctor may ask, "How are you?" to open a conversation, and the usual polite response of "fine" may be recorded as "no pain today."

Patients are often reluctant to complain. They may fail to mention pain to their doctors because they know that time with the physician may be short and their highest priority is to talk about treatment and cure. Many are reluctant to distract the doctor from this mission, or to "bother" or annoy him with their complaints. Some deny the pain in their effort to deny the disease and possibly its progress. If pain has intensified, patients may not want to admit it; instead, they want to tell the doctor they feel better. Or, perhaps they don't want to complain because they believe that their "good" behavior will be rewarded and that "bad" behavior will be punished. Yet information about pain is vital for doctors to know—not only for diagnosing other problems but also because treating pain improves a patient's physical and psychological status. Proper rest, nutrition, and a good attitude, all of which suffer with pain, have never been so important as during a cancer illness and must be preserved.

Complaining about pain is not a weakness and shouldn't be an embarrassment. Patients and families who are reluctant to discuss the cancer pain problem are doing themselves and their doctors an enormous disservice.

COMMUNICATION BETWEEN PATIENT AND MEDICAL TEAM

Often a doctor will prescribe a painkiller, usually a mild one at first, and the patient will passively accept that treatment, whether it works or not. *Patients need to communicate frequently and effectively with their doctor if relief is not obtained. Together they need to persevere until adequate relief is achieved.* Patients also need to realize that their primary doctor is not the only one who can help—oncology nurses, physician-assistants, anesthesiologists, pharmacists, psychologists, and social workers are often part of the primary doctor's team. Their expertise can be invaluable in obtaining advice about problems and options.

Since some non-opioid medications may take several days to even weeks to take full effect, patients and their families also need to learn how long before a prescribed treatment is expected to become fully effective so they can tell the doctor or medical team as soon as possible if the treatment does not seem to be working. Possible side effects should be reported immediately—since the drug may need to be stopped or its dose changed. (Refer to Chapters 5 to 8 for specific information about particular medications and possible side effects.)

PATIENTS OFTEN DON'T TELL THEIR DOCTORS WHEN THEY DON'T FOLLOW RECOMMENDATIONS

Some patients hesitate to take their medications around the clock, on a prescribed schedule, as they should be taken. Instead, they believe, incorrectly, that they should tough it out until the very last moment when the pain is so bad that they just can't endure it any longer. By that time, however, the painkillers are much, much less effective. Rather than achieving steady relief, the patient is on a rollercoaster of pain—the pain escalates until it's intolerable, and then the painkiller may or may not relieve it (because they have waited so long). If the pain subsides, the next wave is around the corner. It is far more effective to maintain a certain level of the painkiller in the bloodstream so that it can act *preventively*. In this way, the patient achieves a more steady level of pain relief. The only way to do so is to take the medication in the manner prescribed, usually regularly, every 4 or 6 or 12 hours, depending on the medication, rather than as needed, after the pain returns. (See Chapter 3 on Pain Assessments and Pain Strategies.)

HOW PHARMACISTS MAY CONTRIBUTE TO UNDERTREATMENT

Another problem that contributes to the cancer pain problem is that some pharmacists have "old-fashioned" ideas about opioids. They may make negative comments to patients about the use of opioids, which could make patients feel guilty about taking them; as a result, patients may be less likely to fully comply with their doctor's instructions. Also, many pharmacists, especially in urban areas, often don't stock morphine and other opioids because they fear theft. In more isolated areas, pharmacies may not stock up on opioids because of relatively few requests for it. The lack of oral morphine in pharmacies makes it very difficult for many unhospitalized patients to get their medicine. It's a good idea, therefore, to call pharmacies in advance to find out who carries the medication, and to order it if necessary.

LAWS INTIMIDATE MANY DOCTORS FROM PRESCRIBING ENOUGH MEDICATION

Unfortunately, cancer pain patients are the innocent victims of the "War on Drugs," a campaign that is supposed to discourage the illegal use of these substances. Although morphine and other opioids are highly effective for many pain problems, they are tightly controlled substances. Regulations are intended to curb abuse and not to interfere with the practice of medicine, yet many doctors find the stringent regulations confusing, inhibiting, burdensome, and threatening. To prescribe opioids in nine states including California, New York, Michigan, and Illinois, doctors must fill out mandatory and time-consuming triplicate prescription forms—one for the doctor, one for the pharmacist, and the third for the state regulators. Such prescriptions cannot be refilled automatically and are carefully monitored. And there are many pitfalls in trying to complete such paperwork. If the patient's name is spelled incorrectly, if a doctor needs to change the quantity of the drug rapidly, or wants to prescribe more than five days' worth of a drug on an urgent basis, there may be delays, frustrations, and fears of being investigated.

Although devised to reduce drug abuse, such restrictions have resulted in fewer prescriptions for pain-stricken patients. Most states that have instituted a multiple-copy prescription program have reported a 50 percent or greater *decrease* in prescriptions, with no evidence of declining drug abuse on the street, says lawyer Robert T. Angarola, a Washington, D.C. expert on the legal impediments to cancer pain treatments.

Angarola reported in 1991 that only one in five doctors in California even had the appropriate prescription pad, which meant that 80 percent of doctors couldn't prescribe morphine and similar drugs. And New York State law mandates that doctors report any "addicts"—defined as a person who is "dependent" on a narcotic—to the Department of Health.

In Texas, before the landmark 1989 Intractable Pain Treatment Act was passed, doctors could have lost their licenses if they prescribed any controlled substances to persons they knew or should have known were "habitual users." The law did not distinguish between drug addicts and pain patients. Although that confusion has been cleared up with the new act, such ambiguous "street talk" is still common in other states and puts doctors in a vulnerable position for simply prescribing adequate pain medication.

Fortunately, the cumbersome triplicate prescription program may be abandoned in the future, but what's next in store may not be much better. Since January 1993, states have been required to have Drug Utilization Review programs in place for Medicaid prescriptions; these are usually electronic programs that pool together all prescription information and that can monitor all kinds of information about the kinds of drugs prescribed. Although now only required for prescriptions associated with Medicaid, medical experts such as Dr. John Ambre, director of the American Medical Association's Department of Toxicology and Drug Abuse, says that chances are such systems will soon be instituted for all kinds of prescriptions.

Although such electronic monitoring and review systems do not prevent physicians from prescribing controlled substances and although some patients need large doses of opioids for adequate pain relief, many doctors avoid prescribing such doses because so many of the laws regulating controlled substances are ambiguous. Although high dosing is necessary for some cancer patients, it is still not the norm. As a result, many doctors are reluctant to prescribe opioids at all, even in low doses, because of fears they may attract the unwanted attention of regulatory agencies. Even if cleared of wrong-doing, such an investigation could be damaging professionally and could incur high legal costs.

EVEN WHEN CURE IS UNLIKELY, COMFORT IS ESSENTIAL

Millions are spent each year on developing cures for cancer, yet only a fraction goes to pain relief research and palliative care—treatment for ill patients who will probably get no better. Many oncologists, medical schools, researchers, and even some of the national and international cancer agencies

Table 1.2. *Reasons Why Cancer Pain Is Often Undertreated*

Society and the Law
- The drug abuse problem has led to stringent laws that can inhibit the medical community's use of narcotics.
- Triplicate prescription forms are cumbersome, time-consuming, and intimidating.
- Ambiguous laws fail to adequately distinguish between addiction and the legitimate medical use of opioids when cancer patients are involved.
- Physicians are afraid to prescribe large doses of narcotics for fear of attracting the attention of authorities.
- Confusion between legitimate and illegitimate use of narcotics is common.

Medical Staff
- Treatments for chronic cancer pain are not emphasized enough in medical school or residency.
- Concerns about addiction in cancer patients are exaggerated and unfounded.
- Respiratory depression and other side effects of treatment are incompletely understood.
- Addiction, physical dependence, and tolerance are terms often confused.
- Misconceptions abound about how tolerance develops and about the need for increasing doses over time.
- Inappropriately low expectations for successful pain relief are harbored by medical staff.
- Many believe that pain needs to be severe before treatment is started.
- Others believe that complaining reflects a weak character that must be strengthened.
- Pain management is given a low priority.
- Undermedication is the norm and so is perpetuated in young, incoming staff.

Patients and Families
- Complaining about pain is viewed as a sign of weakness or an admission that the disease is progressing.
- Distracting the doctor from treatment and cure is feared.
- Addiction is feared.
- When medication does not provide relief, little support exists.
- Holding out or suffering in silence is considered virtuous.
- Patients often fail to comply with instructions.
- The individual wishes to be a "good patient" and not complain.

Health-Care System
- Comfort of the patient who will not get better (palliative care) is not a focus of the medical team, who are trained to focus on cure.
- Patients move among health-care professionals and institutions so much that their care may not be well coordinated.
- Pharmacists are reluctant to stock morphine for fear of theft.
- Triplicate prescription forms inhibit the use of opioids for cancer patients.

have historically overlooked the importance of palliative care and have focused instead on anti-cancer treatments exclusively. This perspective is beginning to change with the recognition that the quality of life of patients could be radically improved if cancer pain relief and palliative care (which deals with the psychological, social, and spiritual well-being as well as physical comfort of patients) were given greater attention. Without such efforts, the suffering of these patients goes unnoticed. Once their active treatment is completed, pain may be overlooked, mismanaged, unnoticed, and sometimes even neglected. Patients should not feel abandoned just because they are not currently receiving radiotherapy or chemotherapy. Health care is still necessary for achieving and maintaining comfort.

RECENT DEVELOPMENTS

Although still an uphill struggle, a movement is afoot that has been gaining ground—a movement of doctors, patients, and health-care activists concerned with improving cancer pain treatments. A few years ago, a book like this could never have been written. More doctors are becoming expert in the basic principles of pain management, so fewer patients will suffer. The attendance at professional meetings and conferences on pain control is soaring. Increasingly, hospitals are pulling together multidisciplinary teams to diagnose and treat pain, including cancer pain. More than 35 states have developed specific initiatives (called Cancer Pain Initiatives) to attack the cancer pain problem, with the Wisconsin Cancer Pain Initiative working with the World Health Organization to take the lead. (See Appendix for more information on these initiatives.) And finally, the hospice movement, with its basic premise of maximizing quality of life for terminally ill patients, is becoming more widely accepted (see Chapter 15).

THE RIGHT TO REQUEST AND OBTAIN
ADEQUATE RELIEF

Yet change is slow, and consumers cannot take for granted that they will receive state-of-the-art pain relief. If pain remains unrelieved or the patient cannot rest and sleep comfortably, family caregivers must persevere and ask for help from the doctor or medical team until comfort is achieved.

To ensure that a loved one does not suffer, consumers must learn what is available and appropriate for their case, and how to be an advocate for the patient and successfully work to see that the pain is relieved. To ensure optimal relief, consumers need to know what to expect in the course of cancer pain treatment.

We must disregard old-fashioned notions about toughing out pain and begin to understand that pain undermines our body's best defenses against disease, not to mention the psychological and emotional suffering and toll on the quality of life that pain extracts. Dr. Schuster's comments bear repeating: "The overriding ethic which must guide our use of the narcotic drugs for the treatment of severe cancer pain is that no patient should suffer needlessly, and no patient should wish for death, because of our failure to use properly our strongest weapons against pain."

2

Understanding Cancer and Pain

In short, the right drug at the right dose given at the right time relieves
80 to 90 percent of pain.
—World Health Organization

A diagnosis of cancer is usually unexpected and is always a frightening and
overwhelming experience. Few families have the knowledge initially needed
to make the many very difficult decisions that will be required, and with
the doctor's office so busy, it is easy to feel bewildered and confused. In
addition to providing basic information about cancer and how it is treated,
this chapter will discuss the various kinds of pain that are associated with
cancer.

WHAT IS CANCER?

In the disease of cancer, a tumor—a mass of abnormal tissue—begins to
grow in some part of the body. The tumor is comprised of many cells distinct from normal cells, and these tumor cells serve no useful purpose. The
growths, known as *neoplasms* (meaning "new growths"), may be benign or
malignant. Benign growths are usually harmless and are not cancerous. Malignant neoplasms, on the other hand, continue to grow and are potentially
deadly.

What makes malignant cells so dangerous is their ability to grow uncontrollably and to spread throughout the body *(metastasize)*, competing with
normal cells for vital nutrients and interfering with the body's normal functions. As a malignancy grows, it may invade or destroy tissues near by or
may spread to distant parts of the body, such as the lungs, liver, or bone.

Understanding the Diagnosis

Cancer is not one disease, but, in fact, a group of more than 100 diseases
that are classified according to where and how the growth occurs, as well as
specific microscopic or other features. Luckily, with the variety of medical

tools now available, doctors can diagnose cancer early in the disease process if a patient is seen early on.

Each type of cancer has certain general characteristics that are used to define the disease:

- *Type and site of cancer.* Where a cancer starts (such as lung, liver, or breast), as well as the type of cell within the growth, defines a cancer. Thus, for example, squamous cell, adenocarcinoma, small-cell, and non-small-cell tumors are all different types of lung cancers, and each tends to behave in a different way. To ascertain the type of cell, doctors will usually need to take a sample of the tumor or cell mass, called a *biopsy*, to have it analyzed in a laboratory to determine if it is a harmless (benign) or cancerous (malignant) growth.
- *Cell growth.* Tumors can be slow growing or may be of a type that grows quickly.
- *Ability to metastasize.* Some tumors are more likely to spread in one way or another compared to other types of cancers.
- *Stage at diagnosis.* Doctors classify cancers as in early, middle, or late phases of the disease. The stage of cancer is defined by how much cell growth is seen in the original site of the disease and how much tissue is involved beyond this site. Whether lymph nodes or distant organs are involved is crucial to treatment.
- *Treatment options.* Certain cancers may be responsive to surgery, chemotherapy, radiation, or all three.

Oncologists use a shorthand to put these characteristics together to define stage and site. T0 to T4 describe the size of the tumor; N0 to N3 describe whether the nearby lymph nodes have been affected; M0 if there are no distant metastases and M1 if there are. And depending on these characteristics, a tumor will be assigned a stage from Stage 0 to Stage IV. For example, a tumor whose local growth is limited to the organ where it started, and which has not invaded the lymph nodes or other organs, might be called a "Stage I (for early disease), T1 (for very small tumor), N0 (no involvement of nearby lymph nodes), M0 (no distant metastases)."

The doctor can explain the exact kind of cancer that has been diagnosed and the nature of its usual behavior. But remember that doctors talk of averages—some people are lucky and do better than average, and some fare worse. Many organizations will provide free educational material to supplement what the doctor explains. (See Appendix for sources to obtain additional information about various types of cancer and their treatment.)

CANCER TREATMENTS

Once a diagnosis is confirmed, treatment is tailored to the particular type of cancer. Site of cancer, cell type, cell growth, and stage of cancer—all are taken into consideration in designing appropriate treatment. The goal of any treatment is to kill or remove as many cancerous cells as possible with as little damage as possible to normal cells. Depending on the type of cancer involved and how advanced it is, doctors may prescribe one or all of the following kinds of treatment.

Surgery may either attempt to remove the entire tumor (curative surgery) or part of the tumor (debulking surgery) when all of it can't be removed. Making the tumor smaller in some cases makes it more responsive to other treatments. Even if a tumor is thought to have been completely removed, chemotherapy, radiation therapy, or both are often prescribed after surgery to try to ensure that individual cancer cells have been destroyed. Surgery may also be used to biopsy the growth (to diagnose whether the growth is cancerous), to determine the kind of cancer present, to prevent further growth of a hormonally dependent cancer (by removing a particular organ that secretes the hormone that is triggering the cancer growth), and in some cases to reduce pain.

Radiation therapy, used in about half of all cases of cancer, uses targeted X-ray, gamma rays, or electron beams to bombard the specific cancer site. Radiation interferes with the ability of cancer cells to continue dividing and spreading by breaking parts of the cell. Relatively common side effects may include mouth soreness, skin changes, and later on, bone marrow problems; less common complications are described later in this chapter (under the section titled Cancer Pain Syndromes Associated with Cancer Therapy; see page 36). Radiation is also often used to reduce pain by shrinking a tumor even when a cure is no longer possible (known as palliative radiotherapy).

Chemotherapy uses drugs, taken either by mouth or through a needle, that destroy cancerous cells or slow their growth while harming as few normal cells as possible. Often used after surgery or radiation to ensure that as many cancer cells as possible have been destroyed, chemotherapy is also sometimes used to relieve pain when tumors press on nerves, parts of the lymph system, or veins. Side effects may include nausea, vomiting, mouth sores, and baldness (alopecia). Again, less common complications will be described later in this chapter.

OTHER IMPORTANT TERMS ASSOCIATED WITH CANCER

When a family faces cancer for the first time, they are usually overwhelmed and may encounter unfamiliar words associated with the disease. Here is a

primer of some of the most important terms; check the Glossary at the back
of the book for others as you read this book.

Metastasize, Metastasis, or Metastases

When cancer cells spread through the body, they are said to be *metastasiz-
ing*. The process of cancer cells spreading to other areas of the body is called
metastasising. When a cancer has originated from one area, say the mouth,
but then spreads to another site, the secondary sites are called *metastases*.
Metastases, however, can be local or distant. Local metastases indicate that
the cancer spread has occurred near the primary tumor. In addition, there
may be local extensions of the tumor. On the other hand, a metastasis may
be to a distant organ, spreading usually through the blood or lymph system,
and most commonly to bone, liver, or lung. Metastasis is a very serious
complication of cancer and usually makes treatment of the disease much
more difficult.

Oncologist or Oncology

A doctor who specializes in cancer is called an *oncologist;* his or her area of
expertise is called *oncology,* the science of cancer. Subspecialties within the
field of oncology include medical oncology, radiation oncology, gynecologi-
cal oncology, surgical oncology, and so on.

Biopsy

A *biopsy* is often a minor surgery or procedure in which a doctor will remove a small bit of tissue from a growth to have it analyzed in a laboratory
to determine whether the growth is benign or malignant. More and more,
biopsies are being performed without surgery. By placing a small needle in
the troublesome area under X-ray guidance, a bit of tissue can be removed
and analyzed. This is now sometimes an office procedure.

Lymph System

The lymph system, like the blood's circulatory system, is distributed
throughout the human body. Lymph can be understood as a fluid in an
intermediate stage between blood and other tissue cells in the body. The
lymph system is a common route through which cancer cells may metastasize.

For other terms, please refer to the Glossary at the end of this book.

WHAT IS PAIN?

Pain is an unpleasant sensation or emotional experience that is triggered by
tissue damage or threatened tissue damage. But how intensely a particular

person will perceive pain depends on his or her psychological state as well as other predispositions as outlined in the following pages.

Basically, pain has two components:

1. A sensory component that involves the transmission of the pain signal (electrical and chemical events) from the hurt or threatened tissues to the spinal cord and brain (which comprise the central nervous system). Upon receiving the pain signals, the brain then perceives the stimulus as pain.

2. A reactive component that involves how the person reacts to the pain, which is dependent on the person's pain threshold and his or her pain tolerance. A person's *pain threshold* is the intensity of the stimulus a person considers painful. *Pain tolerance,* on the other hand, is how intense or how long the unpleasant sensation can persist before the person experiences the sensation as pain. (See Table 2.1.)

People not only have individual differences in their pain thresholds and tolerances, but a person's perception of pain depends largely on how the uncomfortable sensation is filtered, altered, or distorted by that person's thoughts, feelings, and memories. For example, depressed or anxious patients tend to have lower thresholds of pain (see Chapter 14). Other factors may play a role as well, such as age (some research suggests that older people, for example, may need more painkiller to dull pain) and race (research suggests blacks may need less morphine that whites). Also, prior experiences with cancer or pain or the meaning of the pain can influence pain perception. If a woman with breast cancer remembers witnessing a relative with breast cancer die in agony, she may be terrified that she'll end

Table 2.1. *Factors That May Influence Pain Threshold*

Threshold Lowered	Threshold Raised
Discomfort	Relief of symptoms
Insomnia	Sleep
Fatigue	Rest
Anxiety	Sympathy
Fear	Understanding
Anger	Companionship
Sadness	Diversional activity
Depression	Reduction in anxiety
Boredom	Elevation of mood
Introversion	Use of analgesics
Mental isolation	Use of anxiolytics
Social abandonment	Use of antidepressants

Source: From R. Twycross and S. Lack, *Therapeutics in Terminal Care* (New York: Churchill Livingstone, 1990), p. 11. Reprinted with permission.

up the same way and be particularly sensitive to pain. On the other hand, the meaning of pain to a football player who is paid $2 million a year who is mercilessly tackled and badly injured in a game is very different; he may feel much less pain because he is thinking of his bonus or respite in the hospital, and knows his pain has nothing to do with his life span or mortality.

Although pain is the most common ailment for which people consult a doctor, it has been historically a "stepchild" of medicine—something that has always been around but has never been fully accepted as a bona fide medical problem. Fortunately, that is becoming less and less so. In fact, some doctors have been sued for inadequate pain management.

Since pain cannot be measured or directly perceived by an observer, doctors cannot know how much of the pain is derived from physical as distinct from psychological distress—a split that many doctors believe should not be made. In other words, as scientists are becoming aware of how enmeshed mind and body phenomena are, they are viewing pain as real and a medical problem, regardless of whether it is derived from a physical problem or is an expression of anxiety or depression. If a patient complains of pain, it should be taken seriously whether the source is known or not.

HOW PAIN OCCURS AND IS DETECTED

In almost all cases, pain starts with some injury or damage to a body part. Most of the time, the injury is in the periphery—that is, anywhere in the body except the spinal cord and brain (which make up the central nervous system). The skin, muscles, and bones are tissues that respond to usual injuries like cuts, pressure, and burns, which trigger a pain signal. Other tissues, such as those of the intestine, heart, and blood vessels, produce pain signals when internal organs are injured, such as when they are distended (when they are stretched or swollen), twisted, or suffering from a lack of blood, a condition called *ischemia*.

How Pain Is Triggered

Body tissue is made up mostly of cells, and when cells are damaged by some injury, their damaged walls release a variety of chemicals, especially one called *arachadonic acid*. This substance is broken up into a series of chemicals called *prostaglandins*. These chemicals, among others, trigger pain receptors (also called *nociceptors*) to react by sending electrochemical signals to the spinal cord and brain. Prostaglandins make the nociceptors even more sensitive, which is why a finger that's been accidentally cut or banged with a hammer, for example, becomes extrasensitive to touch after it has been hurt. The signals initiated by the nociceptors are like a code, carrying information related to how severe the injury is, what kind of damage has occurred, and where it is located.

The idea of receptors is relatively new. Experts believe they are specialized proteins located on cell walls that react to only very specific stimuli, chemicals, or drugs. When disturbed by injury, they initiate a long chain of events, culminating in pain. The receptor and the chemical or event that activates it (turns it on) have been compared to a lock and key. The receptor is like a lock—its resting state is "closed for business"—it ignores everything around it, preventing the activity that it controls. Only when the receptor encounters the special substance that activates it (the key that fits the lock) does it respond, in this case by initiating a signal that will ultimately be interpreted as pain.

How Pain Is Detected

Once the signal has been initiated, a very complex series of events is set into motion, which is only now beginning to be fully understood. We can imagine a complex matrix of electrical switchboards in which electrical signals travel from the periphery along nerves into the spinal cord. Once received at the spinal cord, the signals release other chemicals, and impulses travel to the thalamus (another waystation) in the brain. The brain acts like a computer, deciphering the encoded message, ultimately interpreting the signal as pain.

How Pain Strategies Interrupt the Pain Signals

One very effective way to relieve pain during this transmission of signals is to prevent the formation of prostaglandins—and that's just what aspirin and other anti-inflammatory drugs, such as ibuprofen, do. They have little effect on the brain and work mostly in the periphery to prevent the nociceptors (pain receptors) from becoming overly sensitive.

The spinal cord and brain contain other paths that can be interrupted or modified to control pain. Morphine and the other opioid drugs help to suppress the pain messages primarily within and to the brain, thereby blunting or diminishing the pain perceived.

Thus, aspirin (and other anti-inflammatory drugs) and narcotic drugs (opioids) suppress pain by two different mechanisms. As we'll see in later chapters, this is why they are often used together to treat cancer pain.

TYPES OF PAIN

In general, the pain of cancer patients (and other patients) may be divided into the following major types:

1. *Acute pain* is usually sharp and intense and is easily identified as coming from a particular spot. It usually comes on suddenly, passes in time, and triggers autonomic (or automatic), bodily responses such as heavy perspiration, rising blood pressure, and faster pulse and respiratory rates. Acute pain may last for several days to up to several months. People suffering from acute pain often grimace or rub the painful area. Acute pain is very responsive to pain treatments.

Acute pain serves a useful, protective purpose. It is a strong message that an injury has occurred and that the body must react in ways to avoid further injury—for example, to remove a burnt hand from a hot pot, or to get treatment for a persistent stomachache. Once the cause of pain has been established, the pain is no longer beneficial, as in the case of cancer, and should be treated.

When pain occurs in a patient with cancer, it is often incorrectly assumed to be due to the tumor pressing on some pain-sensitive structure. This is often not the case—one-quarter to one-third of patients experience acute pain not from the tumor but as a side effect of the cancer treatment itself, such as surgery or the pain of getting on and off a radiation table.

2. *Chronic pain,* on the other hand, starts off as acute pain. But when it persists for a period of months, it is considered chronic. From dull and achy to agonizing, chronic pain is often more difficult for the patient to pinpoint, describe, and cope with; its cause is also more difficult for the doctor to diagnose. Chronic pain differs from acute pain in that it triggers autonomic responses less often, doesn't diminish with time, and is not a part of the healing process.

Chronic pain may be harder to bear because we don't know when it might end. We expect pain after surgery, for example, and knowing that it will lessen and end at some point makes it more bearable. That is why acute pain in the early stages of cancer is usually well tolerated by patients; because aggressive treatment is usually in progress, the pain is more easily ignored. Pain that is chronic and unrelenting with no end in sight, on the other hand, is much harder to tolerate, even when it is not actually more severe than when it started. With time, coping mechanisms wear out; we become frustrated and depressed. Although it may not be as sharp as acute pain, chronic pain can be severe, taking a serious toll on a patient's personality, lifestyle, and activities, affecting his or her mental, emotional, psychological, and sexual well-being, as well as impairing appetite and sleep. Sufferers may show signs of depression and feelings of hopelessness, and may withdraw from social activities altogether.

3. *Chronic and acute pain,* however, often occur together. When cancer patients have pain, the most common situation is that of a chronic pain (low level if treated effectively) with occasional bouts of acute pain. The acute pain episodes may be due to a new source of discomfort, a recently developed psychological condition, bodily movement, or an undermanaged chronic pain condition, resulting from arthritis, for example.

TERMS THAT DESCRIBE PAIN

Doctors will often use other terms to describe pain. Learning these terms will help you communicate more effectively with physicians and their team.

Constant pain refers to pain that doesn't let up—it hurts all the time and should be treated with medication that is taken regularly, around the clock (a-t-c) rather than just when it hurts the most. (The difference between "around the clock" and "as needed," or prn, pain administration is discussed in Chapter 3.) This strategy helps to prevent pain rather than treating it after it has become intense, which is a much more difficult task.

Breakthrough pain is pain that occasionally "breaks" through an otherwise effective preventive medication schedule. When it is related to a specific activity, such as eating, going to the bathroom, laughing, or walking, it is called *incident pain.* Breakthrough pain is best managed by allowing the patient to take an extra dose of medicine when the pain breaks through the medicated comfort; these extra doses are called "escape" or "rescue" doses or may be referred to as a *bolus.* When there is incident pain, that same extra dose can be taken just before engaging in the pain-provoking activity.

End-of-dose failure refers to breakthrough pain that usually occurs just before the next dose of around-the-clock medication is due. This usually signals that the dose of a-t-c medicine is too low and that it is time to raise it, or that it needs to be given more frequently.

Intermittent pain is unpredictable and occurs in an irregular, on-and-off pattern. Taking medication around the clock on schedule may be a problem with intermittent pain because the medication may be inadequate during painful episodes yet cause sedation during pain-free periods. Intermittent pain, therefore, is one of the few instances in which an "as needed" (prn) prescription for medicine is usually best.

WHO HAS CANCER PAIN

Not all cancer hurts. In fact, many cancer patients will experience relatively little pain. In the early stages of the disease, only one out of ten patients has pain that is strong enough to affect mood and activities. In the intermediate stages of the disease, about half of patients will suffer moderate to severe pain. In patients with advanced or terminal cancer, some three-quarters to 90 percent may have chronic pain, often severe to excruciating pain. *But remember: if treated correctly, the vast majority of cancer pain victims—from 90 to 99 percent—can expect satisfactory pain relief.*

WHY CANCER PAIN IS DIFFERENT

Chronic pain that is not related to cancer—such as pain from arthritis, back injuries, or gastrointestinal disorders—is different from the pain of progressive cancer. One reason is that cancer pain responds well to modern treatments while many chronic painful syndromes unrelated to cancer do not. Morphine and other opioids (narcotic drugs), for example, are extremely effective in alleviating cancer pain, and addiction is rare. Morphine is not routinely used for most other forms of chronic pain, both because it is often not effective and because patients may be at risk for addiction. Unfortunately, when chronic pain is not due to cancer, patients often need to be told to live with some or all of their pain because there is no cure. If there is any good news with cancer, it is that the pain can be controlled.

PAIN VERSUS SUFFERING

Before we get into discussing specific cancer pain syndromes, it's important to understand the difference between pain and suffering, two very closely related concepts. Pain has more to do with the actual injury to tissue and the signal that is generated. Suffering, on the other hand, includes pain, but seems more related to our interpretation of the pain signal and the way we respond to it. Psychological, cultural, and socioeconomic factors all play an important role in how we respond to every life event, including how much we suffer when we have pain. *These psychosocial components, however, do not make the pain any less real or valid.* It may explain, however, why the pain from tumor growth or tumor recurrence may be much harder to tolerate than pain that stems from scarring in cancer that has been cured: these pains have different meanings. Suffering, therefore, includes feelings that are linked to the problems of being ill with cancer. Terminal cancer patients suffer more, for example, if they believe their pain can't be controlled. Once it can be demonstrated to them that, in fact, their pain can be relieved, their suffering is diminished to some extent. Childbirth, for example, may hurt but not cause suffering because it may be viewed as uplifting or part of a joyous event. In expressing suffering, patients may exhibit attention-seeking behaviors, such as remaining disabled despite improvement or constantly looking for a different doctor. Other examples of how psychological factors influence suffering include:

- Depression stemming from loss of income, feelings of helplessness, or isolation, fatigue, physical disability, and fear of death.
- Anxiety about treatment, outcome, expenses, and the welfare of family members.
- Anger at being ill; at friends and family for not being as supportive as possible; at doctors for being unavailable or unable to cure them; and at the health-care facilities for delays, blunders, or insensitive treatment.

So although a person's response to pain—their so-called pain behavior (grimacing, crying, asking for help)—may seem to be just a direct result of the damage caused by cancer, it is strongly influenced by psychological factors, a fact that some patients resist acknowledging. But perhaps this is an artificial distinction. Most experts would now argue that you can't have pain without the influence of psychological factors. In fact, more and more scientists are convinced that we cannot separate these mind-body connections, and that treatments, especially those for cancer patients, must consider the mind and body as a whole.

This relationship between pain and feelings or mood is complex. If an underlying depression is effectively treated—for example, either through counseling or through antidepressants, or both—some pain problems can significantly subside. If depression persists, however, even aggressive therapy with morphine or surgery will not relieve pain that has a strong psychological component.

For example, one doctor tells the story of one woman with persistent pain that didn't seem to respond to treatments that should have worked. After days of trying all kinds of things, a member of the staff finally took the time to talk to the patient in more depth. The staff member discovered that the patient was most anxious about what would happen to her poodle if she died. The social services staff pursued the case and reassured the patient that they had found a foster home for her dog. After that, the woman's pain subsided, and she responded to treatment.

On the other hand, persistent pain can trigger depression—cancer patients in pain have been found to have higher rates of depression than cancer patients in no pain in all kinds of cases. When pain is well managed, depression may be significantly reduced.

What's vital to remember here is that regardless of how psychological, emotional, or spiritual factors trigger or influence pain, the pain and suffering are just as legitimate and real to the person experiencing them. In working with a patient who has pain and suffering, therefore, caregivers need to understand how efforts to relieve pain must also take into account the full range of reasons for the patient's suffering. (See Chapter 14 on Dealing with Feelings.)

WHY CANCER HURTS

Tumors themselves do not hurt. Pain is caused either by the effects of the cancer treatments (such as chemotherapy, surgical scarring, and radiation), the effects of the tumor's growth (intruding on neighboring tissues or invading other tissues), or other conditions that are occurring at the same time as the cancer (such as herpes soster, commonly known as shingles, a condition that chemotherapy patients are more susceptible to, or back pain from being bedridden), or side effects from therapies and medications (such as getting on and off the radiation table or constipation or nausea that can cause pain).

Although many of the treatments do cause some toxicity, because in the effort to destroy cancer cells, some healthy cells may be damaged as well, it can be reassuring that many therapies have an excellent chance of helping the patient. After treatment, many patients live long and healthy lives. It is also reassuring that not all the pain associated with cancer is from tumors, but rather may be related to treatments.

Cancer Pain Syndromes Associated with Cancer Therapy

As we've said, one of the challenges of designing the best cancer treatment involves destroying as many tumor cells as possible while preserving normal cells. Still, some injury, either temporary or permanent, usually occurs to normal cells and may produce pain. That is why it is wrong to always assume that more pain in the cancer patient means the tumor has gotten worse. Pain from cancer therapy is, in fact, much more common than is realized, and as we've already mentioned, accounts for pain in about one-quarter to one-third of cancer patients who have pain.

Although we list many of the possible problems that may crop up for a cancer patient, it must be remembered that there is an enormous diversity in the experiences of cancer patients, and although we discuss many different syndromes below, the likelihood of any patient experiencing more than a few is very unlikely. We list many here so that a patient who is having a particular problem can find it described and know that it is not a freak occurrence, but the possible effect of a particular treatment.

Specifically, these pain syndromes include the following:

From Surgery

In addition to the self-limited pain that follows most surgeries, surgery on the chest (thoracotomy), breast (mastectomy), and neck (radical neck dissection), in particular, may cause lasting pain. Usually, pain is from nerve injury and may be described as "numbing" or "shooting." Also, pain after amputation is much more common than was previously thought. In the past, patients used to literally think they were going crazy when they felt sensations in the part of the body that had been removed (called *phantom limb pain*). It has only recently been recognized that similar pain may follow breast or colostomy surgery ("phantom breast" or "phantom anus" pain).

From Chemotherapy

Certain types of chemotherapy are more likely than others to cause pain. Here is another reason to make sure pain is fully discussed with the doctor. This kind of pain can often be relieved or eliminated by adjusting the chemotherapy. *Polyneuropathy* (meaning nerve damage to many nerves), especially common after treatment with the drugs vincristine or vinblastine, is usually first felt as jaw pain, but can also cause tingling sensations in the feet and hands, as well as stomach problems (autonomic neuropathy). When steroids are taken for a long time, they can weaken the bones (called *osteoporosis* or bone resorption) or even destroy the bone, especially the hip joints (called *aseptic necrosis*). If the steroids are withdrawn too quickly, joint pain (*pseudorheumatism*) can result as well. Painful, sensitive mouth sores (known as *stomatitis* and *mucositis*) can be caused by many types of chemotherapy, especially when combined with radiation or bone-marrow transplantation. This kind of pain is usually very severe, but lasts only days to weeks in most cases. The recognition and treatment of mucositis is crucial so that treatment does not interfere with nutrition.

From Radiation

Radiation therapy can cause a variety of symptoms. In addition to fatigue, bleeding problems, skin injury, and diarrhea, there may be pain in the skin, bone, or near nerves. Pain can result from actual injury to these structures, or may be due to indirect causes, like scarring and fibrosis (excessive connective tissue), or injury to blood vessels that supply these structures. The spinal cord is very sensitive to radiation, and occasionally injury here may produce bizarre pain in the lower half of the body, sometimes accompanied by numbness and even paralysis or bladder problems (incontinence). Occasionally, radiation can even produce new tumors on nerves that are included in the treatment field.

Cancer Pain Syndromes Caused by Tumor Growth

Although pain may stem from many other causes, one of the most common sources of pain in the cancer patient is a result of the effects of the tumor growth; it accounts for almost 80 percent of the pain in hospitalized cancer patients and about 60 percent in outpatients. Again, although many different syndromes are listed here, the likelihood of a particular patient experiencing more than a couple are very unlikely.

Specifically, pain from the cancer itself is caused by the cancer:

- Invading nerves, blood vessels, bones, or parts of the lymph system.
- Pressing on nerves, causing compression.
- Obstructing hollow organs such as the gastrointestinal tract, trachea, or ureter.
- Blocking blood vessels, which can cause poor circulation and cause the veins to engorge and swell.
- Killing, infecting, or inflaming tissues.
- Pushing on tissues, causing them to distend.

The type of pain depends on exactly where the tumor damage occurs within the body. The part of the body that is injured will help determine what type of medications will help. Here is a general view of the various pain syndromes associated with cancer:

Bone Pain

Tumor invading bone is the most common cause of cancer pain. It is most often the result of cancer of the prostate, breast, thyroid, lung, or kidney, but can occur with almost any tumor. A test called a *bone scan* is most often used to identify tumors that have spread to the bone, but plain X-rays, CAT scans, and multiple resonance imaging (MRI) may also be used. Although many types of tumors in bone are not painful, when they do cause pain, they often flare up at night and are worse with movement or when the body or body part bears weight. Typically, bone pain feels like a dull deep ache or like a gnawing pain; it may cause muscle spasms or spells of stabbing pain.

Occasionally, headaches are associated with tumors in the bones of the skull. Back pain is often linked with lung, breast, and prostate cancer, which can metastasize to the spine.

Pain Due to Nerve Damage

Pain from nerve damage, which affects 20 to 40 percent of patients, is often described as burning, tingling, numbing, pressing, squeezing, or itching, and may even trigger pain in numb areas. Patients often describe nerve pain as being different from the sensations they usually associate with pain. Nerve pain can be extremely unpleasant, even intolerable.

Usually, nerve pain is constant and steady. Sometimes, in addition to the continuous pain, sudden intermittent pains occur, often described as shooting, like a lance stabbing, electrical or jolting in nature. In trying to understand pain better, doctors have compared these types of pain to a seizure or convulsion, and have found more than a few similarities. Pain does not cause seizures, but researchers have found that their physical nature may be alike in some ways. Both pain and seizure are electrical phenomenon, and, like a seizure, pain from a nerve injury may be sudden and unpredictable in onset and duration. This similarity is the basis for doctors' use of anticonvulsants like carbamazepine (Tegretol) and phenytoin (Dilantin) to treat shooting pain.

Many patients with nerve pain also experience associated problems, such as bladder or bowel weakness or an impaired sense—poor taste, smell, hearing, feeling, or seeing—or motor or reflex problems. Some patients also suffer from what is known as *evoked pain*—that is, an unpleasant abnormal sensation, such as that experienced with shingles, in which a patient exhibits unusual pain sensitivity from something as ordinary as touch, which doesn't normally cause pain; this may result from contact with clothing, bedsheets, or wind.

Unfortunately, nerve pain responds relatively poorly to narcotic drugs such as morphine when they are used alone. Sometimes, however, it can be relieved by using combinations of drugs such as adding certain types of antidepressants (tricyclic ones), anticonvulsants, anesthetics administered orally (sodium channel blockers) or through an intravenous route, and drugs known as alpha adrenergic antagonists. Still, in all these cases, relief is unpredictable and new combinations may be needed every three to four weeks, during which time the drugs are increased steadily to find the right dose. Sometimes, rubbing the painful area with topical medicines that contain aspirin, chlorophorm, or even red peppers (capsaicin) can help nerve pain as well. (See Chapter 8 for more details.)

More invasive techniques such as nerve blocks may provide short-term relief, and sometimes, a series of blocks may provide prolonged periods of relief. In special cases, long-term electrical stimulation of the spinal cord or brain can be used to provide long-term relief as well.

Muscle Pain

Until recently, muscle pain had been underrecognized in cancer patients, largely because even modern tests do a poor job of identifying damage to muscles. When muscles are injured, the pain may be described as dull, aching, and sore, often associated with stiffness and local tenderness. Although it may feel like a cramp, muscular cancer pain is usually more severe and persistent than a typical cramp.

In general, muscle pain does not respond well to morphine and similar drugs, or to muscle relaxants. Typically, doctors treat muscle pain with medications such as the nonsteroidal anti-inflammatory drugs, or NSAIDs as they are commonly referred to (for example, aspirin and ibuprofen), quinine, diazepam (Valium), baclofen (Lioresal), phenytoin (Dilantin), dantrolene (Dantrium), and carbamazepine (Tegretol).

Therapies such as mild exercise, gradual stretching, heat or ice, ultrasound, TENS (Transcutaneous Electrical Nerve Stimulation), and massage may help relieve such pain. (See Chapter 12 for details.) Many patients obtain relief when a local anesthetic and steroids are injected into persistent areas of pain. (See Chapters 9 and 8, respectively.)

Abdominal Pain

Pain originating in the abdomen may stem from several sources. When nerves are involved, the pain tends to be well localized but may radiate out in bandlike patterns and be associated with hypersensitivity and altered sensation. Abdominal pain may also stem from tumors in the:

- Liver which tend to result in constant dull pain and often a feeling of fullness. It may express itself in the midback, or in the right shoulder if the diaphragm is irritated. Such a tumor may also cause nausea and vomiting.
- Pancreas which tend to cause relentless, boring, mid-stomach aching pain that spreads to the midback and often is relieved by curling up into the fetal position and is aggravated by lying flat.
- Stomach which give rise to pain similar to that of pancreatic tumors or a burning pain, like that of ulcers.
- Intestines which may block the bowel, causing colicky pain and bloating.
- Pelvic region which may be caused by bowel, ovarian, or uterine cancer, or tumors in the abdomen that are outside of specific organs. Such pain tends to feel vague and hard to pinpoint, yet causes fullness, pressure, or discomfort on both sides of the body. In some patients, pelvic pain may be intermittent shooting pain or feel like red hot pokerlike pain in the rectum. When a tumor affects the bladder, the pain may be burning and cause a sense of fullness of the bladder.

When blood vessels or areas of the lymph system become blocked by a tumor, pain may also arise. When an artery is blocked, for example, the patient may feel numb or weak in the area; as an area becomes deprived of blood and oxygen because of the blockage, a deep aching pain may be felt. Moving the area may be particularly uncomfortable. When veins or lymph vessels are obstructed, an area may become engorged, causing swelling and tightness; sometimes, the area affected may look bluish red. Some of these conditions are medical emergencies and consultations with a doctor should be made immediately.

Headache

In about 60 percent of patients with brain tumors, headache is experienced. It often feels steady, deep, dull, and aching and is rarely rhythmic or throbbing. It is usually intermittent and may be worse in the morning or with coughing or straining. Usually, the pain is moderate, rarely severe enough to waken patients. Often, such headaches are helped by aspirin or steroids, cold packs, or lying prone. Sometimes, however, headaches have nothing to do with the cancer itself and stem from the stress of having cancer.

Other Head and Neck Pain

Pain in the neck and head area is often triggered by swallowing, eating, coughing, talking, and other movements of the head. Such pains usually respond well to many types of therapies, including radiation, nonsteroidal anti-inflammatories, narcotics, anticonvulsants, and antidepressants. Nerve blocks, neurosurgery, and the administration of narcotics near the brain (intraventricular) may also be effective.

OTHER SOURCES OF PAIN ASSOCIATED WITH CANCER
Other Conditions

Pain may result from other conditions that are occurring at the same time as the cancer. Examples may be arthritis, gastrointestinal disorders, or back pain; they account for the complaints of pain in about 3 percent of hospitalized cancer patients and 10 percent of those at home. Some physicians also consider problems related to the side effects of cancer therapies as another category of pain, such as discomfort due to muscle spasms, constipation, and bedsores. These problems will be discussed more fully in Chapters 10 and 11.

"Benign Pain"

As we've said, patients are sometimes fearful of admitting their pain for fear that it means their condition has worsened. Yet, not all pain associated with cancer means a tumor has grown or reoccurred, or that the cancer has gotten worse. We have already talked about how treatment of the tumor can cause pain by injuring normal tissue; scarring can also cause pain. Doctors sometimes call such a pain "benign pain," even though it can have ill effects if untreated. Muscle spasm is a good example. Spasm is a protective reflex that causes us to hold an injured body part still. Sometimes muscle spasm persists longer than it should, and can become the main source of pain. The pain is not associated with the tumor having gotten worse, and to provide the proper treatment, the doctor would need to know that there was persistent pain. In this case, under doctor's counsel, it may be safe to push through the body's alarm system and to exercise despite the pain. Even though physical therapy or rehabilitation may make the pain worse until the stiffness is gone, no new harm is brewing.

Furthermore, more pain may result from the simple reason that tolerance to painkillers may have developed. Discussing these issues is another reason why patients shouldn't be fearful about admitting pain.

WHY PAIN SHOULD BE RELIEVED: "HOLDING OUT" DOES NOT HELP

Regardless of the source of the pain, it should be treated, not only to make the patient more comfortable, but for other reasons as well.

▪ *Pain is harmful to your health.*

In most cases, pain is hazardous to one's health. Unrelieved pain impacts negatively on all aspects of a person's well-being. Nutrition, rest, and mood—all suffer when severe pain persists, and this is at a time when these aspects of life are of the utmost importance. Pain may also interfere with a patient's ability to follow doctor's recommendations for treatment of the tumor. Radiation therapy, for example, may involve daily treatments on a hard table for several weeks; if each movement causes pain, patients may be less willing to comply with the daily regimen. Worse yet, preliminary research on animals even suggests that "pain can kill": tumors grew much faster in rats when morphine was withheld after painful surgery.

▪ *Pain disqualifies patients for experimental therapy.*

If pain is unrelieved, it can also affect the patient's "performance status," a term doctors use to describe how well someone is getting around. If a performance status is low, a patient may be excluded from qualifying for any experimental therapy, a practice especially common in research hospitals.

▪ *Most times, unwarranted fears interfere with getting treatment.*

One of the key reasons patients give for avoiding painkillers is the fear of drug addiction. It is a tragedy that the rarity of true addiction in cancer patients is seldom emphasized amid the rhetoric of our dramatic "War on Drugs." Well-meaning friends and relatives also may not understand how uncommon addiction is, making the problem worse by discouraging the patient from taking painkillers. Unaware that drug side effects can usually be avoided, patients maintain irrational fears of "becoming a zombie" or "getting a high." Sometimes, patients erroneously believe they have to "save" the strong medication until the pain is "really bad." Patients with this "money in the bank" syndrome don't realize that pain medications do not stop working, even if taken for a long time. Other patients may endure pain to preserve its "warning function," believing that their pain continues to help the doctor track their disease. This is rarely the case in cancer cases.

Often, doctors are the reason why a patient's pain goes unrelieved. As we said in the last chapter, education about pain is inadequate in most medical schools, and doctors may not adequately communicate to their patients that pain can be treated effectively and safely. Not recognizing that "good patients" are reluctant to talk about pain on their own, many doctors may be too busy to ask about pain. Moreover, as we've seen, current drug laws discourage doctors from treating pain aggressively.

Finally, some patients are plagued by what some have called the "stiff upper lip syndrome." This individual wants to "tough it out," either to avoid painkillers altogether or to wait until the last possible minute before taking a painkiller. This attitude can be traced to erroneous social and cultural messages that it is good or virtuous to "suffer in silence," and even to religious beliefs that the pain is punishment for some real or imagined sin.

- *Yet good pain treatment is good cancer treatment.*

Adequate pain relief is vital not only for quality of life, but for energy to fight the disease itself. As we've said, when pain is undertreated, the mind, body, and spirit all suffer. Patients are less likely to have the energy to fight the cancer or to comply with the demanding antitumor therapy required; that means that inadequate pain relief could result in undermining the cancer treatment. Pain may also impair one's ability to concentrate, increase irritability, and trigger feelings of depression, helplessness, hopelessness, and fear of pain and death—all feelings that may compound one's sense of pain. In fact, more than three-quarters of patients in pain complain that they have problems sleeping; trouble concentrating is the next most common symptom. Feelings of anxiety, depression, and irritability, and just outright crying affect about half of all patients in cancer pain.

The important point to remember is that suffering is needless—it only is going to make things worse. Pain treatment should be a front burner issue, not relegated to the back burner. It is as essential to treat pain as it is to treat the cancer itself because the pain can influence the cancer. They should be viewed as inseparable.

Next, we'll look at how to most effectively communicate pain to doctors—a process that is vital to proper treatment.

3

Assessing Pain and Planning Strategies

Inform patients and families that most if not all cancer-related pain can be relieved by a variety of therapies that are now available.

Tell patients and families they should not suffer in silence. "Good patients" do tell their caregivers about their pain.

Convince your colleagues, patients and families that addiction is extremely rare when narcotic analgesics are used to treat the pain of cancer. . . .

Cancer denies life, and the pain associated with cancer denies the quality of life. We cannot yet be victorious over cancer, but it is hopeful and exciting that we can conquer much if not all of the pain of this dread disease. The imperative . . . [is] that we do not fail in this endeavor.
> —Dr. C. Everett Koop, as Surgeon General of the United States, statement on the Occasion of the First National Meeting for State Cancer Pain Initiatives, Madison, Wisconsin, July 7, 1989

This chapter provides an overview of how doctors assess cancer pain, what to expect from a comprehensive pain assessment, and the general approaches doctors take in tackling cancer pain.

STRATEGIES TO RELIEVE PAIN

Doctors use three basic strategies to relieve cancer pain, and each specific technique discussed in this book reflects one of these three strategies.

Strategy 1: Attacking the Source

Whenever possible, the first and best way to relieve cancer pain is to eliminate the source of the pain. The main way to do this is to remove or shrink the cancer, either with surgery, radiation treatment, or chemotherapy (including hormones). These treatments have some limitations, however:

- Each of these kinds of treatments has some risk.
- Many patients are not candidates for surgery.
- Not all tumors respond to radiation and chemotherapy. Even when they do, there are limits as to how much can be administered.

Nevertheless, these strategies are often very effective in relieving pain, even when a cure may be unlikely. They don't work instantly, though; it takes *time* to shrink a tumor and so their benefit for pain relief may accrue slowly. During this time, painkillers may be needed. And even if the pain persists, the treatment still may be working because lingering pain may be from other sources, such as scarring or fibrosis. When these treatments are used to relieve symptoms, without a hope of a "cure," they are called *palliative treatments*. We'll discuss them in more detail later in the chapter.

Strategy 2: Distorting the Message

The second and by far the most common way to relieve pain is to alter the perception of pain in the brain, where the pain message is received and interpreted. This is usually accomplished by using painkillers, called *analgesics*, such as morphine. Even though patients may fear that doctors will view their pain as "in their head," truth is, pain *is* "all in the head." No matter how it aches or where it hurts, all pain *is* ultimately recorded in the brain, which acts like a great computer interpreting the meaning of all the sensations we experience. Morphine and related drugs alter the perception of pain in a selective and reversible way, with no permanent damage or changes. Pain is blunted and individuals can continue to function normally, and often much better, on the properly chosen medication.

Strategy 3: Interrupting the Signal

The third way to treat cancer pain—and the one needed much less frequently—is to interrupt the pain signal somewhere between the tumor and the central nervous system, which is made up of both the spinal cord and brain. This kind of treatment is like cutting an electrical wire to interrupt a circuit. Examples include neurosurgical and anesthetic procedures that actually cut or numb nerves. Nerve blocks, for example, interrupt the pain signal by anesthetizing nerves with chemicals injected nearby. These treatments have some risk and are appropriate for only a small proportion of patients. We'll discuss them further in Chapter 9.

Before doctors embark on any of these approaches, though, they must first assess the situation. Some doctors will ask about characteristics of the pain; others will use formal questionnaires.

Since every person's pain is different, each treatment plan will be different as well. What worked for Aunt Lucy, who may even have had a similar cancer, probably won't work for cousin Harry. Even though similar methods and drugs are used for everyone, they need to be adjusted to match the patient's unique situation. Just as most people can't buy their suits off the rack, drugs must be tailored for an optimal fit.

Regardless of the kind of doctor that is consulted, however, the patient will benefit from conveying effectively to the physician all relevant information about the disease, treatments used so far, the patient's lifestyle, coping styles, activities, and so forth. The following section will help the patient and family best prepare for a consultation whose goal includes pain relief.

HOW TO PREPARE FOR A PAIN ASSESSMENT

Be Prepared with Details

Many assessments begin with a basic history—marital and job status, ability to complete activities of daily living, activity levels, recreational activities, network of support, cultural and ethnic background, the patient's psychological and social strengths, weaknesses, spiritual beliefs, general health, and abilities of the spouse or significant other (including the ability to care for the cancer patient, to drive, etc.), health problems other than cancer, ability of the patient to exercise, allergies to medication, medication use, and prior surgery. *One very useful and time-saving tip is to bring a list of the patient's medications that includes doses, times when taken, and how effective they are. If making a list is too difficult, bring all the pill bottles in a shopping bag.* Patients should also expect the doctor to review their cancer history, of course, and the current status of the disease.

Patients Should Have a Companion

When possible, at least one close relative or friend should accompany a patient to a pain assessment. Ideally, that person should be the one who is identified as being responsible for the patient's overall care, who can serve as the patient's advocate, and who can be an active member in the decision-making process. Many doctors encourage whole families to come so that the understanding, responsibility, and decisions regarding the loved one who is ill can be shared. If patients are ill, distracted by their pain and other concerns, perhaps denying their illness, they may find it difficult to concentrate. It is helpful for the companion(s) to be sure that all the prepared questions have been answered, to take notes on what was discussed, and be prepared to review them with the patient later. Of course, some patients, especially those without a spouse, will prefer to remain independent in consulting with a doctor. If so, the patient should attempt to take notes carefully as she or he may have trouble remembering everything the doctor says.

Give Pain Details

Most people find it hard to talk about their pain. When pressed for details about their discomfort, many people are surprised by the questions and may respond, "It just hurts—I can't describe it." This is a very common response. Like the many words that Eskimos have for snow, pain specialists have more than 75 words for pain (see Table 3.1). Even though one is tempted to just say, "pain is pain," think about the differences between the feelings that go with a toothache, say, versus a burn, a bruise, or a fresh surgical incision.

To best communicate with a doctor about pain, it is advisable that a patient try to use the same types of measures that doctors use. Valid and reliable measures of pain not only help doctors in making an accurate diagnosis of disease, but also help them assess the effectiveness of treatment and side effects.

Basically, measures of pain attempt to assess three dimensions:

1. Pain intensity, location, and character
2. Pain relief
3. Psychological distress or mood

Doctors can benefit from descriptions of pain that cover the following dimensions:

What kind of pain is it?
Is it flickering, pulsing, throbbing, or pounding?
How does the patient feel about the pain?
Is it exhausting, sickening, fearful, or terrifying?
How does the patient view the pain?
Is it annoying or unbearable?

Consult Table 3.1 for a specific vocabulary of pain.

Although pain clinics may use detailed pain questionnaires, most doctors, including oncologists, don't use them. Yet patients can best prepare for an appointment that will include a discussion of pain by reviewing the words

Table 3.1. *How to Describe Pain*

Flickering	Hot	Punishing
Quivering	Burning	Grueling
Pulsing	Scalding	Cruel
Beating	Searing	Vicious
Pounding		Killing
	Tingling	
Jumping	Itching	Wretched
Flashing	Smarting	Blinding
Shooting	Stinging	
		Annoying
Pricking	Dull	Troublesome
Boring	Sore	Miserable
Drilling	Hurting	Intense
Stabbing	Aching	Unbearable
	Heavy	
Sharp		Spreading
Cutting	Tender	Radiating
Lacerating	Taut	Penetrating
	Rasping	Piercing
Pinching	Splitting	
Pressing		Tight
Gnawing	Tiring	Numb
Cramping	Exhausting	Drawing
Crushing		Squeezing
	Sickening	Tearing
Tugging	Suffocating	
Pulling		Cool
Wrenching	Fearful	Cold
	Frightful	Freezing
	Terrifying	
		Nagging
		Nauseating
Pain Intensity Scale		Agonizing
		Dreadful
0 No Pain		Torturing
1 Mild		
2 Discomforting		
3 Distressing		
4 Horrible		
5 Excruciating		

Source: Reprinted from the McGill Pain Questionnaire. Copyright
© 1970 by Ronald Melzack, Ph.D., and used with permission of
Dr. Melzack.

given in Table 3.1 which are part of what is called the McGill Pain Questionnaire. Though lengthy, its many adjectives help describe the pain more specifically. Other common forms used to assess pain include The Brief Pain Inventory (which may take about 15 minutes to fill out but which has psychological questions because psychological factors can have a powerful influence on pain); the short Memorial Pain Assessment Card (MPAC, which is one of the simplest assessment tools and also includes psychological components); or a "visual analog scale" (which shows a line divided into 10 segments and numbered from 0 to 10, where 0 = no pain and 10 = excruciating, worst imaginable pain). (See Figures 3.1 and 3.2.)

For children under 7 and adults who can't use such scales, several tools are used—a series of smiling to frowning faces (see Figure 3.3); the "Oucher" which shows a scale from 0 to 100 and six photographs of a 4-year-old's face depicting different levels of pain; pain drawings or pain maps where children color where they hurt (using four different colors that represent varying intensities of pain); a Poker Chip Assessment in which children are given four red poker chips which represent "a piece of hurt" and are asked how many chips their pain has; and a list of pain words for children and teens (see Table 3.2).

Some of these forms have been reproduced here to familiarize the patient and family with the types of questions asked and to give the patient the opportunity to fill one out before a pain consultation, because while many doctors still don't use these tools, it is important for them to have this kind of information. (See, for example, the Brief Pain Inventory in Figure 3.4, which may help a patient communicate pain to family members, caregivers, and health-care professionals.)

WHAT TO TELL A DOCTOR ABOUT PAIN

The most basic information a doctor will need to treat pain is covered by the following questions. Think about these carefully before meeting with the physician.

- Where is the pain? Is it in more than one place? If so, which is the worst pain? Does the pain ever radiate—shoot or travel—from one location to another? Are there any "secondary pains"?
- Did the pain predate the cancer? Is it chronic pain, like arthritis or migraine pain?
- Is the pain constant (uninterrupted)? Intermittent (comes and goes)? Or is it constant (perhaps at a low level), but punctuated with periods of severe pain (which is the most common mode of all)?

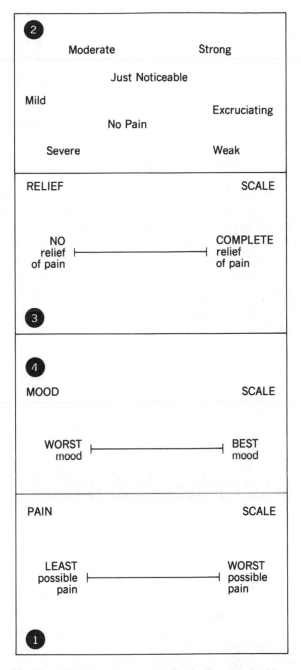

Figure 3.1. *The Memorial Pain Assessment Card. (Reprinted with permission from B. Fishman, S. Pasternack, S. Wallenstein, R. W. Houde, and K. M. Foley, The Memorial Pain Assessment Card: A valid instrument for the evaluation of cancer pain. Cancer 1987: (60) 1151–1158.)*

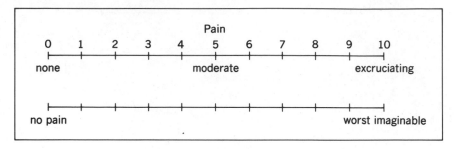

Figure 3.2. *Visual Analog Scale.*

- How severe is each pain on average? How severe when it subsides (least pain experienced)? How severe when it is at its worst? Try using a 0 to 10 scale; zero means no pain, and 10 is the worst pain imaginable.
- What kind of pain is it? What words describe it (burning, aching, stabbing, piercing, etc. (See Table 3.1.)
- When does each pain start (during the night, when getting out of bed, etc.)? How long does it last? Are there any patterns to it?
- What tends to aggravate the pain—for example, what movement or position? What helps relieve it? Does heat, cold, or massage have any effect?

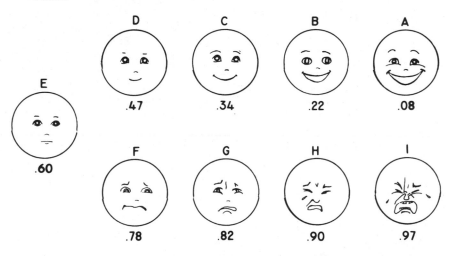

Figure 3.3. *McGrath's face scale. Children are presented with one of three different randomly ordered face sheets. They select the face that best represents how they feel in relation to their pain, from "the happiest feeling possible" to the "saddest feeling possible." This figure is actually the scoring card used to quantify children's responses. The numbers represent the magnitude of pain affect (between 0 and 1) shown in each face based on previous research on children. (From P. A. McGrath,* Pain in Children: Nature, Assessment, and Treatment. *New York: Guilford, 1990, p. 76. Used by permission.)*

Table 3.2. *Pain Word List for Children and Teenagers*

Sensory Words	Like a sharp knife	Itching
Aching	Pinlike	Like a scratch
Hurting	Sharp	Like a sting
Like an ache	Stabbing	Scratching
Like a hurt	Blistering	Stinging
Sore	Burning	Shocking
Beating	Hot	Shooting
Hitting	Cramping	Splitting
Pounding	Crushing	Numb
Punching	Like a pinch	Stiff
Throbbing	Pinching	Swollen
Biting	Pressure	Tight
Cutting		
Like a pin		
Emotional Words	*Evaluative Words*	
Awful	Annoying	
Deadly	Bad	
Dying	Horrible	
Killing	Miserable	
Crying	Terrible	
Frightening	Uncomfortable	
Screaming	Never goes away	
Terrifying	Uncontrollable	
Dizzy		
Sickening		
Suffocating		

Source: From D. Wilkie, W. Holzemer, M. Tesler et al. Measuring pain quality: validity and reliability of children's and adolescent's pain language. *Pain* 1990: (41) 151. Reprinted with permission of authors and publisher.

- How does the pain affect activities, energy level, appetite, sexual habits, movement, posture, mood, and sleep?
- Are there any other changes associated with the pain? Is there numbness or weakness?
- Is there leakage of urine or soiling of undergarments?
- Is the skin near the area ever affected—for example, are there changes in the temperature, color, or texture of the skin?
- Has sweating or the growth of hair or nails changed?
- Have any painkillers ever been used in the past? Were any particularly effective or ineffective? How long were they effective? Were there side effects?
- What would the patient do differently if the pain didn't exist? What new activities would they engage in?

STUDY ID# _____   HOSPITAL# _____

DO NOT WRITE ABOVE THIS LINE

Brief Pain Inventory (Short Form)

Date: __ / __ / __   Time: _____

Name: _____ _____ _____
           Last   First   Middle Initial

1) Throughout our lives, most of us have had pain from time to time (such as minor headaches, sprains, and toothaches). Have you had pain other than these everyday kinds of pain today?

      1.   Yes   2.   No

2) On the diagram, shade in the areas where you feel pain. Put an X on the area that hurts the most.

Right   Left   Left   Right

3) Please rate your pain by circling the one number that best describes your pain at its worst in the last 24 hours.

   0   1   2   3   4   5   6   7   8   9   10
   No   Pain as bad as
   Pain   you can imagine

4) Please rate your pain by circling the one number that best describes your pain at its least in the last 24 hours.

   0   1   2   3   4   5   6   7   8   9   10
   No   Pain as bad as
   Pain   you can imagine

5) Please rate your pain by circling the one number that best describes your pain on the average.

   0   1   2   3   4   5   6   7   8   9   10
   No   Pain as bad as
   Pain   you can imagine

6) Please rate your pain by circling the one number that tells how much pain you have right now.

   0   1   2   3   4   5   6   7   8   9   10
   No   Pain as bad as
   Pain   you can imagine

Figure 3.4. *Brief Pain Inventory (short form). (Reprinted with permission of the Pain Research Group, Department of Neurology, University of Wisconsin-Madison Medical School. Copyright © 1991 by C. S. Cleeland.)*

7) What treatments or medications are you receiving for your pain?

8) In the last 24 hours, how much relief have pain treatments or medications provided? Please circle the one percentage that most shows how much relief you have received.

0%	10%	20%	30%	40%	50%	60%	70%	80%	90%	100%
No Relief										Complete Relief

9) Circle the one number that describes how, during the past 24 hours, pain has interfered with your:

A. General Activity

0	1	2	3	4	5	6	7	8	9	10
Does not interfere										Completely interferes

B. Mood

0	1	2	3	4	5	6	7	8	9	10
Does not interfere										Completely interferes

C. Walking ability

0	1	2	3	4	5	6	7	8	9	10
Does not interfere										Completely interferes

D. Normal work (includes both work outside the home and housework)

0	1	2	3	4	5	6	7	8	9	10
Does not interfere										Completely interferes

E. Relations with other people

0	1	2	3	4	5	6	7	8	9	10
Does not interfere										Completely interferes

F. Sleep

0	1	2	3	4	5	6	7	8	9	10
Does not interfere										Completely interferes

G. Enjoyment of life

0	1	2	3	4	5	6	7	8	9	10
Does not interfere										Completely interferes

Keeping a Pain Diary

One of the most effective ways to sort out some of the answers to these questions is to keep a pain log or pain diary. Such a diary not only helps doctors diagnose a pain problem but also helps measure progress (or lack of progress) in treating the pain. After only a few days' entries, a pattern may emerge, such as a particular time of day or a particular activity that can be associated with the pain when it is at its worst. Using the same numeric scale (0 to 10, with 0 = no pain and 10 the most severe pain imaginable) to measure the pain day after day (and recording it), or using one of the other assessment tools regularly, can help the doctor know whether to increase, decrease, or change the medication. See the sample diary in Figure 3.5.

Although attending to all the details in caring for an ill loved one can become overwhelming, it helps to also log medication use, doctors' visits, toilet habits (for example, last bowel movement), and other problems.

Keeping a journal or old-fashioned diary to record thoughts and feelings also can be helpful, especially for patients and family members who find it hard to express themselves to other people. Life-threatening illnesses are passages in people's lives, both for the patient and caregiver; an openness to what we are experiencing and feeling can help launch gratifying communication with others.

Convey All Symptoms

Cancer has been called a multi-symptomatic disease, which means that it can affect different patients in many different ways. Here is a list of some of the symptoms people with cancer have described; each is important for the doctor to know about.

Systemwide Symptoms
   Loss of appetite (anorexia)
   Weight loss (cachexia)
   Tiredness/weakness (fatigue)
   Poor sleep (insomnia)

Neurological Problems
   Sedation
   Confusion
   Hallucinations
   Headache
   Muscle weakness
   Altered sensations

Respiratory Problems
Difficulty breathing (dyspnea)
Cough
Hiccoughs (singultus)

Gastrointestinal Problems
Difficulty in swallowing (dysphagia)
Nausea
Vomiting
Dehydration
Constipation
Diarrhea

Psychological Problems
Irritability
Anxiety
Depression
Dementia

Urinary Problems
Inability to control bladder (incontinence)
Difficulty urinating (hesitancy)

Other
Bed sores
Dry, sore mouth

The Doctor Should Be Informed of Any of These Symptoms

Knowing the condition of the patient by taking into account the whole person—the well-being of the body, mind, and spirit—will help the doctor determine if something else is going on. Only with this information will your physician begin to sort out what is caused by the cancer, the cancer treatment, or the medications. Painkillers sometimes produce side effects, and in some patients, it is these side effects that keep the doctor from prescribing enough medicine to take the pain away. If the doctor knows about the symptoms, she or he can usually take action to reverse them so that the patient can receive whatever dose is needed to relieve the pain. For example, even though constipation almost always accompanies the use of painkillers, it should not limit how much painkiller is taken because the dose of laxative should be increased along with that of the painkiller.

Many of the symptoms that people put up with, thinking that they must, can, in fact, be reversed or reduced. Often by simply adding an anti-nausea medication during chemotherapy treatment or a laxative when an opioid is

Figure 3.5. *Daily Pain Diary*

Date: _____	Pain Level, 0 to 10	Activity That Triggered Pain	Medication Taken, Including Dose	Other Pain or Relief Methods Used	Pain Level, 0 to 10, after Medication	Other Comments (other symptoms, moods, problems)
Midnight 12 AM						
1:00 AM						
2:00 AM						
3:00 AM						
4:00 AM						
5:00 AM						
6:00 AM						
7:00 AM						
8:00 AM						
9:00 AM						
10:00 AM						
11:00 AM						

Noon 12 PM				
1:00 PM				
2:00 PM				
3:00 PM				
4:00 PM				
5:00 PM				
6:00 PM				
7:00 PM				
8:00 PM				
9:00 PM				
10:00 PM				
11:00 PM				

being used, the patient can easily achieve relief. Even problems such as fatigue, weight loss, and sedation—which are often difficult to treat—may soon be better managed with products and methods currently being researched.

Be Prepared for Psychological Questions

As discussed in Chapter 2, suffering is more than physical discomfort—the suffering a patient endures usually includes psychological factors, among them moodiness, anxiety over family and financial burdens, and fears about the illness, pain, disfigurement, loss of mental and physical control, and death. To treat pain comprehensively, doctors need to address psychological concerns. They may ask about a patient's personal or cognitive style (how the patient explains the world to him or herself), whether the patient feels depressed or anxious, whether these feelings were persistent before the illness (preexisting) or brought on by the illness, whether there is any history of excessive concern about health and illness (hypochondria), or a preoccupation with one's looks and attractiveness (body image), and so forth. Doctors also need to be apprised of any history of drug or alcohol use because these patients may have a different tolerance to drugs and may respond differently to analgesics compared to others. (See Table 3.3.)

THE GOALS OF THE PAIN TREATMENT

The overall goal of any pain treatment is to enhance quality of life, improve the patient's ability to maintain or resume normal activities, and allow the patient to focus on the things in life that give it meaning. The priorities of a pain strategy are:

1. To Provide a Good Night's Sleep

One of the very first goals should be to boost the hours of pain-free sleep at night. This is important because research shows that when sleep is ab-

Table 3.3. *Patient and Family Checklist for Doctor's Appointment*

BRING TO THE APPOINTMENT
- A companion who is prepared with questions, paper, and pen
- A list of important events in medical history
- A summary of cancer treatment so far
- A list of medications (or the bottles in a bag) and allergies
- Pain questionnaire filled out
- List of problem symptoms
- Notes on patient's outlook and emotional well-being

normal we become less tolerant to pain, and it becomes more bothersome. Also, if patients don't sleep well at night, they will be fatigued during the day and will nap often. This, in turn, makes it harder to sleep the next night. Reversing this cycle is crucial to restoring well-being.

2. To Relieve Resting Pain

The next step is to soothe pain that occurs when the patient is resting but awake.

3. To Relieve Pain Triggered by Movement

The next goal is to relieve pain that occurs when the patient performs a particular activity, such as getting out of bed, turning over, taking a bath, and so on.

These priorities are usually addressed in this order, with getting a good night sleep being paramount. Once that is accomplished, the doctor will then attempt to relieve the pain that persists during rest and finally will tackle that which accompanies movement.

DRUG THERAPY IS THE CORNERSTONE OF PAIN TREATMENT

Although removing the tumor itself is the primary goal for both cancer treatment and pain relief, medications are often needed to attack pain either during treatments or afterward. And as we'll see later in the chapter, those cancer treatments—surgery, chemotherapy (including hormone therapy), or radiation—are not only used to remove or shrink the tumor in an effort to cure the cancer, but are sometimes used for the sole purpose of relieving pain as well.

Pain medications are used commonly for acute or chronic pain—for patients of all ages, including infants—and will relieve pain in up to 90 percent of cases. The World Health Organization (WHO) has revolutionized cancer pain therapies by establishing the following recommended ladder of medications, which recommends the appropriate sequence of therapies. It suggests that doctors treat mild cancer pain with mild painkillers and progress to more potent ones as needed, adding supplemental medications that can enhance pain relief or relieve side effects from the medications where necessary.

THE BASIC PAIN STRATEGY: THE PAINKILLER LADDER

WHO's basic pain strategy, now used worldwide to treat cancer pain, suggests the following steps:

Step 1: Non-steroidal Anti-inflammatory Drugs (NSAIDs)

These drugs, useful for mild to moderate pain, include aspirin, acetamino-phen (Tylenol, etc.), and ibuprofen (Advil, Motrin, Rufen, Nuprin, Medi-pren, among others). In fact, there are almost 20 different types of NSAIDs. It's confusing because, like most medicines, they each have two names: a generic or chemical name, such as ibuprofen, and a trade name that the manufacturer uses for its product of ibuprofen, such as Advil or Motrin.

The various NSAIDs do not differ greatly, but a doctor may still suggest trying different types, because one may work better for one person than another. Unfortunately, there's no way of knowing which will be better for a particular person until they are taken and tried.

Surprisingly, these medications, when taken in the right dose (not too high or too low) at the right time (around-the-clock, as directed) are often effective for even severe pain—especially pain that stems from bone tumors or bone metastases.

Often, an *adjuvant medication,* a complementary medication that is known to amplify pain relief, such as an antidepressant, anticonvulsant, muscle relaxant, or other drug, may be prescribed to enhance the effects of pain killers. Medications to prevent nausea or constipation may also be pre-scribed.

If taken on schedule continuously, relief can occur quickly, within 24 hours. If these medications don't help within 48 hours, or if side effects such as stomach problems or blood-thinning effects occur, then the doctor should be informed and the pain strategy should escalate to the next step.

Even when they aren't strong enough to control the pain, as long as there are no serious side effects, the NSAIDs should probably still be continued along with a stronger (opioid) medication. Since they work by different mechanisms, they can produce an additive or synergistic benefit, so that less opioid medication is needed.

Step 2: "Mild" or "Weak" Opioids

Codeine is the prototype and most familiar example of this drug class, with dextropropoxyphene (Darvon, Darvocet) the most common alternative. Other weak opioids are usually preferred and include oxycodone (Percodan, Per-cocet), hydrocodone (Vicodin, Lortab, etc.), and dihydrocodeine (Synalgos-DC). Most of the "weak" narcotics come combined with aspirin or acet-aminophen. This limits how much can be taken (usually to two tablets every three or four hours)—not because of the narcotic, but because too much aspirin or acetaminophen can cause serious problems.

Some experts have suggested that the importance of these medicines is not so much medical, but social or cultural. As a society, we are "drug-phobic"—so overconcerned about prescribing morphine—that doctors would rather prescribe (and patients would rather take) weaker drugs, even though they are not as effective. *One of the most common mistakes that occurs is that a patient stays on these weaker medicines when a stronger one would better relieve the pain and is no riskier.* If the pain is not controlled with a mild opioid, a doctor or nurse should be consulted.

Often, a combination product will be prescribed, such as codeine with acetaminophen (Tylenol #3), oxycodone with aspirin (Percodan), or acetaminophen (Percocet). Again, adding an adjuvant medication can improve pain relief without having to increase the narcotic dose and can reduce the likelihood of side effects such as nausea, sedation, and constipation. When pain relief fails at maximum doses and pain persists for more than 24 to 48 hours in spite of increasing doses, the next step should be considered.

Step 3: Strong Opioids

Morphine is the first choice and the most commonly used and recommended drug for this step. It is the "gold standard" against which all other cancer pain treatments are compared. But when a patient has a problem with morphine, such as nausea, patients may be switched to similar drugs such as fentanyl (Duragesic), hydromorphone (Dilaudid), methadone (Dolophine), and oxymorphone (Numorphan). When pain relief is inadequate, more morphine (or the similar narcotic being used) may be given—there are no maximum or "ceiling" doses. Again, adjuvant drugs are often prescribed as well as medication from Step 1, such as aspirin, ibuprofen, or acetaminophen, to enhance the pain relief without having to increase the narcotic dose. Other adjuvant drugs may be used to reduce anxiety or control side effects. In spite of the effectiveness of pain relief on this rung of the ladder, some 10 to 20 percent of patients will still need more invasive techniques to control their pain. If so, doctors proceed with other treatments.

Step 4: Surgical and Other Anesthetic Measures

Although WHO's ladder covers only pharmacological approaches, some patients will need additional treatments that go beyond medication to achieve pain relief. Even though WHO does not use another step, we will.

These more advanced techniques are discussed in-depth in Chapter 9, and include short- and long-acting anesthetics, nerve blocks, nerve stimulation, trigger-point injections, and surgical procedures to interrupt the transmission of the pain signal to the brain.

Throughout these treatments, other practices may help as well, including psychological/behavioral procedures, such as hypnosis, relaxation, and imagery techniques, psychological counseling, physical therapy including the use of splints, massage, braces, and other measures such as acupuncture and nerve stimulation. These techniques may be integrated throughout the sequence of analgesic therapies and will be discussed in greater detail in Chapter 12.

HOW DRUG THERAPIES ARE PLANNED

Even though a prognosis for curing cancer may not be what we hoped for, the prognosis for controlling the pain is usually quite excellent. But effective pain treatment is not a hard-and-fast science that is determined in one visit to the doctor. The first prescription and dose may, or may not, work. If it does, chances are that it will only work optimally for a limited time until the illness recedes or progresses, or the patient builds a tolerance to the medication.

Charting the Course of Treatment—Trial and Error

The road to good pain control is not an exact science and we are learning more and more about the body, mind, and pain every day. Nevertheless, basic principles are used, though applying them can be complicated. A person's particular route on the road to good pain control is not always clear; there are usually a few detours or bumps, maybe even a few "deadends," as the treatment is getting started and the doctor discovers what is the best medication and dose for the patient at that time. Don't get discouraged. Good pain control involves some trial and error to determine the best method or drug. Prescribing the correct dose is not always an easy task for the doctor. Often, a doctor will start at an initial "test" dose, and depending on a patient's degree of illness, personal tolerance levels, and other factors, the dose will need to be increased until it relieves the pain. Sometimes, just a day or two is adequate to determine whether the dose should be boosted; with some drugs, however, a week or two is needed to determine if the dose is correct. (See Chapters 5 to 7 which discuss dose and expected relief time for the primary drugs prescribed for pain.)

Whenever a new drug is started, patients should be sure to ask about when the drug should take effect. They will need to contact their doctor if the pain is not relieved within the specified period. Frequent communication with the doctor or health-care professional who is working on the doctor's behalf, therefore, is essential to any effective pain treatment program.

Don't get overly concerned about the trial-and-error process—it is the norm. Remember each person is different and medication must be tailored to take into consideration age, drug tolerance, level of activity, and other factors. Occasionally, a drug or dose won't work, either because it doesn't relieve the pain or because it produces an unpleasant side effect. Remember, it is a temporary, reversible treatment—unlike surgery—and can easily be modified. A lasting side effect is rare—and in fact, most side effects go away in a few days. The important thing is to keep in touch with the doctor or nurse so they always have the vital information they need to refine the treatment.

To Ensure Maximum Relief

▪ Ask how long a particular medication may take before the patient should expect significant relief. Can the dose be raised or taken more frequently without contacting the medical team? If yes, then by how much and how often. Call the medical team if relief does not occur. (Refer to Chapters 5 to 8 for expected time to relief for particular medications.)

▪ Ask what to expect from each new drug and be prepared to call the team about any side effects so they can be treated immediately. If symptoms occur, can the doses be tapered without calling the medical team; if so, by how much?

▪ If the drug does not seem to work or causes serious side effects, no one is to blame; and the failure of one drug is no indication that another won't work.

▪ Using a problem-solving approach, the team should continually monitor the pain and drug's effectiveness. As soon as pain relief wanes or side effects cannot be controlled by one medication, the team should be contacted to either raise the dose (if pain is the problem, this is usually the preferred and first route), add an adjuvant medication (to treat side effects or to reduce the dose of painkiller which should reduce side effects), or switch medications.

▪ Be sure to communicate all changes in the patient's condition—physical, psychological, emotional, and so forth. Insomnia should be treated most vigorously!

▪ If the patient is accustomed to having an alcoholic drink occasionally or regularly, be sure to ask the doctor whether that routine is still acceptable with the given medication. In most cases, an occasional drink will be okay except when beginning a new medication or adjusting a dose. Many doctors feel that once a medication is stabilized, a glass of beer or wine may even be beneficial to help relax the patient, help ease the pain, boost appetite, reduce anxiety, and even promote a good night's sleep. Alcohol in combination with a narcotic, however, will enhance the narcotic's sedative effect, so be sure to discuss this with the doctor.

▪ Ask the doctor about other nonprescription medications that the patient may want to take, such as cold medications and analgesics for headache or menstrual cramps. Some medications contain aspirin which should be avoided by patients on chemotherapy. Others, such as those for allergies, may induce drowsiness and compound the sedative effects of narcotics. To be safe, ask the doctor.

▪ Communicate all decisions to the patient, whether the caregiver thinks the patient understands or not.

▪ Communicate all symptoms to the team and be sure they are treated (e.g., nausea, constipation, dry mouth, etc.). Each affects the comfort and well-being of the patient.

▪ All possible medications should be considered before more invasive techniques are used.

▪ Drugs should be administered by mouth whenever possible to preserve the patient's mobility and independence. Only when patients can no longer take medicine by mouth, perhaps because of mouth sores or the inability to swallow or digest, should other routes be explored, such as rectal suppositories, administration through a small needle just under the skin (subcutaneous), and so on.

▪ Be prepared for increasing doses of opioids as time goes on. There is no single right dose for many analgesics; the appropriate dose will vary from patient to patient and over time. "Recommended" or "maximum" doses used in textbooks were not intended for cancer pain; these doses are often used as useful starting points, but more will usually be required. Once a drug, or combination of drugs, is prescribed, if it is not relieving the pain, its dose should first be increased until a "ceiling" dose is reached (which will not occur with the opioids) or until side effects are unmanageable. The ceiling dose is a level after which increases in the medication no longer provide added pain relief but only increase toxicity. The opioids usually have no ceiling. If a new medication is needed, the patient should then be switched to a stronger medication—not one of equal analgesic effect.

▪ Expect drug combinations to be prescribed; ask about them if they are not. (See Chapter 8.)

▪ A laxative should be prescribed as soon as opioid therapy (Step 2) begins. *Ask for it if it is not offered.*

▪ Anti-nausea medications (anti-emetics) will be needed in up to 40 percent of cancer patients, at least for a time. Anticipate their need and have nausea treated as soon as possible, should it develop.

▪ Medications should generally be prescribed on a regular basis, not as needed. Discuss this with the doctor if they are not. (See the following section on "as needed" versus "around-the-clock" prescriptions.)

Frustrations and Problems

A concerned and knowledgeable doctor, from any specialty, can help up to 90 percent of patients achieve good control of pain. This process can be time consuming and frustrating, though, for the patient, their family, and the doctor. It is okay to communicate that frustration to the doctor. No doubt the doctor is just as frustrated. The key is to accept in advance that rarely can a doctor get it right the first time, through no fault of his. Continue to work with the health-care team until you are satisfied.

Consider whether it makes sense to ask the doctor about consulting a pain specialist or a local or regional pain clinic. (See the Appendix for where to find pain specialists.)

"AS NEEDED" VERSUS "AROUND-THE-CLOCK" PRESCRIPTIONS

Many studies have shown that far too often doctors prescribe doses of painkillers that are both too low and given too infrequently. To compound the problem, nurses may then cut down on the already deficient doses that have been prescribed. These doctors and nurses are not heartless (far from it), but are responding to antiquated concerns about addiction and insufficient teaching in medical and nursing schools.

As Needed (prn) Prescriptions: A Questionable Approach to Cancer Treatment

A traditional means of prescribing pain medication for cancer patients, no longer regarded as appropriate in most cases, is prescribing it on a prn basis (from the Latin *pro re nata*) which means that analgesics may only be taken "as needed" at specified intervals. Some patients try to tough it out, thinking that they should be stoic or that delaying their medication will help them somehow, such as in preventing addiction. Other patients, if hospitalized, must wait for a certain number of hours to pass if medication is prescribed on a prn basis, and then they must specifically *request* pain medication in order to receive it. Although still an effective way to control some kinds of pain, it not only is ineffective for most cases of cancer pain, but may make matters worse!

With the prn method, patients must wait for the pain to return before they can request additional medication. Since doses are often too low or too widely separated, patients may become preoccupied with their pain, becoming "clock watchers," anxious and fearful that their pain will return before the next dose is allowed.

When a patient is hospitalized, such an order can trigger a confrontation between the patient and nurse who incorrectly expects morphine, for example, to last four to six hours. Yet patients often experience the return of pain earlier than expected and may be in agony, pleading for the next dose. Because of exaggerated fears of addiction, the nurse may postpone the dose of painkiller as long as possible. By the time the pain is finally treated, however, it may be so severe that a much larger dose may be needed to relieve it, which also boosts the chances of triggering a side effect, such as nausea or mental confusion.

It is ironic that this clockwatching, brought about by undertreatment and prn dosing, is often interpreted as addictive behavior. The appearance of the very problem we are trying to avoid (addiction) seems to be triggered by undertreating, not overtreating, the pain. Actually, when undertreated cancer patients seek additional medication, it is not really addiction but is a *pseudoaddiction*, a problem that is caused by the treatment itself (*iatrogenic*). These unfortunate individuals are actually seeking relief from pain, not more medication, and will usually stop taking pain medications altogether if the pain disappears.

Prolonged prn treatment is like a rollercoaster ride—the patient's level of comfort is always changing—periods of relief occur, but often with side effects, and the pain always returns. Even after more effective therapy is started, patients may maintain an anticipation and memory of pain that is very hard to shake.

Around-the-Clock Prescriptions

Most often, pain from cancer is relatively constant. Isn't it, then, logical that around-the-clock pain is best treated with around-the-clock medication? By staying slightly ahead of the pain, the patient's comfort is much more uniform. Less medication is actually needed to prevent pain than to treat it once it is allowed to become severe.

This more humane and effective approach of taking medicine on an appropriate schedule "around the clock" actually prevents severe pain from returning. Each dose is given before the effect of the last dose wears off completely. As a result, studies have shown that dosing pain at regular intervals and at levels high enough to prevent severe pain ends up with overall lower doses being needed, which also wards off undesirable side effects. (See Figure 3.6.)

Cancer pain specialists now recommend that adequate doses of all the analgesics—including aspirin, acetaminophen, ibuprofen, and morphine—as well as the medications to control constipation, nausea, and vomiting, be prescribed and taken before pain or symptoms worsen. Once pain or symptoms have occurred, medication to prevent them should be prescribed around the clock.

HOW DRUGS ARE CHOSEN

Although cancer pain specialists will follow the order of the WHO analgesic ladder, which drug they prescribe on each rung of the ladder will depend on the individual patient and doctor. Doctors will take into account age, type of cancer, analgesic history (what worked in the past to relieve pain, what didn't), and a doctor's familiarity with particular medications. No one drug on each rung is better than another. What one patient can easily tolerate, another may get sick on; the same patient may do well when switched to a similar, equally potent medication.

UNDERSTANDING PALLIATIVE THERAPY

When cancer causes pain, the first thing a doctor will try to do is to treat the cause of it. One of three treatments—radiation, surgery, or chemotherapy (which sometimes includes hormone therapy)—alone or in combination, is usually used to eliminate a cancer or the source of the pain. The primary goal, as we've said, initially is to remove or shrink the tumor com-

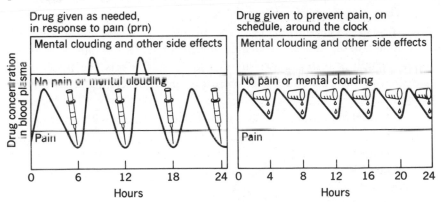

Figure 3.6. *"As needed" versus "around-the-clock" dosing. "As needed" (prn) dosing, usually in the form of an injection, results in patients becoming anxious about the pain returning, and then needing large doses to relieve the pain. As a result, the side effects such as confusion and nausea are greater. "Around-the-clock" (a-t-c) scheduled dosing (every 4 hours or every 12 hours), on the other hand, prevents pain from returning or growing and results in overall lower doses and few side effects. (From R. Melzack, The tragedy of needless pain. Scientific American, February 1990, Vol. 262, No. 2, p. 28. Used by permission.)*

pletely, and although the patient's comfort and symptoms are important concerns, they are only secondary to the primary objective, which is to cure the patient of the cancer. Often, high doses or major surgery are required to eradicate the tumor and surrounding tissue and to maximize the chance of a patient's survival. This initial treatment is called *radical therapy*—the patient and physician must do whatever is necessary to storm the cancer.

Since this book is about pain, however, our discussion of surgery, chemotherapy, and radiation centers around these treatments as procedures to alleviate pain and other symptoms; what we refer to here is *palliative therapy*. These procedures are also used as methods to help cure the patient of cancer. We make no distinction and no prognosis as to the survival of patients reading this book—our main emphasis is on conquering their pain.

Although cancer can't always be completely "cured" or eliminated completely, it can be managed and people can live with cancer that is arrested or in remission for many years. Palliative therapy refers to treatments that enhance the patient's comfort and improves the quality of life when the cancer cannot be completely eliminated. Although many cancers are incurable, few are untreatable. Often, doctors will treat a cancer and its accompanying pain and continue to treat them for years. A patient with breast or prostate cancer, for example, may undergo surgery and radiation treatment and have several years with no problems; a few years later, a painful bone metastasis may develop and need to be treated with radiation and painkillers again. Years may pass before another problem arises and needs to be treated. Thus, palliative treatment does not necessarily mean the patient is succumbing to the illness; it merely means that comfort and quality of life take a high priority; treatments that incur side effects and toxicity are minimized as the goal shifts from cure to enhancing comfort and quality of life.

Palliative treatments are usually for pain, but can help with other symptoms as well. For example, sometimes persistent cough or difficulty breathing or swallowing can be reduced with radiation, chemotherapy, or other medications. (See Chapters 10 and 11 which discuss the treatment strategies for various side effects.)

Palliative Radiation

Radiation can be a very effective way to reduce pain, especially when the cancer is causing a localized pain. Radiation therapy is prescribed and administered by a specially trained doctor called a *radiation oncologist*. Radiotherapy is particularly effective for:

- Bone pain, especially when it stems from breast, lung, or prostate cancer
- Pain from a brain or spinal tumor
- Pain stemming from a tumor pressing on nerves or growing into nerves
- The control of bleeding due to tumors
- Reducing the pain and discomfort from tumors that ulcerate the skin, such as certain breast cancers, head and neck cancers, and skin cancers
- Relieving difficulty in breathing (dyspnea), coughing, or chest pains due to tumors blocking the bronchial tubes, esophagus, or trachea
- Reducing the pain caused by large liver tumors
- Relieving pain from tumors pressing on the spinal cord, causing back pain, leg weakness, shooting pains, sphincter problems, or numbness
- Relieving headaches due to inoperable brain tumors that cause too much pressure in the skull
- Shrinking tumors that are blocking hollow organs or tubes, such as the bronchial tubes, esophagus, bile ducts, ureters, lymph channels, blood vessels or gynecologic, gastrointestinal, or upper digestive tracts, or those causing problems because the tumors are growing in small, constricted spaces

Treatments should be convenient and efficient for patients so that they need not spend a great deal of time and energy going to and from therapy.

Palliative Chemotherapy

Although systemwide treatments with chemotherapy and hormone therapy for malignancies are a common line of attack in radical therapy to eradicate the cancer, they are often overlooked in treating cancer pain. One reason may be that doctors tend to divide cancers into "curables" and "incurables," and then treat the disease accordingly. And "incurable" is not commonly linked with chemotherapy—a systemwide approach. Although cases vary widely, by the time the pain of advanced disease requires an aggressive pain strategy, many oncologists rule out systemwide chemotherapy because they know that it is futile in terms of a cure. Even without a cure, palliative chemotherapy (or hormonal therapy) can alleviate pain from a growing tumor, although usually slowly.

Who Can Benefit?

Among the cancers that respond most promptly to palliative chemotherapy or hormonal therapy are:

- Small-cell lung cancer, which comprises about one-quarter of lung cancers, is particularly responsive to systemic chemotherapy.

- Multiple myeloma, a kind of cancer that often affects the bone marrow, is almost always treated with chemotherapy, and often with radiation.
- Colon cancer, the third most common cancer among adults, responds to chemotherapy.
- Cancer of the testes responds well to chemotherapy.
- Any kind of bone cancer (metastases), spine pain, or headache may be treated with chemotherapy.

Hormone Therapy

Hormone therapy, a type of chemotherapy, changes hormone levels in hormonal-responsive cancers and can provide excellent pain relief with few side effects. Often two or three different hormones need to be tried, especially in prostate or breast cancer, before getting a response. Cancers that respond particularly well to palliative hormonal therapies are:

- Breast cancers that have spread widely (metastasized) to the bone or vital organs (lungs, liver) are often treated with hormonal therapy. In particular, patients with a type of breast cancer (referred to as being progesterone-receptor positive) have a high likelihood of responding well to hormonal therapy. Similarly, traditional chemotherapy can play an important role in patients with all types of breast cancer.
- Prostate cancer, the third leading cancer among men, often is first treated with spot radiation or by surgery. If it has spread to the bone and causes pain, it tends to respond well to hormonal therapy. Doctors will sometimes recommend surgically removing the testicles to change hormone levels and diminish pain.
- Endometrial cancers are another type of cancer that responds to hormone treatments. In about one-third of these cancers, the pain can be significantly relieved with hormonal therapy.

Concurrent Therapy

Even though palliative treatment with radiation or chemotherapy can be chosen, most patients will still need to take medication for pain, at least until the effects of the treatment become established.

When to Start

Difficult questions arise, however, when considering a course of chemotherapy or hormonal treatments for pain. All medical treatments have potential risks and benefits, and these must be weighed carefully with each new recommendation. How strong will the toxic effects be and how well can the patient, at that particular time, tolerate them? If there's not a good chance of a significant improvement, then the net result may only be uncomfortable, perhaps devastating side effects—nausea, vomiting, fatigue—and a diminished quality of life. Families and physicians may find it difficult to justify marginal to mild benefits against the certainty of some toxic effects. Another dilemma is that the patient's response to chemotherapy and ability to cope often decrease with each successive treatment. So when the cancer is incurable and not causing a problem, it is sometimes best to wait and see how the disease progresses. Some cancers will not cause problems for months or years, and although the family may feel an urgency "to do something," it may be best to reserve a systemwide approach until it's needed to reduce pain and discomfort later on. Although this may sound contradictory to earlier statements made about not putting off pain medication, in this case we're talking about putting off chemotherapy for when it might be most effective.

When pain does become a problem, and stems from a tumor that is known to respond well to chemotherapy, if the tumor is localized and can just as easily be treated by radiation or even surgery, that's usually, though not always, the better way to go; the systemwide approach is then reserved in case it is needed later.

A logical, stepwise approach cannot be described here because each treatment is extremely individualized; when considering palliative treatments for pain, doctors must take into account the age of the patient, the type of tumor, how much it has spread, whether it is responsive to chemotherapy or radiation, and so on.

When to Stop

Once chemotherapy is being used, a common pitfall is that doctors tend to "see it through," sometimes failing to stop treatment even when it becomes clear that it is doing no good. That's because there is no clear signal to the doctor that the patient has had an adequate treatment, or that the patient wants to stop. Although there are accepted regimens for typical chemotherapy treatments for particular cancers, they vary widely from center to center, and from tumor type to tumor type. When chemotherapy is used to palliate pain, the variation in protocols is even greater. Relief will take time, if it occurs at all.

On rare occasions, a patient may be given chemotherapy for "psychological" reasons, so the patient and family feel that something is being done. Since palliative chemotherapy may result in only a small boost in the quality or length of life, it's very important that the family continually assess the risks versus benefits, and to express their wishes to either further treatment or to stop treatment.

Palliative Surgery

Though not very common, surgery may be the best way to relieve a particular pain. But surgery should only be considered if there is a reasonably good chance that it will significantly improve the quality of life of the patient or reduce high doses of medication that are triggering unpleasant side effects. In general, there are four kinds of palliative surgery:

- Direct palliative surgery which removes the source of the problem (such as the removal of a breast) or improves the outcome of radiation or chemotherapy because the mass is smaller to treat after the surgery.
- Indirect palliative surgery which removes an organ that aggravates the cancer, such as the endocrine glands or ovaries to prevent hormone-dependent breast cancer from getting worse.
- Mediate palliative surgery which opens access to an area for chemotherapy or radiation treatment.
- Surgery which interrupts the pain signal. (This type of surgery will be discussed in Chapter 9 in the discussion of "high-tech" neurosurgical procedures.)

Palliative surgery is commonly performed in the following situations:

- The intestines are blocked, producing nausea, vomiting, and pain. If a patient's medical condition is stable, a bypass or colostomy may relieve these symptoms.
- The biliary system is blocked, producing an obstruction of bile from the liver and causing pain and jaundice (yellow skin). If the patient is stable, a bypass may be performed.
- The urinary system is blocked, producing pain and other problems. A urinary diversion (called nephrostomy, ureterostomy, or cystostomy) may be performed, either with surgery or in the radiology suite.
- A buildup of fluid in the abdomen (ascites), around the heart (pericardial effusion), or in the lung (pleural effusion) occurs. In some cases, the fluid can be drained surgically.
- The veins of the circulatory system are hard to find and treatment is planned. An intravenous catheter or port may be inserted to gain access to a vein.
- Access to an artery is blocked. Occasionally, chemotherapy is administered through an artery and surgery may be necessary.
- When a tumor is large and causing pain. In this case, surgery may be the answer, especially if the tumor is unresponsive to radiotherapy and chemotherapy, ulcerates, produces pain, gets in the way of daily activities, and causes psychological distress. In the case of abdominal pain,

for example, a surgeon may go in and "debulk" a tumor if its size was such that it was causing pain from pressing on other organs.

- Tumors have weakened bones so much so that a fracture occurs or is imminent. In these cases, surgically inserted pins or prostheses can relieve the pain and improve function.
- Tumors compress the spinal cord. In this case, a procedure called a *decompressive laminectomy,* if done early, may prevent paralysis.

WHEN CONSIDERING PALLIATIVE TREATMENTS

In deciding whether to pursue any of these palliative treatments, patients and their families should consider:

- How active is the patient, and how likely is the patient to become more active as a result of treatment?
- What is the risk of major organ failure (lungs, kidney, or liver) with and without the treatment?
- Is the patient willing or reluctant to cooperate?
- Have previous radiation or chemotherapy treatments made another treatment less likely to be effective?
- How do the short-term discomforts compare with the potential benefits?
- How demanding is the treatment? Is hospitalization required? How long will it take to expect results (sometimes radiation is given daily for weeks)?
- What about options? For example, sometimes radiation therapy must be given over a period of weeks, but it may be possible to recalculate in a way so as to allow fewer hospital visits or even to provide all treatments in a single dose.
- How long is the life expectancy, with and without the treatment?

To maximize the efficacy of any treatment, whether for the cancer or pain, or both, patients and their caregivers must be active participants in their treatment. Care should be tailored to the needs and problems of each particular patient, but can only be done so when the patient or family communicates clearly and effectively with the health team. Next, we'll look at just how to maximize that communication.

4

On Being an Active Health-Care Consumer

January 1987

I watched a person who was very close to me suffer needlessly from cancer pain. The nurses refused to give the person the prescribed pain-killer more than every five hours, even when the medication was effective for only one hour and eventually became totally ineffective. The nurses refused to call the doctor. . . . [They] were concerned about addiction. . . . How could anyone who is in the last stage of terminal cancer live long enough to become addicted?

It is shocking to think that street addicts can get narcotics while inno cent victims of cancer who are dying in pain are denied access to them because there are so many ignorant doctors and nurses in this crazy world.

It is very perplexing to me that millions of people suffer needlessly from cancer pain every day while our nation has the most advanced technol-ogy of any nation in the world. Has this problem been ignored because families don't speak out and the dying don't have the strength to speak out? . . . I saw this happen and I haven't gotten over the shock of the experience.
—Name withheld

How effectively pain is controlled will depend on two major factors: (1) the strategy used by the doctor, and (2) the patient's relationship with the doc-tor. Even an effective strategy will fall short if communication with the doctor is poor, because then the patient's changing needs can't be met. This chapter will help families:

- Determine what to look for in a doctor.
- Assess their doctor's attitude toward pain and pain management.
- Encourage a doctor to take pain problems more seriously.
- Teach you to be a good consumer of health care.
- Learn strategies to communicate pain problems.

- Cope with doctors who are reluctant to medicate pain adequately.
- Help doctors to be most effective in helping you.

WHY IS IT DIFFICULT
TO DISCUSS PAIN WITH DOCTORS?

Although they may be excellent physicians, many oncologists are likely to be very busy and may be preoccupied with treatment decisions. They also may minimize the importance and impact of their patients' pain or inaccurately judge its severity. In many cases, how a nurse, doctor, or oncology fellow assesses a patient's pain has little relationship to the patient's own self-scoring of pain intensity.

Doctors sometimes prescribe pain medication but may have an inappropriately low expectation for satisfactory relief and then pass those low expectations on to their patients; some overlook their patients' discomfort once they've prescribed a medication. Study after study has shown that far too many doctors—including the majority of oncologists—end up giving their patients far too little pain medication or are unfamiliar with proper dosing or alternatives when basic pain relief treatments don't work. A recent survey conducted by the Eastern Cooperative Oncology Group (a national network of more than 250 institutions in the United States and Canada supported by the U.S. National Cancer Institute to track promising new cancer treatments for large-scale clinical trials) of 12,000 medical oncologists, for example, demonstrated that 50 percent of these cancer specialists felt that the pain treatment was inadequate in their own cancer centers. Only 10 percent remembered being taught about cancer pain in medical school and only 20 percent in residency (more on this study later in the chapter). And a 1991 Northwestern University survey of more than 1,100 cancer specialists showed that 85 percent felt that cancer pain was undermedicated; only 11 percent said their medical school training for treating cancer pain was adequate.

Chronic pain can also slip by a doctor's notice if the patient doesn't speak up. Acute pain is easier to recognize because the autonomic responses are triggered: the heart races (tachycardia), blood pressure goes up (hypertension), the patient sweats (diaphoresis), may turn pale, and the pupils may dilate. The body adapts, however, to pain over time and the autonomic responses are no longer triggered. Although an inexperienced doctor may say the patient doesn't "look as if he is in pain," doctors should never doubt or second-guess a patient's experience of pain. Studies have shown that doctors, nurses, and even spouses often underestimate the amount of pain a patient has. Without any sort of "pain detector"—a blood test or X-ray that indicates pain levels—experts insist that the patient is the best authority on how much pain there is, should be asked frequently about it, and always believed. Whether the doctor can determine the source of the pain or not, analgesics should be started to make the patient comfortable as soon as possible.

Another common problem in medicine is that even though new information is always emerging and doctors are besieged with it in new textbooks and at meetings, because of its sheer volume, it may not be recognized. Like many professionals, doctors feel most comfortable practicing medicine as they were taught it. Once someone is in practice, their habits are slow to change, even with continuing education. That leaves much of the responsibility for instituting change up to the consumer of health care.

A similar situation occurred several decades ago when researchers found that an annual pap smear could prevent many cases of cancer. Professional societies tried to educate doctors with mailers, courses, and lectures; a few years later, studies found that many doctors still were not doing the exam annually. Instead of targeting doctors, the societies launched a public education campaign. It was only when patients asked for and even demanded a pap smear that doctors finally made the transition to today's standard practice. The situation with cancer pain is quite similar. Even though doctors have read that cancer pain can and should be treated aggressively, many are still reluctant to do so, holding on to yesterday's practices. Fortunately, public education about the treatability of cancer pain is starting to take hold. As patients become more knowledgeable about what is the proper way to treat cancer pain, doctors will become more accommodating and get over their fears of prescribing larger doses than those they were taught were "normal."

ON BEING A "GOOD" AND RESPONSIBLE PATIENT

Patients have a choice: they can either suffer in silence or speak up, even though it may be uncomfortable, and express their need for more aggressive pain management. Patients and families need to call their doctor's attention to their needs. Some patients try to be "good" patients, thinking that if they complain, ask too many questions, don't respond well to a particular medication or treatment, or express other problems, their doctor will view them as a "difficult" patient and not feel as positively toward them. Many of these things are beyond anyone's control, and though not hoped for, are anticipated in a proportion of patients.

A good health-care consumer and a responsible patient means working effectively as a partner with the doctor—working *with* the physician, not *against* the physician. That means doing the little things that count toward making treatments more successful and satisfying. These include working to understand the problems and complexities, being knowledgeable about the condition that is being treated by reading what you can, including materials in doctors' offices, cancer centers, and libraries, and those available from the American Cancer Society and other associations (see Appendix).

COMPLYING WITH THE DOCTOR'S RECOMMENDATIONS

Doctors expect that patients will follow their recommendations, and that if they don't, they will tell the doctor what they didn't do and why. Yet only half of patients follow their doctors' recommendations. In their sincere attempts to help patients, doctors will become frustrated when patients don't comply and don't tell them. Patients need not follow blindly whatever the doctor asks, but the responsible thing to do is to tell the doctor if the patient or family disagree or find it too difficult to comply. Doctors will find it frustrating to find out at the next appointment that a recommendation was not followed and that up to a month may have been lost. Patients and families need to speak up immediately if they do not agree with or do not understand a recommendation. The doctor will have the opportunity to help the patient understand it better, or to make an alternate recommendation that suits the patient better. Once home, if the doctor's recommendations can't be followed for whatever reason, inform the office so that an alternate plan can be made.

Not complying with the doctor's instruction can end up being a dangerous thing. Even something simple, like not taking a laxative regularly when prescribed, can end up as an emergency. Although it may be difficult for patients to make the transition from being independent well persons to being ill patients with a shopping bag full of medications, it is still very important that patients follow their doctor's instructions or inform the doctor why they can't.

Try not to cancel, miss, or be late for appointments. Doctors are busier than ever today, and oncologists are often faced with "squeezing in" emergencies. Try not to get frustrated if the waiting time for an appointment seems unreasonable or even if an appointment is cancelled—more than likely, the doctor is treating an urgent case, and families should be able to put themselves in another's shoes and consider that if that were their emergency, they would be ever grateful to the doctor for giving the loved one the time when he needed it. If the family is very bothered by the waits, it is okay to express that frustration, but realize that it may be beyond the doctor's control.

Keep track of the patient's treatments. The doctor has many patients, and paperwork may fall behind. Save valuable time for discussion of pressing matters and difficulties by bringing a list of the medications to visits with specialists unfamiliar with the patient's records.

Determine the degree to which the doctor would like the family to stay in touch with his or her staff between visits, and let the staff know how the patient is doing.

ON BEING AN ACTIVE HEALTH-CARE CONSUMER

Having cancer or helping a loved one with cancer is one of the most stressful events you will likely experience, and you may very well have feelings of anger and frustration. Times will be trying, and doctors may be rushed. Since patients and their families are eager to discuss treatments, they need to be careful that in their efforts to be "good patients," they do not neglect to explore questions related to pain, and to advocate the need or desire for aggressive pain management.

Even though most doctors are very caring people, sometimes they may just seem not to understand what the patient and family are going through. Try to help them understand, but don't be too frustrated if they seem distracted. After all, no matter how caring, no one can really get under the patient's skin and feel what she is feeling. In fact, many doctors pride themselves on their "objectivity"—maintaining a distance from their patients so they can be more scientific. This style may suit a patient and family, or they may prefer a doctor with a more humanistic style, who has time for an occasional hug. Just as people have different styles in interacting with others, so do doctors in dealing with patients.

Ironically, with all the information consumers have on how to be better health-care consumers, many fail to become one. And yet, they invest much time, energy, and research into decisions like buying a new car, mulling over questions such as, Is it the right one for me? Can I afford it? What are the problems usually experienced with such-and-such a model? How is it better than others in the price range? What do the consumer magazines in the library have to say about this model or that one?

One reason consumers haven't been giving the same time and energy to their medical problems is because the traditional doctor-patient relationship has been a paternal one—patients were expected to blindly accept doctors orders without question. But this is slowly giving way to a more equal relationship based on the growing recognition that patients have rights. In fact, most hospitals require that a patient's "Bill of Rights" be posted prominently. Patients have a right to understand their alternatives, to assess potential benefits and risks of each alternative, and to have a second opinion.

THE BENEFITS OF BEING A RESPONSIBLE
AND ACTIVE CONSUMER

Actively taking a role in one's own health care or the health care of a loved one has numerous advantages. First of all, taking an active role helps patients feel as if they have some control over the treatment, and this may diminish their sense of helplessness that the disease may have triggered. Exerting control, for example, over the time of day of a radiation treatment so that it is convenient to the patient or even the timing of a bath if the patient is very ill can have psychological rewards at a time when they are badly needed.

Families that track their own medical care can also help prevent careless mistakes. A doctor may prescribe a medication that has a side effect of aggravating an ulcer, for example; although a patient's ulcer may be ten years old and not on the front page of the medical chart, a family member who checks on the medication (say, by checking the library's copy of the *Physician's Desk Reference,* a standard reference book of medications that lists contraindications, or conditions to watch out for with each medication) can take an active role, alongside the patient. Caregivers may discover particular concerns regarding the patient's medical history or dosage inconsistencies that should be brought to the doctor's attention.

Furthermore, sometimes doctors may change the medication or dose for a patient on the telephone and that change may not be entered onto the patient's chart. A patient or caregiver who can rattle off what medications are being taken and the doses, rather than describing "a pink pill in the morning and a blue one at night," will be a tremendous help during any consultation. Moreover, doctors may get ill themselves and have a substitute who is unfamiliar with the patient and his or her chart. Patients or family members who can clearly convey the vital information will prove extremely helpful.

WHAT TO EXPECT FROM DOCTORS

In the best of all worlds, doctors would welcome informed patients who ask good questions so that they can make responsible choices about their care. Unfortunately, this is not always so. Doctors are pressed for time, and regrettably may dread seeing an inquisitive, informed patient, simply because it means it will take more time.

Although it may be difficult for a patient or caregiver to take such an active role when a doctor seems to be discouraging it, consider doing it anyway. When you or a loved one's life and well-being are at stake, it may well be worth taking the heat.

Doctors also may sometimes shy away from discussions because they are uncomfortable talking about unpleasant topics, or may feel that patients are not prepared to engage in such discussions. Most doctors chose their profession to help people, to save lives; it can be frustrating for many doctors to deal with cancer, because so many people don't get better.

Yet doctors should welcome discussions about controlling the pain and other symptoms because they have remedies for many such complaints. Even if they are reluctant to use strong medications because of training or prejudices, it is unlikely that the family's concerns will fall on deaf ears. But the tide is turning, and doctors everywhere are beginning to understand that the pain can, and should, be controlled. However, if the family fails to bring up pain problems, there still is a good chance that the doctor will not bring them up and they will not be addressed.

If the doctor doesn't seem to understand, or doesn't take the complaints of pain seriously enough, there are things patients and families may do; they will be discussed later in this chapter.

WHAT TO LOOK FOR IN A DOCTOR

One of the first things any cancer patient should do is to be sure that he or she consults an *oncologist*, a doctor who specializes in cancer. Before any appointment, patients and their families should prepare their list of questions and concerns. To find out the doctor's attitude and aggressiveness in treating cancer pain:

- Ask about the doctor's expectations for being able to relieve pain.
- Ask about the doctor's strategy in treating the pain.
- Ask the doctor if addiction or tolerance to narcotics will be problem. (If he or she says yes, chances are the doctor is not well informed about modern cancer pain treatments.)
- Express the family's attitudes and expectations about treating pain aggressively.
- Ask about the doctor's team—is there a nurse or other professional on the team who can take the time to talk more about the family's concerns about pain management if the doctor is busy?
- If pain has persisted despite treatments, ask whether the doctor has any training from specialized cancer units or in cancer pain treatments.
- Ask whether the doctor's philosophy for pain treatment is "as needed" or "around the clock." If it is "as needed," the doctor may not be well informed about modern cancer pain treatments.
- In asking about contingencies or other treatments if the pain medication doesn't work, if the physician does not mention morphine, as much

as needed, chances are the doctor is not up to date on the latest techniques and pain relief philosophies.

HOW DOCTORS DIFFER IN TREATING CANCER PAIN

When the Eastern Cooperative Oncology Group (ECOG) surveyed their own doctors in 1990 about attitudes and knowledge about cancer pain and its control, the results were shocking. Together, the 1,177 cancer specialists (86 percent were board certified in oncology) had treated more than 70,000 cancer patients in the previous six months. Here are some of the findings:

- Only half the doctors felt that the pain management in their own practices was good or very good.
- Only 11 percent remembered having any medical school training in cancer pain management, and only one-quarter said their residency training in pain management was good to excellent.
- Although all cancer pain specialists recommend using complementary medications, known as *adjuvant medications* (see Chapter 8), to amplify the painkilling effect of the basic analgesic (painkiller), very few doctors in the survey actually considered doing so.
- In responding to a case study of a patient with persistent pain, 14 percent failed to include a strong opioid as part of their "most aggressive" strategy.
- Although many drugs are available to control the expected side effects from opioids, such as nausea and constipation, less than 1 percent of the surveyed doctors prescribed them for the case study.
- Although all cancer pain specialists recommend morphine or a similar narcotic as the first-choice drug for prolonged moderate to severe pain, only 38 percent of the surveyed doctors rated such a drug as their first choice.
- Even though cancer pain specialists promote the use of as much painkiller as necessary that can be tolerated to soothe severe cancer pain, 31 percent of the doctors surveyed said they would not recommend maximum tolerated analgesic therapy for severe pain unless the patient had a prognosis (what the doctor predicted to be the patient's outcome from the illness) of less than six months to live. Their primary reasons were concerns about side effects (which can be managed with appropriate drugs) and concerns about patients building too much tolerance (an erroneous concern, according to cancer pain specialists).

In another study at the University of Wisconsin Medical School's Pain Research Group, the researchers found that doctors who treated cancer fell into two groups:

1. "Liberals" who treat patients according to the WHO guidelines and the philosophy of other cancer pain specialists. Such doctors, who treat cancer pain properly, only comprise one-fifth (21 percent) of doctors who treat cancer. These doctors correctly believe that:
   - Patients should be given as much analgesia as they need and can tolerate, even if it is early in the disease process.
   - Patients should be given some control over giving themselves a dose of painkiller if needed.
   - "Successful" pain treatments are those that eliminate the pain or reduce it to minimal discomfort.
2. "Typical" doctors, four out of five doctors (79 percent), who appear to undermedicate cancer pain. These characteristics describe this group:
   - Sixty percent of this group wouldn't use as much painkiller as necessary to soothe the pain unless the patient had less than six months to live.
   - Only half felt it was okay for patients to ask for analgesia for mild pain (versus 80 percent of the liberals).
   - Only 60 percent of this group felt that the patient was the best judge of pain intensity (versus 80 percent of the liberals).
   - Far fewer of the doctors in this group prescribed alternative therapies that have been found to reduce cancer pain, such as nerve stimulation, relaxation techniques, nerve blocks, and so on. (See Chapters 9 and 12.)

The researchers found that only two factors distinguished the two groups of doctors: (1) age of the doctor, and (2) their training on specialized oncology units. The bulk of the liberal doctors were younger and had training on such units.

And unfortunately, being treated at a major medical center is no guarantee of better pain treatment. In a 1992 study of 1,063 cancer outpatients at 80 clinics across the country, neuropsychologist Charles Cleeland of the University of Wisconsin, a leading cancer pain expert, found that women and the elderly, in particular, were being undertreated for their cancer pain. Of the women younger than 50 years old, half were not receiving adequate relief and some 45 percent of men and women over 71 were undermedicated. Interestingly, patients at the large teaching hospitals and cancer centers were no more likely to have their pain adequately managed than patients at other smaller facilities. Cleeland and others say that women and the elderly may be at higher risk because doctors tend to take women's complaints less seriously, and the elderly may be more reluctant to express their discomfort.

CHECKLIST FOR CHOOSING A DOCTOR FOR PAIN MANAGEMENT

Patients and their families can identify whether their doctor will treat the cancer pain adequately by exploring several issues. Be particularly wary if the doctor:

- Minimizes the importance of the pain or expresses any doubts about the patient's pain.
- Has low expectations for relieving severe pain.
- Prescribes analgesics "as needed" rather than "around the clock" (although there are exceptions to this general rule).
- Does not create an open environment in which the patient feels free to express needs, anger, and fears and to ask questions.
- Discourages the family from bringing or presenting a prepared list of questions.
- Doesn't seem to take pain complaints seriously or with full attention or interest.
- Doesn't encourage the patient or family to get back to a member of the doctor's team as soon as possible if the current prescription is ineffective.
- Is concerned about tolerance, addiction, or physical dependence.
- Doesn't reassure the patient and family that many pain treatments are available.

WHEN THE DOCTOR DOES NOT TAKE PAIN SERIOUSLY

If a family discovers that its primary doctor is one of the many doctors who is overconcerned about the side effects of an aggressive pain management strategy or has a less aggressive philosophy about treating pain, the family members might try:

- Discussing their concerns openly with the doctor. In the course of a busy day, the physician may just not have realized that the patient wasn't getting what she or he needed. In the best of situations, a good frank conversation like this will clear the air, allowing for things to get better.
- Asking about the possibility of consulting a pain specialist or a pain consulting service, such as the Pain Management Information Center or the hotline of the National Cancer Institute (see Appendix). A family might tell their doctor that although he or she may be an outstanding oncologist, they'd like to take advantage of the recent strides in cancer pain management, an emerging subspecialty; while they understand how oncologists can't be expected to stay abreast of every development, the family would, nevertheless, appreciate access to state-of-the-art techniques.

■ Even if the doctor has proven to be humanistic, sensitive, and caring, he or she may still be unable to manage the pain adequately. To ask for a second opinion, try something like, "We hope you don't mind us asking, but since this illness is of such profound importance to us, we really want to seek all the information we can. It's not that we doubt your opinion, but we need reassurance that this is the way to go. Would you mind giving us the name of a colleague with whom we could consult for a second opinion?" Free referrals can also be obtained through the National Cancer Institute (see Appendix).

■ Asking whether there are any pain specialists in the area with whom the family could consult.

■ If the doctor's answers indicate that he or she is not a proponent of aggressive pain management, is defensive about the subject, or tries to talk the family out of seeking a second opinion, the family should be aware that more aggressive pain management is available elsewhere. (Check the Appendix for other resources in obtaining a referral.)

ACCEPT NOTHING LESS THAN SATISFACTORY RELIEF

Cancer is bad enough, and families need to be as assertive as necessary in asking for pain relief and in communicating frequently with their doctors. Although most consumers will spend hours in choosing a car, they fail to be good consumers in choosing their doctors or in looking for a second opinion. Cancer can be a life-and-death situation—families need to remember that they choose their physicians and need not accept anything less than the best when it comes to being treated—not only for the disease, but for the pain that often accompanies the disease.

It is the patient's and the family's responsibility to report the pain and to expect the best pain relief possible. Consumer demand will be the most powerful factor in getting more doctors to take their patient's pain seriously and to treat it as aggressively as possible. The goal is for a painless-as-possible illness, and if the time should come, a painless death. We should accept nothing less.

Part II
THE PAINKILLERS

5

Understanding Mild Pain Relievers

GENERAL GUIDELINES

For mild to moderate pain, the first step in a typical treatment is to use non-narcotic pain relievers. This approach is advocated by the World Health Organization's analgesic ladder and leading cancer pain specialists. These are the *non-steroidal anti-inflammatory (NSAIDs)* drugs, of which aspirin, ibuprofen, and acetaminophen (such as Tylenol and Anacin-3) are the best known examples. (Some of these products actually have a weak anti-inflammatory effect but are usually categorized in this group because they are non-narcotic analgesics.) Non-narcotic analgesics are also often called non-opioid analgesics. They are the pain relievers that are not derived from opium and opium-like substances and do not cause many of the side effects commonly associated with the opioid analgesics (e.g., morphine), such as drowsiness.

If the doctor prescribes a medicine that you already know, which may even be available over-the-counter (without a prescription), don't be concerned that he is not taking the pain seriously. When taken in the right dose at the right time and for the appropriate circumstances (described here), these medications can be surprisingly effective for even severe pain—pain such as that from bone metastases. If the NSAIDs prove ineffective in quelling pain, then other stronger medications should be started which will be described in the next two chapters.

The NSAIDs relieve pain in the tissues rather than in the brain or central nervous system. They work by inhibiting an enzyme that is important in producing substances called *prostaglandins.* Certain prostaglandins cause pain and make pain receptors more sensitive. By inhibiting prostaglandin production, the NSAIDs reduce pain and decrease the activity of the pain receptors. They also inhibit inflammation, a process in the body that causes redness, local heat, swelling, and pain.

Unlike opioids, whose doses can be increased to very high levels if needed, the NSAIDs do have "ceiling doses." The ceiling dose is the dose beyond which no additional pain-relieving effect is achieved and only increased side effects occur. Ceiling doses, however, vary among individuals. As a result, the doctor may increase the initial dose of an NSAID, but there will be limits. Moreover, the side effects of the NSAIDs are very different from those of opioids—NSAIDs have little to no effect on alertness, mood, nausea, tolerance, or physical dependence. Most NSAIDs, though, may aggravate sensitive gastrointestinal conditions, such as gastric ulcers and bleeding.

Although the NSAIDs are used frequently to soothe mild to moderate pain, they may also be very useful for more severe pain when prescribed in combination with stronger drugs—in other words, the weak and strong opioids. The combination of an NSAID with an opioid provides an additive pain-relieving effect because, as we've seen, NSAIDs and opioids soothe pain through different mechanisms. By prescribing a non-opioid together with a weak or strong opioid, the pain is attacked on two fronts—one cutting pain off on the peripheral level (in the tissue), and the other intercepting the pain message en route to the central nervous system (brain and spinal cord).

Such combinations are also used because the NSAIDs allow lower levels of opioids to be taken, which reduces the risk of side effects.

Although able to relieve many types of pain, the NSAIDs are particularly effective for bone pain and the pain resulting from inflammation; in addition, they help reduce stiffness, swelling, and tenderness.

GENERAL DOSE GUIDELINES

Typically, doses should be started low and increased gradually every few days until the ceiling dose for the particular patient is obtained. If the patient is more comfortable after a recent increase in dose, then doctors usually assume that the ceiling dose has not been reached and higher doses and greater relief may still be achieved when needed. Once a higher dose no longer has any added effect, the ceiling dose has probably been exceeded and the dose may be lowered to the previous level. At high doses, NSAIDs can have toxic effects, so experts recommend that usually no more than two times the standard dose ever be used. With the NSAIDs, the objective is to find the lowest dose possible to achieve the greatest degree of relief.

If a patient finds relief with one of these drugs and stays on a higher-than-standard dose for more than a month, she should be monitored closely (usually every one to two months) with certain tests to check for any problems. These tests may include stool, urine, and blood samples.

What most people don't realize is that the NSAIDs do more than one thing. They are painkillers (analgesics), but also reduce inflammation, which affects pain, too. The analgesic effect of these medications may show up after just a few doses, but it sometimes takes several weeks for their full anti-inflammatory effect to exert itself.

If the pain is mild or moderate, be patient with a doctor's request to stay on NSAIDs even if it's not clear that it's helping. After a week, if there are no side effects, then an ineffective dose can be boosted, or another NSAID tried, since patients often respond differently to different NSAIDs. Also, many NSAIDs may take up to two weeks to reach peak effectiveness.

However, if the pain is severe, ask about using a stronger medication first (an opioid). Do not feel that the patient must work his way up slowly from NSAIDs to opioids when the pain is severe.

Be sure to take these medications at scheduled, regular intervals—"around-the-clock." Don't underestimate their effectiveness even if they are over-the-counter medications. When taken on a regular basis, they can be powerful pain relievers. In fact, studies of cancer as well as postsurgical, postbirth, and oral surgical pain have found that aspirin is just as effective as the weak opioids, such as codeine, which will be explored in the next chapter. Weak opioids can become more effective when they are taken in combination with acetaminophen or aspirin or other NSAIDs.

A few general precautions: for the elderly, the kidney-impaired, liver-impaired, and those on certain other medications, NSAIDs may have more side effects, and so should be used cautiously, often at lower starting doses, or not at all.

It should also be noted that these substances tend to mask a fever, which can be particularly important for patients with low white-blood counts.

All of these medications should be taken with a full glass of water and after food (if even only a cracker) to minimize gastrointestinal irritation.

WHEN ALTERNATIVE NSAIDs SHOULD BE CONSIDERED

In general, NSAIDs have very similar pain-relieving results. Which drug is chosen will depend on:

- The patient's prior history or experience with specific drugs. For example, whatever might have worked well a few years ago for a sprained ankle without side effects will probably be a good choice and should be mentioned to the doctor.
- Whether the patient is particularly vulnerable to gastrointestinal irritation, kidney, or liver problems. Trilisate or Disalcid may be gentler on the stomach than some others. Newer (usually more costly) drugs may be associated with lower rates of ulcers, but can still cause an upset stomach and diarrhea.
- Whether the patient has a condition for which thinning of the blood or

prolongation of blood clotting (which would increase the time a person would bleed) would be a danger (such as having hemophilia or recent chemotherapy or already being on a blood thinner such as heparin or Coumadin). Again, Trilisate does not usually thin the blood as much as other NSAIDs.

- The doctor's experience with the drug. New drugs are released all the time. It is hard to keep up, so the doctor might not yet be experienced with the latest addition. Remember however: the newer drugs are not necessarily better, and usually cost much more.
- Scheduling considerations. In patients who are already taking many other medications, it can be beneficial to prescribe an NSAID that only needs to be taken once or twice a day, like piroxicam (Feldene) or nabumetone (Relafen). They seem to work just as well.
- And cost. In the absence of other factors, probably the least expensive NSAID should be selected, and in most communities, this is ibuprofen.

Table 5.1 offers some guidelines as to which medication might be particularly useful, or potentially harmful, in particular situations.

THE NON-STEROIDAL ANTI-INFLAMMATORY (NON-OPIOID) DRUGS

The following list of medications represents the choices most often prescribed for cancer pain, which are either used alone or in combination with a weak or strong opioid. These are general guidelines and are no substitute for a doctor's care and judgment.

Aspirin

Brand Names
Many, too numerous to mention.

Dose Range
650 milligrams (mg) four times a day is the standard dose, although a few studies suggest that 900 or 1,000 mg may lengthen how long the relief will last (its duration) or improve pain relief.

If doses are 1,000 mg or higher, GI problems usually occur.

How Long It Takes to Reach Peak Effect
About 2 hours.

Table 5.1. *NSAIDs by Side Effect*

Good choices for patients sensitive to gastrointestinal side effects or with a history of ulcers or bleeding
    Acetaminophen (Tylenol, Datril, Panadol)
    Choline magnesium salicylate (Trilisate)
    Salsalate (Disalcid)
    Nabumetone (Relafen)
Bad choices for patients sensitive to gastrointestinal side effects
    Suppositories of any of the NSAIDs
    Aspirin
    Indomethacin (Indocin, Indocid, Indomethine)
    Flurbiprofen (Ansaid)
Good choices for patients who take blood-thinning medication (anti-coagulants)
    Indomethacin (Indocin, Indocid, Indomethine)
    Naproxen (Naprosyn, Naprosine, Proxen)
    Ibuprofen (Advil, Motrin, Nuprin, Rufen)
    Piroxicam (Feldene)
Bad choices for patients who take blood-thinning medication
    Aspirin
    Phenylbutazone (Butazolidin, Antadol, Phebuzine)
Bad choice for patients with brain tumors
    Most NSAIDs
Good choice for patients with brain tumors
    Acetaminophen
Bad choice for patients with severe kidney problems
    Most NSAIDs
Good choice for patients with kidney problems
    Sulindac (or Clinoril)
Good choices for children
    Ibuprofen (Advil, Motrin, Nuprin, Rufen)
    Naproxen (Naprosyn, Naprosine, Proxen)

Source: Modified from E. C. Huskisson, "Non-narcotic Analgesics," in P. D. Wall and R. Melzack (eds.), *Textbook of Pain.* New York: Churchill Livingstone, Inc., 1984, p. 510. Used with permission of the publisher.

Equivalent Pain Relief

A standard dose of aspirin is equivalent to 2 mg of morphine when injected into muscle (that is, intramuscularly or IM). A dose of 600 mg of aspirin is about equivalent to 60 mg of codeine.

Comments

- Used as the standard for comparison. The NSAIDs are the first rung of the WHO ladder, and are compared to aspirin to rate their effectiveness.
- Inexpensive and available over the counter (doesn't require a prescription).

- Ceiling dose reached very quickly.
- Often used in combination with opioid analgesics.
- Rectal suppositories available.
- The other NSAIDs are usually better tolerated; they don't have the same long-lasting effects of increasing bleeding time—that is, the time it takes for the blood to clot.
- To minimize side effects, take with a glass of milk, after meals, or with antacids, or take the specially coated (enteric) tablets intended to minimize gastrointestinal irritation. Regularly scheduled doses for several days are needed to determine whether it is effective or not.

Precautions

- Can irritate gastrointestinal (GI) tract, causing bleeding. In fact, a single dose may double the time a person bleeds, and this effect can last up to 3 weeks; antacids can help with GI symptoms.
- Can also cause nausea and general GI discomfort.
- Use often limited when patients are involved in chemotherapy and radiation treatments, because they already are more likely to bleed longer.

The Story of Aspirin

One of the most commonly used drugs in the world, aspirin—known as acetylsalicylic acid by chemists—is so mundane, so readily available, and inexpensive that many underestimate it. In fact, it is one of the most powerful substances in the medicine cabinet.

Although aspirin has been available since the turn of the century, its predecessors were originally derived from willow bark and used by Hippocrates as early as 450 B.C. Rediscovered in the mid-1700s and synthesized by the Bayer Company in Germany in the 1800s, aspirin has been gaining popularity ever since. Today, some 80 million tablets are taken in the United States every day—1,200 tons every year around the world.

Among Its Powerful Benefits

- Can reduce fever.
- Has been shown that regular low doses can reduce the risk of heart attack, at least in men.
- Relieves aches and inflammation.
- Reduces the risk of certain kinds of strokes.

Among Its Potential Benefits

- May help prevent colon, stomach, esophageal, and rectal cancer.
- May help prevent migraines from recurring.
- May help prevent gallstones and cataracts.
- May even help boost immunity to infection.

- Avoid with use of steroids to prevent stomach bleeding.
- Avoid with severe kidney problems.
- Avoid during pregnancy.
- Ringing in the ears (tinnitus) is an early warning sign that the patient is getting a toxic response to too much aspirin.
- If taken with alcohol, can increase likelihood of GI bleeding.
- If taken with Dilantin, becomes more toxic.
- If taken with Coumadin (a blood thinner), increases bleeding.
- Aspirin-sensitive asthma can occur.

Choline Magnesium Trisalicylate

Brand Name
Trilisate.

Dose Range
Usually 1,000 to 1,500 mg, twice a day; available as a pill and as an elixir (in liquid form).

In children, a typical dose is 25 mg a day (usually prescribed by child's weight).

How Long It Takes to Reach Peak Effect
1 to 2 hours, longer when suppository.

Equivalent Pain Relief
Not known.

Comments
- Has minimal effect on blood clotting and GI system, yet has a strong anti-inflammatory effect so may be particularly good for those with history of ulcer or stomach bleeding.
- May be particularly beneficial for bone pain.

Precautions
- May cause problems in patients who have severe kidney problems or GI disturbances, such as gastric ulcers or gastritis.

Acetaminophen (paracetamol in the United Kingdom)

Brand Names
Tylenol, Tempra, Anacin-3, Datril, Panadol, among others.

Dose Range

Usually 650 mg is the standard dose, every 4 hours.

In children, a typical dose is 10 to 15 mg (usually prescribed by child's weight).

Equivalent Pain Relief

The equivalent doses of morphine and codeine are about the same as those for aspirin. The standard dose of acetaminophen (650 mg) is about equivalent to 60 mg of codeine or 2 mg of morphine.

Comments

- Has proven just as effective as aspirin in relieving pain; yet it is a safer drug and does not require a prescription.
- Not actually considered an anti-inflammatory drug because its anti-inflammatory effects are very weak.
- Does not cause GI problems, bleeding, ulcers, thinning of blood, or aspirin-sensitive asthma.
- Rectal suppositories available for children and adults, also available as an elixir, syrup, or solution.
- Good alternative to aspirin when patient is sensitive to aspirin's blood-thinning effect or GI tract irritation, including patients with peptic ulcer.
- Not a first choice for bone pain because its anti-inflammatory activity is very weak.
- Safest choice for those with serious kidney problems.

Precautions

- Large overdoses can cause serious or fatal liver damage. Normal dosing is usually not a problem, except for alcoholics and those with active liver disease.

Ibuprofen

Brand Names

Motrin, Rufen, Advil, Haltran, Ibuprin, Medipren, Midol 200, Nuprin, Trendar, Aches-N-Pain, Dolgesic, Genpril, Ibren, Ibumed, Ibupro-600, Ibutex, Ifen, Pamprin, Profen, among others.

Dose Range

Usually up to 800 mg, three times a day.

In children, a typical dose is 10 mg (usually prescribed by child's weight).

How Long It Takes to Reach Peak Effect
1½ to 2 hours.

Equivalent Pain Relief
Not known.

Comments
- Usually provides more pain relief than aspirin, with fewer GI problems.
- Available over the counter in low doses (200 mg).
- Chemically similar to naproxen (taken every 12 hours), fenoprofen, ketoprofen, and flurbiprofen.
- Like most other NSAIDs, this medication may increase bleeding by thinning blood (though less so than aspirin) and may cause gastrointestinal upset. It should be taken with food and used with caution in patients with kidney or liver problems.

Diflunisal

Brand Name
Dolobid.

Dose Range
Usually 500 to 1,000 mg as the initial dose. Then 500 mg, two or three times a day.

How Long It Takes to Reach Peak Effect
About 1 hour.

Equivalent Pain Relief
Not known, though 500 mg of diflunisal will usually offer more pain relief than a standard dose of aspirin, and lasts longer.

Comments
- Less irritating to stomach than aspirin.
- Can take doses just twice a day.
- Lasts longer than ibuprofen, and is stronger than aspirin.

Precautions
- Occasionally can irritate gastrointestinal tract and even cause bleeding, particularly when taken for long-term periods (more than six months).

- May cause bleeding in susceptible individuals, although less so than aspirin.
- If eye complaints occur, patient should consult an eye doctor (ophthalmologist).
- Other occasional side effects include drowsiness in some but insomnia in others, dizziness, ringing of the ears (tinnitus), rash, headache, and fatigue.
- Should be taken with food.

Salsalate

Brand Names
Disalcid, Amigesic, Diagen, Mono-Gesic, Salcylic Acid, Salflex, Salgesic, Salsitab.

Dose Range
Usual starting dose is a 1,500-mg dose, followed by 500 mg every 12 hours, up to 4,000 mg a day.

Comments
- Same as choline magnesium trisalicylate (see previous listing).
- Often recommended for those with a history of ulcer or stomach bleeding, because this medication has minimal effects on blood thinning and usually does not cause gastrointestinal irritation.

Precautions
- Extra caution should be taken with patients having kidney or ulcer problems.
- Occasional side effects include ringing in the ears, nausea, hearing impairment, rash, and dizziness.
- Should be taken with food.

Piroxicam

Brand Name
Feldene.

Dose Range
Usually 20 to 40 mg a day.

How Long It Takes to Reach Peak Effect
May take five to seven days to reach its peak effect.

Comments
- Only has to be taken once a day.

Precautions
- If severe kidney or liver problems are present, may cause problems because it accumulates in the system.
- Higher doses, those above 20 mg a day, for longer than three weeks are linked to higher rates of ulcer problems, especially in the elderly.
- Like most other NSAIDs, this medication may increase bleeding by thinning blood (though less so than aspirin) and may cause gastrointestinal upset. May also cause fluid retention.
- Should be taken with food and used with caution in patients with kidney or liver problems.

Nabumetone

Brand Name
Relafen.

Dose Range
Usually 1,000 to 2,000 mg per day, in either one or two doses during the day.

How Long It Takes to Reach Peak Effect
May take up to two weeks to reach maximum effectiveness.

Comments
- Has only recently been released in the United States.

Precautions
- Like most other NSAIDs, this medication may increase bleeding by thinning blood (though less so than aspirin) and may cause gastrointestinal upset, but ulcers and gastrointestinal bleeding are less common.
- Should be taken with food and used with caution in patients with kidney or liver problems.

Etodolac

Brand Name
Lodine.

Dose Range

Usually 800 to 1,200 mg per day and split up into doses taken every six or eight hours.

How Long It Takes to Reach Peak Effect

May take up to two weeks to reach maximum effectiveness, which is the case for many NSAIDs.

Comments

- Has only recently been released in the United States.

Precautions

- Like most other NSAIDs, this medication may increase bleeding by thinning blood (though less so than aspirin) and may cause gastrointestinal upset.
- Should be taken with food and used with caution in patients with kidney or liver problems.

Diclofenac

Brand Name

Voltaren.

Dose Range

Usually 75 to 200 mg per day and split up into doses to be taken every 6 hours.

Comments

- Tablets are enteric-coated to minimize gastrointestinal problems, although they still sometimes occur.

Precautions

- Like most other NSAIDs, this medication may increase bleeding by thinning blood (though less so than aspirin) and may cause gastrointestinal upset.
- Should be taken with food and used with caution in patients with kidney or liver problems.

Flurbiprofen

Brand Name

Ansaid.

Dose Range

100 to 300 mg per day, usually split up into doses that are taken every 8 or 12 hours.

Comments

- Similar to other NSAIDs in its analgesic effect.

Precautions

- Like most other NSAIDs, this medication may increase bleeding by thinning blood (though less so than aspirin) and may cause gastrointestinal upset.
- Should be taken with food and used with caution in patients with kidney or liver problems.

Ketoprofen

Brand Name

Orudis.

Dose Range

Usually from 150 to 300 mg per day, split up into doses to be taken every 6 to 8 hours.

Comments

- Similar to other NSAIDs in analgesic effect.

Precautions

- Like most other NSAIDs, this medication may increase bleeding by thinning blood (though less so than aspirin) and may cause gastrointestinal upset.
- Should be taken with food and used with caution in patients with kidney or liver problems.

Meclofenamate

Brand Names

Meclomen, Meclofen, Meclodium.

Dose Range

Usually 150 to 400 mg per day and split up into doses to be taken every 6 or 8 hours.

Precautions
- Somewhat higher rate of gastrointestinal problems than other NSAIDs.
- Should be taken with food and used with caution in patients with kidney or liver problems.

Mefenamic Acid

Brand Name
Ponstel.

Dose Range
Usually 400 to 1,000 mg per day and split up into doses to be taken every 6 hours.

Comments
- Usually not recommended for cancer pain because, compared with other NSAIDs, mefenamic acid has a higher rate of causing gastrointestinal problems after one week of use.

Precautions
- Should be taken with food.
- Should be used with caution in patients with kidney or liver problems.

Suprofen

Brand Name
Suprofen.

Dose Range
Usually 600 to 800 mg per day and split up into doses to be taken every 6 hours.

Comments
- In general, same as other NSAIDs.

Precautions
- Like most other NSAIDs, this medication may increase bleeding by thinning blood (though less so than aspirin) and may cause gastrointestinal upset.
- Should be taken with food and used with caution in patients with kidney or liver problems.

Ketorolac

Brand Name
Toradol.

Dose Range
Usually 120 to 240 mg per day and split up into doses to be taken every 4 or 6 hours.

Comments
- Also available for intramuscular or subcutaneous administration.

Precautions
- Like most other NSAIDs, this medication may increase bleeding by thinning blood (though less so than aspirin) and may cause gastrointestinal upset.
- Should be taken with food and used with caution in patients with kidney or liver problems.
- Oral form recommended for only short-term (less than three weeks) use.

Tolmetin

Brand Name
Tolectin.

Dose Range
Usually 600 to 2,000 mg per day and split up into doses to be taken every 6 to 8 hours.

Precautions
- Like most other NSAIDs, this medication may increase bleeding by thinning blood (though less so than aspirin) and may cause gastrointestinal upset. May also cause fluid retention.
- Should be taken with food and used with caution in patients with kidney or liver problems.

Sulindac

Brand Names
Clinoril, Arthorobid.

Dose Range

Usually 300 to 400 mg per day and split up into two doses to be taken every 12 hours.

Comments

- Seems to have less adverse effects on kidney function than other NSAIDs.

Precautions

- Like most other NSAIDs, this medication may increase bleeding by thinning blood (though less so than aspirin) and may cause gastrointestinal upset.
- Should be taken with food and used with caution in patients with kidney (though less so than other NSAIDs) or liver problems.

Oxyphenbutazone

Brand Names

Tendearil, Rapostan, Rheumapax, and Oxalid.

Dose Range

Usually 300 to 400 mg per day and split up into doses to be taken every 6 to 8 hours.

Precautions

- Like most other NSAIDs, this medication may increase bleeding by thinning blood (though less so than aspirin) and may cause gastrointestinal upset.
- Should be taken with food and used with caution in patients with kidney or liver problems.

For a variety of reasons, the doctor may choose to prescribe any of these NSAIDs, or a number of others too numerous to mention. We have listed the most common NSAIDs here, as well as the most common brand names.

ADDING AN NSAID TO WEAK OPIOIDS

If more pain relief is needed than can be offered by the NSAIDs, then the next step is to add a weak opioid to the current therapy. There is a growing trend, however, to proceed directly to a stronger opioid analgesic, like morphine, much earlier than doctors used to. We will next look at the weak opioids, the next rung on the WHO recommended ladder.

6

Understanding the Weak Opioids

When pain is moderate and can't be controlled by the non-opioid (non-narcotic) drugs, the next step is to use a weak opioid, of which codeine is the most well known. Like the strong opioids, these drugs typically cause constipation, which can be prevented with laxatives (such as senna [Seno-kot-S], Metamucil, Milk of Magnesia, Dulcolax, or suppositories), stool softeners (such as Colace), or enemas as needed (see Chapter 10). Nausea and vomiting are also sometimes a side effect, although these side effects usually last only a few days with consistent use of these medications. Although physical dependence (which means withdrawal symptoms would occur if the drug were stopped suddenly) and tolerance (which means that, as the body adapts to the dose, more is needed to achieve the same pain-relieving effect) sometimes occur, they are usually not important problems when the weak opioids are used for pain. These drugs are not really "weak"; they are just considered weaker than the "strong" opioids (such as morphine) because their dosage is limited by the other compounds with which they are formulated, such as Tylenol or aspirin. Because the dosing guidelines and side effects are so different for the so-called "strong" opioids, a fuller discussion of their use will be explored in the next chapter.

As with other drugs discussed, these medications should usually be taken on schedule, around the clock (a-t-c)—not as needed (prn).

Note that although meperidine (Demerol; Pethedine in Britain) is an effective pain reliever after surgery, it is not recommended for cancer pain because of its short duration and potentially toxic side effects. Moreover, many of the medications listed here may require triplicate prescription forms in the states that require such forms.

THE WEAK OPIOID DRUGS

As mentioned earlier, most of the "weak" opioids come combined with aspirin or acetaminophen. This limits how much can be taken (usually to two tablets every 3 or 4 hours)—not because of the opioid, but because too much aspirin or acetaminophen can cause serious problems. Some experts have suggested that the importance of these medicines stems from the fact

that our society is so "drug-phobic" and overconcerned about using morphine, which is on the next rung of medication. The weak opioids provide
a step between the NSAIDs and the strong opioids. We know in fact that
doctors and patients would rather use weaker drugs, even though they are
not as effective. One of the most common mistakes that doctors make is to
keep patients on these weaker medications when stronger ones would better
relieve the pain and are no riskier.

The following are the drugs most commonly prescribed for moderate to
severe cancer pain, when non-opioid drugs no longer are effective. However, often, doctors will maintain the use of a non-opioid medication to be
used in combination with a weak (or strong) opioid because, when used
together, the pain-relieving effect is enhanced. As a result, lower doses of
the opioid may be used with a lower risk of side effects.

Again, the following information is to be used as a guide only, and should
not be used as a substitute for a physician's care and judgment.

Codeine

Brand Name
Codeine.

Combination Products
Empirin (aspirin) with codeine; Empracet (acetaminophen) with codeine;
Phenaphen (acetaminophen) with codeine; Tylenol (acetaminophen) with
codeine: Tylenol #1, #2, #3, and #4, and many others.

Dose Range
Usually 30 to 80 mg, every 4 hours (may be supplemented with 250 to 500
mg aspirin or 500 mg of acetaminophen, every 4 or 6 hours).

In children, prescriptions are based on a child's weight. Usually prescribed as a liquid for children, the dose range is typically 5 to 10 milliliters
(ml) per day; 1 to 2 teaspoonfuls, 3 or 4 times a day, are recommended for
children over 3 years of age, when the solution is comprised of 120 mg of
acetaminophen and 12 mg of codeine phosphate per teaspoon, or 5 ml.

How Long It Takes to Reach Peak Effect
1 to 2 hours.

Equivalent Pain Relief
A dose of codeine provides slightly more pain relief than a standard dose of
aspirin or acetaminophen. A 130-mg dose of codeine IM or 200 mg of co-

deine by mouth (about 7 standard tablets) is equivalent to 10 mg morphine IM.

Comments

- Even though codeine is probably the most commonly prescribed weak opioid, usually as a product in combination with aspirin or acetaminophen, some doctors feel that it is more constipating and nauseating than some of its alternatives. If constipation or nausea are persistent problems on codeine, ask the doctor to select a related compound.
- Take codeine medications with milk or water; never on an empty stomach.
- Not available for intravenous (IV) use, but occasionally given IM.
- Almost always used in combination with aspirin or acetaminophen, which enhances its pain-relieving effect.
- These combination products do not require special or triplicate prescriptions in New York, for example, and some of the other states that require such forms. This may be a reason why doctors try to stick to these medications rather than more readily switching to a more powerful medication for more severe pain.
- Can be used until 3 tablets every 4 hours fail to relieve the pain.
- Although there is no ceiling dose per se, higher doses cause side effects, which limit the dose. As a result, it is often prescribed with aspirin or acetaminophen.

Precautions

- Constipation is extremely common with codeine and preventive measures must be used. And the higher the dose, the more laxative is needed.
- As dose is increased, nausea and sedation may occur, but these effects usually do not last. While they are occurring, they may need to be treated. Codeine may also cause drowsiness, dry mouth, light-headedness.
- Extra care should be taken when given to patients with poor breathing, asthma, increased brain pressure, or liver failure.

Propoxyphene

Brand Name

Darvon (propoxyphene hydrochloride).

Combination Products

Darvon with ASA (aspirin), Darvon-N (propoxyphene napsylate and aspirin), Darvocet-N (with acetaminophen), Darvon Compound (with aspirin, caffeine), Wygesic (with acetaminophen). Others include Dolene, Dora-phen, Doxaphene, Profene, Pro Pox, Propoxycon.

Dose Range

65 to 130 mg every 4 to 6 hours. When combined with aspirin (250 to 600 mg) or acetaminophen (500 mg), the pain relief will be greater than if both drugs were taken individually.

This drug is not recommended for children.

Equivalent Pain Relief

65 mg of propoxyphene by mouth is same as 600 mg of aspirin.

How Long It Takes to Reach Peak Effect

1 to 1½ hours, though may take two to three days of regular treatment to reach full effectiveness.

Comments

- This is the weakest of the mild opioids, and less effective than aspirin or acetaminophen. But interestingly, it can cause problems. It used to be prescribed often because of doctors' unwarranted fears of using stronger drugs. Its use should be discouraged in treating cancer pain.
- Effects of propoxyphene may be cumulative over time.
- Side effects will limit increasing doses.
- Some studies suggest that doses on the high side, of about 130 mg, are effective for mild to moderate pain.
- Most effective when used with aspirin.
- Take with food and water.

Precautions

- Can cause hallucinations, confusion, and even convulsions at high doses.
- Can become toxic when used over time at high doses.

Hydrocodone

Brand Name

Not available in its pure form but only in combination with other drugs (aspirin, acetaminophen).

Combination Products

Vicodin, Vicodin ES, Bancap HC, Hydrocet, Hy-phen, and Co-Gesic. All of these products contain acetaminophen. Other combination products are also available.

Dose Range
5 to 10 mg (1 or 2 pills) by mouth three or four times a day.

Equivalent Pain Relief
Slightly weaker than oxycodone-combination products (see next section), but stronger than codeine products.

Comments
- Hydrocodone (as well as the very similar drug, dihydrocodeine [Synalgos-DC, which comes with aspirin and caffeine]) is similar to codeine, but is about one-third stronger. Its combination products are used commonly, because (like codeine-combination products) not all states with restrictive prescribing practices require a special or triplicate prescription for them. Most experts feel that one of the most common mistakes doctors make is to overprescribe these drugs to avoid the hassle of triplicate prescribing.
- Available in the United States only as a combination product.
- Also a good cough suppressant.

Precautions
- Because several of the combination products have relatively high levels of acetaminophen (Anexia and Vicodin), taking them too often or taking too many may cause the toxic effects of acetaminophen. Patients should therefore be switched to a stronger drug rather than be prescribed large doses of this medication.

Oxycodone

Brand Name
Roxycodone.

Combination Products
Percodan (with aspirin), Percocet, Tylox, Roxicet (when combined with acetaminophen).

Dose Range
5 to 30 mg by mouth usually every 4 hours.
  In children, the dose is based on the child's weight.

How Long It Takes to Reach Peak Effect
15 minutes to 45 minutes—faster than Darvon or codeine.

Equivalent Pain Relief

30 mg of oxycodone is about the same as 200 mg of codeine given orally or 10 mg of IM morphine.

Comments

- Similar to codeine, but significantly stronger. Even though a triplicate prescription is required in some states, most experts prefer this alternative over the previously mentioned drugs. Oxycodone was formerly only available when combined with aspirin and acetaminophen (Percodan, Percocet), like its cousins mentioned above, but it is now available as a single medication (Roxycodone), in liquid or tablet. This new form permits the dose to be raised without fear of toxicity from too much aspirin or acetaminophen. Research is ongoing to produce a variety of oxycodone that only needs to be taken twice daily.
- When used alone, should be considered a strong opioid.
- Not available for IM or intravenous (IV).

Precautions

- Same as codeine.
- Do not take on empty stomach.

A CLASS OF DRUGS CALLED AGONIST-ANTAGONISTS

The opioids mentioned so far are those that are considered "pure agonists," meaning that they reduce pain by the same mechanism, by binding to opioid receptors. Another class of narcotics are called *agonist-antagonists,* and these tend to produce more mind-altering side effects than the weak opioids already described. In addition, they can cause withdrawal symptoms in narcotic-dependent patients. The use of this entire class of drugs is *strongly discouraged* in cancer patients, especially if they are taking an agonist at the same time. One of these drugs is *pentazocine* (Talwin). It is the only oral agonist-antagonist available in the United States; if a doctor prescribes it, you should probably seek a second opinion. *Buprenorphine* (Temgesic) is a partial-agonist and a stronger narcotic (see Chapter 7). It is available both by injection and as an under-the-tongue medication in Canada and parts of Europe.

When pain is severe, or these "weak" opioids are not controlling pain adequately, doctors will turn to a stronger group of medications known as the strong opioids. Next, we'll look at general guidelines in using these medications and discuss the medications in detail.

7

Understanding the Strong Opioids

Misconceptions about the effects and side effects of morphine, the most well known of the strong opioids, are the primary reasons morphine and similar drugs are incorrectly used. Unfortunately, these misconceptions lead to the undermedication of patients with cancer pain around the world. Yet, with a proper understanding of these drugs, pain can be adequately relieved with a minimum of side effects in most patients.

When pain is moderate to severe, and mild opioids are unable to relieve it, the next course of action is to try morphine or a similar opioid. Most of what is said about morphine, the standard strong opioid against which all others are compared, is true about the other strong opioids mentioned in this chapter, unless otherwise noted.

GENERAL GUIDELINES FOR THE USE OF OPIOIDS

In the past, doctors believed that strong opioids like morphine were not very effective when taken in pill or liquid form, and some doctors will still begin morphine medication in its injectable form even though it is not usually needed. Morphine and other similar drugs, given orally, however, work extremely well as long as higher doses are used to make up for incomplete gastrointestinal absorption. So if strong opioids are needed, whenever possible, they should be given by mouth or through a new skin-patch system that works well. This avoids the need for injections and allows people to remain more independent.

General Guidelines

- Although the dose needed to relieve pain will vary widely among patients, doctors usually start with a low dose (such as 5 to 10 mg intramuscularly (IM) or 20 to 30 mg by mouth of morphine), assuming the patient has been on weak opioids already. The dose is then increased as needed, usually as soon as the evening of the first day and certainly during the second day, if pain is not relieved. The limiting factor is if the patient cannot tolerate a higher dose of the drug because of side effects *that can't be controlled.* If so, another opioid can be tried. Sensitivity to one drug's side effects does not mean the patient will be sensitive to a similar drug's side effects.

▪ Patients on high doses of potent opioids who must switch to another narcotic should not receive a low dose to start. Different doses of the various opioids have equivalent pain-relieving effects. This is called the *equianalgesic dose.* When switching, patients should start with at least one-half the equianalgesic dose of the new medication. This is because tolerance is not always complete between drugs (meaning that when a patient grows tolerant to one drug—needing higher doses to get the same pain relief—they've probably grown somewhat, though not completely, tolerant to a similar drug). Incorrectly calculating the proper dose of a similar drug, known as the equianalgesic dose, is a leading cause of undermedication. (See Table A.3 at the end-of-book section titled More Information on Medications.)

▪ The elderly, those who are malnourished, and those with kidney or liver disease are usually given about 25 percent less than the standard doses to start. Children's doses are calculated by body weight.

▪ Persons 40 years or younger may need more frequent doses than older persons because they metabolize morphine more quickly and, therefore, the pain-relieving effect may not last as long in these younger patients.

▪ Whenever possible, opioids should be taken by mouth (tablets or liquid) for convenience and mobility. If the patient can't take medication orally because of dry mouth, sores, difficulty swallowing, or other problems, many other forms are available and are discussed later in the chapter.

▪ Fixed doses should be prescribed on a schedule, around the clock. Be sure that a *rescue dose,* also called an *escape dose* or *bolus,* is prescribed "as needed" in addition to the standard dose. A rescue dose, usually 5 to 15 percent of the total daily dose, allows the patient to take extra medicine as needed should the pain break through between normal fixed doses. When the patient needs more than two or three rescue doses a day, then it is probably time for the doctor to increase the fixed dose. (See more on rescue doses below.) So, even with all the earlier talk about how cancer pain medications should be given in fixed doses around the clock, sometimes "as needed" dosing is appropriate. Its main role is to relieve breakthrough pain once the around-the-clock medication schedule is established. But there are two other cases when "as needed" dosing may be necessary. When the patient's pain status is rapidly changing—for example, during radiation treatments for a tumor of the bone—or when pain only occurs intermittently (the exception, not the rule).

▪ Expect that the opioid will have to be increased periodically—because of tolerance, pain escalation, disease progression, or increases in psychological distress.

▪ Expect that a combination of drugs will be prescribed—either another analgesic (a non-narcotic one), or an adjuvant (complementary) drug, which will enhance the pain-relieving effect of the opioids or control side effects. (See Chapter 8 for details.)

▪ Be prepared for side effects that may include nausea, vomiting, sedation, constipation, dry mouth, and difficulty expelling urine. (See Chapters 10 and 11 for a discussion of these side effects.) Although these side effects sound rather bad, it must be considered that all medications have the potential for side effects—and in the case of morphine and drugs in its family, they are predictable and can usually be easily managed. Many side effects often do not occur when the initial dose is low (as most doctors prescribe) and is brought up gradually. Even when they do occur, it is rare that a side effect cannot be treated, and most go away in a few days. Obviously though, any problems must be mentioned to the doctor so they can be addressed.

▪ That the drug is being taken "before it gets really bad" should not be a concern, yet this misconception is so common that some have even developed a name for it—the "money-in-the-bank syndrome." Patients think they need to "save" the morphine for when they *really* need it. We now know that morphine doesn't stop being effective; the doses just need to be increased over time. In fact, many people stay on the same dose for weeks or months, even years. As pain worsens, the dose can be increased accordingly. Since there's no "ceiling dose," there's no cause for concern when morphine is started early, before "things get really bad."

▪ The patient should take appropriate medication when it is needed and before pain intensifies, not putting it off until the pain gets really bad. By keeping pain low early on, patients can stay stronger to deal with the other problems associated with cancer.

▪ Although many patients don't need morphine until they are very ill and close to death, that doesn't mean that taking morphine necessarily signals the "beginning of the end." Some patients do not have severe pain until their illness is very advanced and so do not need morphine earlier. Others may take morphine for weeks, months, even years. Many cancer patients need treatment with morphine even though their cancer is under good control for a long time. Taking morphine does not have any kind of negative effect on the course of the disease. In fact, many doctors believe that patients on morphine live longer because they are better able to rest, eat, and sleep, are more interested and active in the life around them, and, therefore, able to use their natural ability to fight the disease more rigorously.

MORE ABOUT RESCUE DOSES

Actually, once pain becomes established as a consistent problem, most patients will be taking not one, but two narcotics. Here's why. As we said before, cancer pain is usually relatively constant, occasionally flaring up from time to time. These flareups are, as described in Chapter 2, called *break-through pain*. When they occur with a specific activity, they are called *incident pain*. Because such pain exists, it makes good sense to always keep some medication in the bloodstream by giving most of it on an around-the-clock schedule (at a *fixed dose*, also called a *basal dose*). This around-the-clock medication is usually a long-acting opioid like controlled-release morphine (MS Contin, Oramorph), transdermal fentanyl (Duragesic), or sometimes even methadone. Since the body is always getting rid of some of the drug in its wastes, we must keep doses constant. Imagine a bucket with a slow leak. To keep that bucket full, you would have to dribble an amount of water in constantly. Similarly, a regularly scheduled dose helps keep the medication level from getting too low (which would allow pain) or too high (which could trigger side effects).

We said before that taking medicine as needed (prn)—in other words, waiting till the pain is bad before taking something—is usually undesirable. One time when it makes perfect sense (and is recommended by most experts) is when the long-acting drug is taking care of the majority of pain on an around-the-clock schedule, but the pain occasionally flares up (breakthrough or incident pain). A short-acting drug in prn doses, known as *rescue doses*, are usually prescribed, perhaps as often as every two to four hours, if needed. Usually a short-acting drug like immediate-release morphine (such as MSIR or Roxanol), hydromorphone (Dilaudid), or oxycodone are prescribed because they work quickly (in 15 to 45 minutes) and don't build up in the system to as great an extent as the long-release preparations.

Ideally, patients will take their around-the-clock medication as directed, and its dose will be high enough so that they will only need occasional rescue doses (2 to 3 a day). If patients are taking their rescue dose much more frequently, it is simply a sign that it is time to increase the dose of around-the-clock medication.

This may seem complex, but if you think about it, it makes sense. Actually, the situation is very much like that of insulin—doctors often use a long-acting (regular) insulin and a short-acting (NPH) dose for the same patient to control blood sugar.

HOW DOSES ARE DETERMINED

Doctors take prescribing medications very seriously and go to great pains to get the dosage right. A problem with pain medications, however, is that, until recently, reference books quoted only the doses used for acute or postoperative pain and didn't talk about cancer pain. We know now that, when prescribing for cancer pain, analgesics shouldn't be prescribed in rigid, fixed doses—as is the case for antibiotics. The dosing is more like that of insulin—the drug is prescribed in the amount necessary to control the problem, and that dosing is known to differ from patient to patient and from time to time. If the doctor seems reluctant to increase the dose, or if the dose is increased very slowly or minimally for moderate to severe pain, try discussing the reasons, pro and con, for larger doses. If you remain uncertain about how the pain is being handled, you may consider seeking a second opinion on pain management (see Appendix for resources).

HOW OPIOIDS ARE CHOSEN FOR EACH PATIENT

The potent opioids work by similar mechanisms. In general, they all offer the same kind of relief and they all have the same kind of potential side effects. Morphine is the best known of these medications and is the standard against which other drugs are compared. Doctors, however, may select from among the many strong narcotics for any of the following reasons.

- The doctor may be more familiar with one drug than another.
- Cost may be an important consideration.
- The patient may need a longer acting drug (controlled-release morphine, methadone, levorphanol, Duragesic) or shorter acting drug (immediate-release morphine, hydromorphone).
- The patient is sensitive to one opioid that causes nausea, vomiting, or another side effect, but may not be to another.
- If a patient becomes very tolerant to one narcotic, the doctor may switch to another because cross-tolerance between narcotics is often not complete—meaning that the patient won't be as tolerant to the alternative drug and lower doses can be used.
- The oral form of medication (pills or liquid) may not be suitable because of nausea and stomach problems, or because so many pills would need to be taken that it becomes inconvenient. The doctor will then consider a form of medication to bypass the particular problem. Examples include transdermal fentanyl (Duragesic), which is a patch placed on the skin (usually on the collarbone or shoulder), rectal suppositories, and medication injected under the skin, in a vein or near the spine. The injected medications are usually given at home through a portable pump (see discussion later in this chapter).
- If a fast-acting drug is needed to prepare a patient for a painful test or surgical procedure, meperidine (Demerol or Pethedine) or fentanyl may be prescribed, usually as an injection.
- And, finally, if a particular drug has worked well, or poorly, for a patient in the past, the doctor should strongly consider that history when choosing a pain medication.

UNDERSTANDING TOLERANCE, DEPENDENCY, ADDICTION, AND WITHDRAWAL

Many doctors, nurses, other health-care providers, and consumers are overly concerned about the potential of opioid addiction in cancer patients. Once the differences among tolerance, physical dependence, and addiction are understood, it will be clear why these phenomena should not be limiting factors for cancer pain patients.

Addiction is a psychological problem in which a person craves a drug for its euphoric effect. Addiction is extremely rare in cancer patients—no greater than one-tenth of 1 percent of cancer patients, according to experts. A person who is addicted takes the drug (it could be almost any drug) for recreation, fun, or a way to escape—not for legitimate pain control. The addict becomes compulsive about taking drugs, expends much of his energy seeking drugs, and uses the narcotics for purposes such as "getting high" (euphoria) rather than for controlling pain. Often, the person will try to get the drug any way he can, such as stealing drugs or the money to buy them, selling drugs, going to several doctors to get prescriptions, and so forth.

Addicts take the drug and become less functional. Cancer patients with pain, on the other hand, take pain medication to become more functional. When cancer patients are medicated properly, unlike addicts, they get back into the mainstream of life. Moreover, cancer patients using opioids rarely report getting a "high" from morphine; in fact, some feel just the opposite of euphoric, reporting dysphoria (an unpleasant state in which the patient doesn't feel like himself).

Even though patients, family members, and health-care providers still fear addiction, studies have shown just how rare it is in cancer patients. It is very unusual for a cancer patient to try to get more pain medication if the pain should go away because of, for example, successful treatment of a tumor. In fact, it is probably more common for cancer patients to stop their pain medication too quickly (it should usually be tapered, or decreased gradually) when their pain source is treated and their pain relieved.

The fear of opioid addiction should not be a factor in treating cancer pain.

Tolerance means that larger doses of a medication (like an opioid) are required over time to achieve the previous pain-relieving effect. Tolerance is an expected phenomenon that occurs in many patients on an opioid for at least several weeks. Tolerance has nothing to do with addiction. Its presence is usually first signaled when the patient notices that the last dose of medication didn't last as long as it used to. To counter tolerance, opioids are often prescribed with non-opioid pain relievers to keep the opioid dose low. Or patients may be switched to an alternative opioid (because tolerance to one drug may not carry over completely to another). This is not, however, the preferred way to treat tolerance.

The more appropriate way to treat tolerance is to increase the pain medication, which is expected and safe, because there is no ceiling effect. In other words, patients don't "use up" the pain-relieving effect of a drug. And just as patients may become tolerant to the pain-relieving effects of a medication, they become tolerant to side effects as well. So while larger doses are needed over time, they do not lose their potency to treat the pain, but they usually do become less likely to trigger unwanted side effects. We needn't worry about saving the morphine until it is "really needed" because it will keep working even if tolerance to a given dose occurs.

Physical dependence and *withdrawal* occur with the chronic use of opioids, but are not psychological phenomena and, therefore, are different from addiction. Physical dependence means that physical symptoms—most notably *withdrawal symptoms*—might occur if the drug were suddenly stopped. These symptoms include anxiety, irritability, alternating chills and hot flashes, excessive salivation, tearing eyes (lacrimation), runny nose, nausea, vomiting, abdominal cramps, insomnia, sweating (diaphoresis), and goose bumps (piloerection). Physical dependence is easily treated, thereby avoiding withdrawal, by gradually decreasing the doses of the opioid, such as reducing the daily dose by 10 to 25 percent. Once a low daily dose of morphine (20 mg orally) is reached, the opioid can be discontinued without withdrawal occurring.

Understanding How These Terms Are Related

Thus, most people who take morphine (and similar drugs) for more than a few weeks will grow tolerant and physically dependent on the medication because that is how the body reacts to opioids. Tolerance and physical dependence should not be a barrier to good pain management since they are expected and can be managed by the doctor just as other side effects are controlled (for example, nausea and constipation).

Tolerance and physical dependence have nothing to do with addiction, which is a psychological dependence. Although a person who is addicted almost always is also physically dependent on the narcotic, the opposite is not true: a person who is physically dependent is not necessarily addicted.

WAYS TO TAKE OPIOIDS

Although taking opioids by mouth is preferred, patients can't always swallow pills or liquids. This may be because too many pills are required, patients mouths are too dry, they are nauseated, their intestines are blocked, or they are unable to swallow. Many patients whose cancer is in advanced stages will probably use at least two different methods for receiving medication; about one-quarter will make use of three different methods as their condition changes. Various methods are available for taking these drugs.

Oral Medication (by Mouth or PO)

Oral forms of medication—using liquid, syrup, or tablets—are usually preferred because it is the most economical, convenient, and safe way to take medication. Although doses may take a little longer to take effect initially, they last about as long as drugs given in other forms.

Transdermal (Transdermal Therapeutic System, or TTS) Medication

Transdermal forms of medication are fairly new. For the treatment of pain, a relatively new system uses skin patches (its trade name is Duragesic and it is much like a Band-Aid) that release fentanyl, an opioid, through the skin where it is absorbed and taken up by the blood to the rest of the body. Fentanyl is more potent than morphine and so is dispensed in the much smaller unit of micrograms (1,000 micrograms, or mcg, equal 1 milligram) instead of milligrams (as is morphine). The fentanyl patch, which is available in four sizes to release 25 mcg, 50 mcg, 75 mcg, or 100 mcg of medication an hour, when effective does away with the need for needles and pumps. At times, several patches may have to be used to achieve the correct dose. The patches must be replaced every 72 hours in most patients, and they take from 12 to 24 hours to become fully effective, during which time other pain relievers should be used. This system still needs to be supplemented with a short-acting drug (orally or rectally) for breakthrough and incident pain. Also, if a side effect occurs, it will persist for up to 24 hours, even after the patch is removed. The patch system is very convenient and its use is on the rise.

Rectal Medication (by Rectum, or PR)

When patients are vomiting or can't swallow medication, suppositories of morphine, oxymorphone, and hydromorphone may be used. When suppositories aren't available, enemas using 10 to 20 mg of water with morphine, opium, or hydromorphone can also be effective.

Suppositories, however, are better in some circumstances than others. Adolescents, for example, may be embarrassed by using the rectal forms of medication and tend not to like it. The rectal forms may also be ruled out if there is diarrhea or hemorroids, or if changing position to insert the suppository is painful. Because of these and other problems, the rectal medications are often used (as is MS Contin, controlled-release morphine, though not formally approved for this route) for short periods, especially when doctors want to avoid injections.

Subcutaneous Infusion (or "sub-q")

Intravenous or intramuscular injections used to be the most popular way to give shots, but the subcutaneous method is gaining in popularity because it is easily managed by patients inside or outside of the hospital once the oral medications have been abandoned. Sub-q, as it is called, avoids the use of painful repeated injections, and the response to this form is the same as if the drug were taken intravenously. This route involves the use of a portable, battery-powered, computerized pump (about the size of a portable tape player) that can be rented. This programmable pump introduces opioids continuously through a small needle (called a *butterfly* because of its shape), which is inserted just under the surface of the skin, where it is left in place. Patients may stay at home and yet have a continuous drip of medication. Some of these pumps are patient-controlled, meaning that the patient can decide, within limits set by the doctor, when to give himself or herself an infusion (see below) or extra dose.

However, to save on the cost of using a programmable pump, many hospices and hospitals may leave a butterfly in place, where it is hooked to a short tubing when needed; the drug is then given manually with a syringe into the tubing. This is much cheaper than using the automatic pump.

Intramuscular Injection (IM)

In this form of administering medication, the drug is given by needle into the muscle tissue. Although drugs given by this route take effect more quickly than those given by mouth, shots can be painful and do not last long. Thus injections are generally not recommended for long-term management of pain. Moreover, patients who have lost weight may not respond well to this form of medication.

Intravenous (IV) Medication

In this form of administering medication, the drug is placed directly into a vein through a needle. Although IV routes are sometimes necessary initially to quickly adjust the dose or to provide immediate pain relief, they are no more effective or quicker to act than sub-q doses and are now used less often than in the past. The main reasons to use IV medication in the long term are if the oral forms of the drugs are no longer suitable, and if a patient already has a permanent IV (a "plug" that is surgically inserted, called a *port* or *catheter*) that was put in place for chemotherapy, nutrition, or antibiotics.

Patient-Controlled Analgesia (PCA)

This route of drug administration has become increasingly popular in recent years. It allows the patient to decide when—within limits set by the doctor —to push a button and receive a preprogrammed dose of painkiller—subcutaneously, intravenously, or epidurally (see below). Usually, the patient will be receiving a regular dose of painkiller around the clock, and the PCA is used to deliver a rescue dose for breakthrough pain or a preventive dose before a particularly painful activity.

When PCA was first introduced about a decade ago, doctors were initially slow to use it because many feared that PCA would give patients too much control and they would abuse the opioid. Studies show, however, that patients do not tend to give themselves more medication than needed. As PCA has proven successful over the years, more and more doctors are accepting and advocating its use. One built-in safety measure is that if a patient ends up giving herself too much medication, chances are she will fall asleep and stop pressing the button.

PCA pain relief also gives patients control at a time in their life when they often feel so helpless; it also eliminates the need for the patient to have to inappropriately negotiate for more painkiller with family members or health-care professionals, or to have to wait for relief. While doctors are the best authorities on which drug to prescribe for which patient on what schedule, patients are the best authorities on their pain and when it hurts. Therefore, it makes sense that they should have the control to do something about it when it hurts. Thus, if pain medication has been prescribed to be given by pump, doctors may decide the patient can take an active role in administering medication. If a patient has been given a pump without their own button to push, they may wish to discuss PCA with their doctor.

Sometimes, when appropriate, PCA becomes parent-controlled analgesia (although PCA is being used successfully in younger and younger children) or spouse-controlled analgesia. When someone other than the patient is pushing the button, however, and the patient is unable to communicate his or her pain, family members may find it difficult to determine whether to push the button for a "rescue" dose at every grimace. Does every grimace mean pain? Is the family treating pain or anxiety? Sometimes, families may need to ask themselves if they are treating their own anxiety. If these questions arise, it may be useful to discuss them with the doctor or hospice nurse; they will know the condition of the patient and the extent of the cancer, and will have experience in understanding grimaces, anxiety, and expressions of pain.

Buccal Administration

This route involves putting a tablet or liquid inside the cheek or between the gums and a cheek when the patient can't swallow tablets or liquid directly, allowing the medicine to be absorbed in the mouth rather than be swallowed. At this time, however, bitter flavors, irritation, and poor absorption often limit the usefulness of this method, but it has promise for the future.

Epidural and Intrathecal Routes

Although various controversies abound, such as the best time and site for treatment, or the best type of catheter (drug tubing) to use, morphine and other opioids can be administered through special catheters placed near the spine. When the needle is placed within the spinal canal but outside the sac that contains the spinal cord and its fluid, it is called an *epidural*. When the needle enters the sac and the drug is mixed with the spinal fluid, it is called *intrathecal, subarachnoid,* or *spinal administration*. Using these methods, pain relief lasts a long time with small doses (5 to 10 mg morphine can last 18 hours or longer). These procedures may be particularly useful for patients with pain in the lower abdomen or back for whom systemwide dosing causes a problem with side effects. While administering opioids near the spine often results in fewer serious side effects, tolerance may develop.

The main advantage of epidural and intrathecal medication is that more relief is obtained with less drug because the drug is placed right where it works (near pain receptors). These advantages must be balanced against some drawbacks—like the risk of infection and the need for minor surgery.

Intraventricular Administration

Intraventricular drug administration is like the epidural methods, except instead of near the spine, the medication goes directly into the fluid of the brain. The need for this type of treatment is infrequent, but it can be useful for some kinds of head and neck pain (see Chapter 9).

Intranasal Methods

This route involves putting the drug into the nostrils. It is still experimental.

Inhaled Medications

With this experimental method, the drug is breathed into the lungs.

Sublingual Methods

Sublingual drug administration involves putting the drug under one's tongue for absorption. Effective for the drug buprenorphine, this medication is not available in the United States. Although not approved for this route, many hospices use liquid morphine this way in patients who can't swallow, instead of starting a pump.

Brompton's Cocktail

In the past, a drink called a *Brompton cocktail* was often given to cancer patients, especially between morphine doses. It gets its name from the location where it was first developed, at Brompton's Chest Hospital in England.

Consisting of a combination of heroin or morphine with cocaine, phenothiazine (a tranquilizer and anti-nausea medication), alcohol, and chloroform water, these drinks were frequently used to help control pain. Yet studies in the late 1970s showed that only the morphine was providing the pain relief. In recent years, therefore, the use of Brompton Cocktails has been discontinued in favor of oral morphine (or substitutes as needed) because doses can more easily be tailored (or titrated) to the patient's needs. If the patient is given a Brompton cocktail these days, consider a consultation with another doctor or pain specialist, since using Brompton cocktails is an old-fashioned, less effective pain reliever than the more modern methods described in this book.

The following information on opioid medications is meant as a guide only, and should not be used as a substitute for a doctor's care and judgment.

THE STRONG OPIOIDS

Morphine

Morphine is the most widely used opioid drug and is available in various forms and concentrations. They vary so much that some doctors consider them different medications.

Brand Names

MSIR and Roxanol are immediate-release formulations (in liquid and tablet forms) that are taken by mouth usually every 2 to 4 hours.

MS Contin and Oramorph are controlled-release formulations that are taken by mouth (and should never be cut, chewed, or crushed), but usually last for 12 hours, though sometimes only for 8 hours.

Sterile morphine solution, a generic term, is used for intramuscular, subcutaneous, and intravenous forms of administration.

RMS is the form of morphine taken as a rectal suppository. Preservative-free morphine (Duramorph, Astramorph, Infumorph) is used for intraspinal use.

For a more complete description of morphine products, see Table 7.1.

Dose Range

Starting doses vary considerably but are generally as follows: 20 to 30 mg if by mouth, every 3 or 4 hours.

5 to 15 mg if administered subcutaneously, intramuscularly, or intravenously, every 1 to 4 hours until an adequate dose that lasts for 4 hours is achieved. Intraspinal doses vary.

30 mg if controlled-release morphine, twice a day.

When switching from injection to oral morphine, or vice versa, the oral dose should be two to three times the injected dose. Conversely, the oral dose should be cut to one-half to one-third if being switched to an intramuscular, intravenous, or subcutaneous dose. This ratio, however, applies to patients who have already been taking morphine for some time. When new to morphine, the ratio may be closer to 1 to 6 rather than 1 to 3. When a patient is switched from IM to oral medication, or vice versa, families may find it helpful to refer to the equianalgesic doses given in the Appendix on page 322.

The Story of Morphine

Opium is the powder derived from the milky juice of split, unripe seed capsules of the oriental poppy. Long renowned for its powerful narcotic effects, opium has been used as a pain reliever for centuries.

As early as 6000 B.C., the Sumerians carved stone tables with pictures of the poppy and were evidently aware of its mind-altering and pain-relieving effects. The Ancient Greeks mentioned it in their writings, and its constipating effect warranted its use in the treatment of dysentery in the Middle East. The Chinese, Egyptians, and Romans all referred to opium as a cure for a variety of maladies.

So lulling was its effects that the painkiller started being used recreationally in the 1600s. Its use peaked in the 1800s when even hyperdermic syringes were available by mail order. Widely available, opium was used freely, and users bore no stigma. Word has it that occasional to frequent users included Lord Byron, Shelley, Keats, Coleridge, Dickens, Turner, Freud, Darwin—even Florence Nightingale and the fictional Sherlock Holmes.

By the early 1800s, chemists had synthesized a substance from opium that was ten times stronger than the original substance. It was dubbed morphine—for the god of sleep, Morpheus—because it could induce sleep. By the late 1800s, a stronger derivative was marketed by the Bayer Company. It was promoted as being as strong as a legendary hero—twenty-five times stronger than the opium resin—and so the Bayer Company called it heroin.

Although heroin and its related compounds are now being abused throughout the United States, Europe, and elsewhere, the World Health Organization recognizes how important these substances, particularly morphine, are in the treatment of cancer pain. They have launched an international campaign to fight the confusion and misconceptions that inappropriately inhibit its medical use.

How Long It Takes to Reach Peak Effect
About 1 hour if by mouth.

Less than an hour if subcutaneous, intravenous, or intramuscular injection.

About 1½ to 3 hours if slow release.

Equivalent Pain Relief
2 mg of IM morphine is equivalent to 650 mg aspirin.

Comments

- Morphine is the standard against which other opioids are compared. If the current (or starting dose) dose doesn't relieve the pain, then the dose should be increased by 30 to 50 percent. But starting doses can be difficult to calculate: if the patient becomes very sedated after the first dose and has no pain, then the next dose should be cut by 50 percent. On the other hand, if pain relief is inadequate in the first 24 hours after consistent around-the-clock dosing, then the dose should be raised by up to 50 percent (in the meantime, if breakthrough pain is experienced, the dosing schedule should be changed to every two or three hours, rather than every 4 hours, to achieve pain relief).
- Morphine comes in different concentrations. In liquids to be taken orally, for example, concentrations range from 2 mg per millimeter (a milliliter [ml] is about one-thirtieth of a fluid ounce) to 20 mg per ml. Concentrations of liquid morphine for subcutaneous or intravenous pumps, on the other hand, usually range from ½ mg per ml to 50 mg per ml.
- Immediate-release morphine tablets (which work relatively quickly for a relatively short period) are available in 15 and 30 mg strengths. Controlled-release morphine, which takes a longer time to work but remains effective for up to 12 hours, is available in 15, 30, 60, and 100 mg. Again, long-acting, or controlled-release, tablets should not be broken, cut, crushed, or chewed but swallowed whole. They should not be taken more often than every 8 hours, though every 12 hours is the recommended frequency.
- Rectal suppositories are available commercially in strengths of 5, 10, 20, and 30 mg. A specially trained pharmacist may manufacture higher doses when needed. Even though the manufacturer does not specifically recommend it, controlled-release morphine has also been shown to be effective and safe when given rectally. If switching from oral to rectal administration, the same dose is usually used rectally. There have even

been some clinical reports of these medications being used vaginally and with colostomy patients.

- Morphine solutions should be stored in cool areas, away from direct sunlight. Solutions used in warm climates should have antimicrobial preservatives.

- Close contact with the doctor, pharmacist, or nurse who is monitoring the medication should be maintained, especially during the first 24 hours and then 72 hours later. Ideally, contact between the health-care provider and the patient or his or her family should be maintained regularly, at least every few days or more frequently if conditions change. Patients need to be monitored for side effects, unresponsiveness, and psychological complications.

- The drug should be taken on schedule, around the clock. If patients awake during the night and this is undesirable, a 50 percent increase or even a double dose (100 percent increase) can be taken at bedtime (with the doctor's approval). If the patient is taking 60 mg or more every 4 hours though, the patient will have greater trouble sleeping through the night and a middle-of-the-night dose will probably be recommended. Sustained-release morphine is ideal in these situations.

- Although most patients take between 5 and 30 mg every 4 hours, doses range enormously, with no ceiling, or top, dose. A few patients require as much as 1,000 mg an hour or more.

Precautions

- Constipation is extremely common, so laxatives should be taken, preferably at night, right from the start to prevent it. In fact, some doctors warn that preventing constipation may be more difficult than preventing pain (see Chapter 10), and so suggest that "the same hand that prescribes for morphine should also prescribe a laxative."

- Nausea is initially quite common when a patient begins to take morphine, but usually does not persist. About one-third of patients need a medication (an *anti-emetic*) to prevent nausea (see Chapter 10), but usually for only a short time (often less than a week).

- Vomiting sometimes occurs along with nausea and requires treatment with an anti-emetic. Vomiting (and the need to treat it) does not usually persist, but depending on how severe it is, anti-emetics and painkillers may have to be given by rectal suppository or injection, again usually for just a few days. After several days, the anti-emetic usually can be tapered off while the morphine use continues.

- Drowsiness, confusion, dizziness, unsteadiness, and sedation are very common during the first three to five days after starting treatment or

Table 7.1. *Morphine Products*

Generic Name	Route	Brand Name (manufacturer in parentheses)	Comments
Immediate-release morphine	Tablets	MSIR (Purdue Frederick) Morphine (Lilly and Roxane)	Must be swallowed with liquid; will be bitter if the patient can't swallow quickly. Rapid onset, short duration.
	Liquid	Roxanol (Roxane) MSIR (Purdue Frederick) OMS Concentrate (Upsher-Smith)	Rapid onset, short duration.
Controlled-release (long-acting) morphine	Tablets	MS Contin (Purdue Frederick) Oramorph (Roxane) Roxanol SR (Roxane)	Long-acting (controlled-release) tablets, lasting 8 to 12 hours. More expensive. Don't break, chew, or crush.
Morphine suppositories	Rectal	RMS (Upsher Smith) Roxanol suppositories (Roxane)	For rectal administration when patient cannot take medication by mouth.

Note: When switching forms of medication from oral (liquid or tablets) to subcutaneous or other needle-administered routes, how to calculate the appropriate dose is controversial. When just starting with morphine, studies suggest using a 6-to-1 ratio for equivalent pain relief; that is, 6 mg of oral morphine would be equivalent to 1 mg parenteral (subcutaneous, intramuscular, or intravenous). But when the patient has already been using morphine and has developed some tolerance to the medication, a stronger 2-to-1 or 3-to-1 ratio, oral to parenteral, is suggested.

Products for injections (including subcutaneous pumps) and epidural and intrathecal use are also available. They include Astramorph PF (by Astra), Duramorph (by Elkins-Sinn), and Tubex (by Wyeth-Ayerst).

For more details about equianalgesic doses, recommended schedules, formulations, toxicity, and alternative opioids, see the Appendix.

raising a dose, and usually clear up within a week. Persistent sedation can sometimes be alleviated with stimulants, such as strong coffee, dextroamphetamine, or methylphenidate (see Chapter 8).

- Respiratory depression (the slowing of breathing) is rare in cancer patients but often erroneously cited as a reason for not giving enough pain medication.
- Remember, these problems are side effects, not signs of allergy, and

can usually either be waited out (until the patient becomes tolerant to the side effects) or managed with another medication (laxative, anti-emetic, or stimulant) prescribed by the doctor. True allergy to morphine is extremely rare.

- Tell your doctor if any of the problems mentioned here occur so that helpful treatments can be prescribed to deal with them. Side effects only occur in a proportion of patients, so there is a good chance you won't have these problems. Still, it is good to know what to look out for. Finally, if a side effect is not getting better, the doctor may consider trying a different opioid (such as transdermal fentanyl, hydromorphone [Dilaudid], or another medication) which may better agree with the patient, or the doctor may consider a whole new method of treatment (see Chapters 8 to 11).
- Other less frequent side effects include severe sweating (diaphorcsis), hallucinations, difficulty breathing (bronchoconstriction), urinary retention, and twitching.
- And remember: addiction is *not* a problem when treating cancer pain.

Transdermal Fentanyl

Brand Name
Duragesic.

Dose Range
Usually 25 to 100 micrograms per hour (may use multiple patches).

How Long It Takes to Reach Peak Effect
Usually 12 to 18 hours.

Equivalent Pain Relief
Onc 25-microgram patch equals about 60 mg of oral morphine per day.

Comments

- This skin-patch form of medication, recently released, is now widely used since many patients find this a particularly convenient form of treatment. The patches contain fentanyl, an opioid that is about 100 times stronger than morphine (which is why it is prescribed in micrograms; one microgram is equal to one-thousandth of a milligram).
- Patches come in four sizes, and more than one patch can be used if necessary.

- The drug must be absorbed through the skin, so it may take about 12 hours after the first application until pain relief starts.
- Once treatment is started, relief is steady. Patches need to be changed every 72 hours, occasionally, every 48 hours (with a doctor's permission). Short-acting opioids will usually still be needed for breakthrough pain.
- Patches should be applied to nonhairy skin on the upper body. They must adhere well to work, and can be reinforced with tape.

Precautions

- Side effects are similar to those for morphine; the medicine, however, stays in the body for about 12 hours after a patch is removed, so if there are side effects, they will persist for a bit.
- Patches should be kept away from children and be disposed of in the toilet after use.

Hydromorphone

Brand Name
Dilaudid.

Dose Range
6 to 7½ mg if oral, every 3 to 4 hours.
1½ mg if IM, every 3 or 4 hours.

How Long It Takes to Reach Peak Effect
½ to 1 hour if by mouth.
1 to 2 hours if IM.

Equivalent Pain Relief
Six times more potent than morphine.
1½ mg of hydromorphone IM or 7½ mg by mouth is equivalent to 10 mg of morphine IM.

Comments

- Hydromorphone is used quite commonly as an alternative to morphine.
- Hydromorphone is relatively inexpensive and is available in a variety of forms (oral, rectal, and by injection).
- It works relatively quickly, and because it doesn't accumulate in the system, it is safe for patients with liver or kidney problems.

- Hydromorphone doesn't last very long, so it usually needs to be administered frequently (as often as every 3 hours).
- It is particularly useful for subcutaneous injections (usually given by a portable pump) because it is so soluble (in other words, it is possible to dissolve a great deal of the drug in a small volume of fluid).

Precautions
- See under morphine.

Methadone

Brand Name
Dolophine.

Dose Range
Although doses are highly variable and difficult to predict, the usual starting dose is 5 to 20 mg if by mouth, at intervals varying from every 4 to every 12 hours.

If given by intramuscular injection (IM), 5 to 10 mg, every 6 hours.

How Long It Takes to Reach Peak Effect
Several days (4 to 14 days) may be required before a "steady state" is reached. The way the body breaks down and disposes of methadone is less predictable than with most opioids, so one to two weeks of use may be required before the best dose and schedule are determined.

Equivalent Pain Relief
10 mg of methadone given IM or 20 mg by mouth is equivalent to 10 mg morphine in intramuscular form.

Comments
- Methadone has a long "half-life" which means that the medication may stay in the bloodstream for up to 100 hours after a single dose. As a result, there is some risk that the buildup of the drug in the body may be excessive and that side effects, even serious ones, might prevail. This is more likely in elderly patients and those with kidney or liver problems.
- If the doctor chooses to treat with methadone, he or she will probably observe the patient closely for problems during the first few days and weeks, after which the chance of serious side effects is minimal.
- We have discussed how around-the-clock (a-t-c) treatment is usually

preferred to as needed (prn) treatment, but since methadone is needed as frequently as every 4 hours in some patients and as infrequently as every 12 hours in others, many authorities recommend a different way of initiating treatment. They may start with prn administration, and only switch to an a-t-c dose when a given patient's best schedule is established.

- Most authorities agree that it takes more skill and closer observation on the doctor's part to administer methadone effectively and safely than morphine and the other opioids. For this reason, it is recommended that methadone *not* be used as a first choice. Still, the doctor's choice of methadone may reflect his familiarity with it, and he may prefer it because it is much cheaper than alternatives, especially controlled-release morphine and transdermal fentanyl.

- Methadone is very commonly used in "methadone-maintenance programs" as a method to manage addiction in street addicts. This alternate use should not be confused with its medical use as an analgesic. Just like morphine and other opioids, when methadone is used to treat cancer pain, addiction is extremely rare.

Precautions

- Methadone is not usually used in an elderly or confused patient, or in those with respiratory, liver, or kidney problems.
- Methadone can cause sedation if it accumulates in the body, especially during the first days of treatment.
- See precautions listed for morphine.

Levorphanol

Brand Name
Levo-Dromoran.

Dose Range
2 mg orally, usually every 4 to 8 hours. (Like methadone, dose interval is variable.)
2 to 4 mg IM every 4 or 6 hours.
1 mg IV.

How Long It Takes to Reach Peak Effect
½ to 1½ hours if IM.
1½ to 2 hours if oral.

Equivalent Pain Relief

Five times more potent than morphine by mouth.
2 mg of levorphanol IM is equivalent to 10 mg of morphine IM.

Comments

- Levorphanol lasts longer than morphine and so a patient would need fewer doses per day.
- Levorphanol is often useful for elderly patients who can not tolerate morphine.

Precautions

- See under morphine and methadone.
- Like methadone, levorphanol may accumulate in the body over time and lead to toxicity.

Oxycodone (without aspirin or acetaminophen)

Brand Name

Roxicodone.

Dose Range

30 mg by mouth, every 3 to 6 hours.

How Long It Takes to Reach Peak Effect

About 1 hour.

Equivalent Pain Relief

30 mg of oxycodone by mouth is equivalent to 10 mg morphine IM.

Comments

- The same medication is available premixed with aspirin or acetaminophen as Percodan or Percocet. Oxycodone is used with aspirin or acetaminophen for moderate pain.
- For moderate to severe pain, oxycodone is used alone, and can only be administered by mouth.
- This drug is particularly useful for patients with sensitivity to aspirin or acetaminophen or those who need more oxycodone than can be given in combined form (because of toxicity resulting from the aspirin or acetaminophen).

Precautions
- See under morphine.

Oxymorphone

Brand Name
Numorphan.

Dose Range
1 mg if IM, every 4 hours.
10 mg if by rectal suppository.

How Long It Takes to Reach Peak Effect
½ to 1 hour if IM.
1 to 2 hours if rectal.

Equivalent Pain Relief
1 mg of oxymorphone IM or 10 mg in suppository is equivalent to 10 mg of morphine IM.

Comments

- Oxymorphone is not available in oral forms, but only as an IM injection or as a suppository.
- It is relatively long acting, usually lasting from 4 to 6 hours.

Precautions
- See under morphine.

Heroin

Brand Name
Diamorphine.

Dose Range
5 to 20 mg IM, every 4 hours.
60 mg by mouth.

How Long It Takes to Reach Peak Effect
1 to 2 hours if by mouth.
½ to 1 hour if by intramuscular injection.

Equivalent Pain Relief

5 mg of heroin IM is equivalent to 10 mg morphine IM.

Comments

- Heroin is not available in the United States.
- Because of so much interest in heroin as a pain reliever, the U.S. government recently sponsored several clinical research programs to compare it to other strong pain relievers. At both the Vincent T. Lombardi Cancer Research Center at Georgetown University (supported by the National Cancer Institute) and at the Memorial Sloan-Kettering Cancer Center in New York (supported by the National Institute on Drug Abuse), researchers concluded that heroin was no more effective than morphine and that the side effects were no milder. In fact, the pain-relieving effect of heroin has been found to be due to its being broken down into morphine in the body; researchers believe, therefore, that it is an inefficient way to give morphine; its only advantage is that a smaller quantity needs to be administered.

Precautions

- See under morphine.

Although there are other classes of strong drugs (known as mixed agonists-antagonists, which are more fully described in Chapter 6), they are generally not recommended for cancer pain because of their potential to cause hallucinations and confusion (psychotomimetic effects) at higher doses. Also not recommended for chronic cancer pain is meperidine (Demerol or Pethedine), which is a frequently prescribed analgesic used for acute pain, such as that experienced after surgery. Its long-term use, however, is linked with muscle jerks, confusion, agitation, and seizures. These side effects appear to be more common in patients with kidney problems.

The opioids and non-opioid drugs described thus far are frequently prescribed with other drugs that enhance the pain-relieving effect of these pain-killers. Next, we'll turn to a discussion of these so-called adjuvant medications.

8

Understanding How Adjuvant Drugs Relieve Pain and Suffering

In addition to the basic pain relievers already described, often other medications are prescribed to enhance the patient's comfort. These drugs, called *adjuvant drugs* or *co-analgesics*, are auxiliary medications that were developed for conditions other than pain. However, they have been found to have pain-relieving properties in certain instances, may enhance the action or minimize the toxic effects of the primary pain reliever, or may help relieve symptoms that are contributing to the pain.

For example, nerve pain or pain resulting from muscle spasms can often be further relieved when a drug primarily used as an anticonvulsant (antiseizure), antidepressant, or corticosteroid (a type of steroid) is added to or used instead of the pain reliever. In other cases, the cancer patient may not only be suffering from pain, but also from depression or anxiety, which can contribute to pain; in these instances, antidepressants, antianxiety (anxiolytics), or antipsychotic (neuroleptics) drugs may be helpful.

Although it may sound odd to put a cancer patient in pain on an anticonvulsant or antidepressant when he or she is not suffering from convulsions or depression, experienced physicians have found it does make sense. More often than not, drugs have multiple effects, sometimes up to a dozen different ones. When drug companies develop and test a new drug, they focus on whatever property they think will be most marketable, but doctors may then choose to use the same drug for an alternative purpose.

For example, if a company were working on a drug that had antidepressant, analgesic, sedative, and antiseizure effects, it would analyze which effect was most needed at that time. Let's say the company chose the drug's ability to prevent seizures—that is, its anticonvulsant property. They would then focus their very costly research efforts on that action. They would test it only as an anticonvulsant, and get it approved by the Food and Drug Administration as such, and subsequently market it as an anticonvulsant. Yet, the drug would still be an effective analgesic, antidepressant, and sedative and can still be prescribed for any of these uses at any time. And let's say that over time, physicians had discovered that its analgesic properties were particularly useful for nerve pain, which is often unresponsive to morphine. They might, therefore, decide to prescribe the so-called anticonvulsant for pain.

GENERAL COMMENTS ABOUT ADJUVANT DRUGS

▪ The dose of the adjuvant drug is tailored to the individual patient, depending on symptoms and type of pain.

▪ Adjuvant drugs are usually used in addition to the more standard opioid drugs, but may also be used alone.

▪ In many cases, the usefulness of these drugs has not been thoroughly tested in well-controlled clinical trials. Nevertheless, in an individual patient a trial of some of these medications may be of great value. The following information is a guide to some of those medications, but should not be used as a substitute for a doctor's care and judgment. (See Table 8.1.)

Table 8.1. *Adjuvant Drugs or Co-analgesics: Drug Classes That Enhance Pain Relief*

Antidepressants
Anticonvulsants
Oral local anesthetics (also called sodium channel blockers)
Anti-anxiety drugs
Muscle relaxants (good for muscle spasms)
Antihistamines
Stimulants
Corticosteroids

Adjuvant Drugs for Cancer Pain
ANTIDEPRESSANTS

The use of the antidepressants in patients with cancer pain is a complex topic. Like the other drugs discussed in this chapter, the antidepressants have more than one use. Primarily, the antidepressants are used in cancer patients:

- To treat depression.
- To treat pain.
- To treat insomnia.

They are often used for patients:

- Who are depressed but do not complain of pain.
- Who have nerve pain, but are not depressed.
- Who have both depression and pain.

These drugs are among the most misunderstood of the painkillers. If an antidepressant is prescribed to control pain, many patients feel offended at their doctor's recommendation because they may feel that their doctor thinks their pain is not real, is in their head, or is only a reflection of their poor mood. In fact, these medications work to control pain directly, and this pain-killing effect is totally independent of any effect on mood. In fact, the doses usually prescribed to control pain are quite low—much lower than would be prescribed for someone who is depressed. And these lower doses which are effective in controlling pain usually do not even affect mood. When depression is a problem, much higher doses would need to be prescribed.

When Depression Is Not a Problem:
Antidepressants and Nerve Pain

One class of antidepressants—those known as the *tricyclic antidepressants*—act by altering the amount of certain neurotransmitters (serotonin and norepinephrine) within the body. Since these neurotransmitters are involved in pain transmission, these drugs are particularly useful for pain due to nerve injury. In fact, a prescription of an antidepressant (with or without other pain medications, such as the opioids) is considered the treatment of first choice for patients with nerve pain. It is particularly useful for pain that is experienced as burning, itching, tingling, or numbing, as well as other types. This kind of pain may be a facial pain, postsurgical pain, or may be due to shingles (herpes zoster), or any tumor that presses on nerves. The tricyclic antidepressants may be more effective for pain that is relatively constant, while the anticonvulsants (see below) may be tried first for pain that is episodic (comes and goes). Also, it is not uncommon for these and other medications to be used together to get the best effect.

When Depression Is a Problem

In many patients, pain and depression do go hand in hand, and more than half of cancer patients who are depressed say that pain is their main problem. Patients in chronic pain also show similar symptoms as those who are depressed: they suffer from poor sleeping and eating patterns as well as mood problems, among others. In fact, pain and depression exhibit some similar physiological characteristics with regard to brain chemistry, specifically changes in levels of neurotransmitters.

Although sadness and a low mood are natural responses to having cancer, in about one-quarter of patients, these feelings become so overwhelming that they may represent a full-blown depression and should be treated medically. Patients need to know that such feelings are common, so they should not be ashamed to admit having them. Sometimes working hard to suppress them is the worst thing to do, because that not only takes energy but they usually come back. If patients are afraid to talk about feeling low because they don't want to upset their loved ones, they should tell their doctor, who can recommend a counselor.

The relationship between pain and depression is complicated, though, and like the chicken-and-egg, it is difficult to determine which came first. Pain is usually the main problem, however. People may become depressed simply because they have had intolerable pain for a long period of time—so much so that they may even consider suicide. In cases like this, the depression often gets better once the pain is resolved. In other cases, the main problem may be depression rather than pain. Because persons are depressed, their attitude is bad, their pain threshold is low, and they may complain a great deal about pain. The pain complaints may in fact be a less upsetting way of getting attention than admitting they are feeling low. In cases like this, the depression usually needs to be resolved before the pain will get better. The difficulty here is that it is hard to know which came first, the pain or the depression, and so it is hard to know where most of the treatment should be directed.

Whenever possible, the pain and depression should be considered separately. All pain should be assumed to be "real" (meaning that it is related to physical injury), and although pain has psychological components, it should never be taken lightly and thought of merely as a mental process. When depression seems to be an important part of the patient's problem, then treatment with an antidepressant may be warranted. The same antidepressants that are used to treat pain are usually used to treat depression as well, but in considerably higher doses. (For a fuller discussion of depression and its treatment, see Chapter 14.)

General Comments

A variety of antidepressants are commonly used to treat pain. Like other pain medications, several different types may need to be tried before the most suitable one for a given person is found. Antidepressants that seem to be most effective in controlling pain are those in the class of drugs called the *tricyclic antidepressants*. They include amitriptyline (Elavil, Endep), imipramine (Tofranil, Antipress, Imavate, Prexanuben SK-Pramine), doxepin (Sinequan, Adapin), desipramine (Norpramin, Pertofrane), and nortriptyline (Pamelor, Aventyl). Because they all promote drowsiness to varying degrees, they are all usually prescribed in a single nighttime dose to help sleep. Low doses are used to start, and are gradually increased as needed and as tolerated. Although insomnia may improve immediately, treatment for one to three weeks may be needed before pain gets better.

Most of these medications have *anticholinergic* effects, meaning that they may cause dry mouth, constipation, difficulty urinating (urinary retention), heart-beat irregularities, sweating, drowsiness, delirium, dizziness, low-blood pressure upon standing up suddenly, and possibly tremors. However, with the exception of dry mouth, these side effects are uncommon with the low doses used for pain.

A new group of antidepressants has recently been introduced that includes fluoxetine (Prozac) and sertraline (Zoloft). They are more likely to perk people up than to make them tired, so they are usually prescribed during the day. Their effects on pain have not yet been well studied. The psychostimulants (Ritalin, Dexedrine; see later in this chapter) also have antidepressant effects, but this is not their main use.

Antidepressants most commonly used for pain include the following.

Amitriptyline

Brand Names
Elavil, Endep, Emitrip, Enovil.

Dose Range
For pain relief, starting doses range from 10 to 25 mg by mouth, taken at bedtime, up to a daily dose of about 50 to 125 mg within one to four weeks, to further relieve pain and improve sleep.

For the elderly, the starting dose is about 10 mg.

To counter depression, daily doses may need to be much higher: usually 150 to 300 mg.

How Long It Takes to Reach Peak Effect

Amitriptyline may take from one to four weeks to achieve its full pain-relieving effect.

Comments

- Amitriptyline is particularly good for nerve pain and for improving sleep patterns.
- It is also recommended for treating anxiety.
- It can help ease depression.
- It may be effective in treating phantom-limb pain.
- It may be effective in treating pain near a surgical scar.
- Children's doses are based on body weight.
- Available as IM injection or as rectal suppository.

Precautions

- The most common side effect of amitriptyline is dry mouth, which often diminishes within one to two weeks.
- Morning drowsiness is relatively common and also tends to subside within a few days to a week, once the dose is held constant; if it doesn't abate, the condition may be relieved by taking the evening dose even earlier in the evening.
- Sedation may occur but usually diminishes within several days.
- Other side effects may include constipation, difficulty urinating (urinary retention) particularly among elderly men, light-headedness, confusion, weight gain, and low-blood pressure upon standing (orthostatic hypotension).
- It is not to be used in patients with glaucoma.
- Rarely, the drug may trigger hyperexcitability in the patient.

Several alternatives are available that may be prescribed in place of amitriptyline. They include:

Doxepin

Brand Names
Adapin, Sinequan.

Dose Range

The usual starting dose is 25 mg at night. This may be gradually increased to up to 300 mg at night. (Lower dose ranges for pain; higher dose ranges for depression.) May take several weeks to reach full effect.

Comments

- Doxepin is similar to amitriptyline, but causes dry mouth and constipation less frequently.
- It is available in liquid form, unlike most of the other antidepressants.

Precautions

- See under amitriptyline.
- It should not be used with patients who have glaucoma or urinary retention problems, especially older patients with these conditions.
- Doxepin may cause drowsiness.

Imipramine

Brand Names

Tofranil, Janimine, Tipramine, Tofranil-PM.

Dose Range

Usually from 25 to 300 mg a day. (Lower dose ranges for pain; higher dose ranges for depression.) May take several weeks to reach full effect.

Comments

- See under amitriptyline; causes less severe dry mouth and less sedation.
- Imipramine may be associated with weight gain.

Desipramine

Brand Names

Norpramin, Pertofrane.

Dose Range

Usually from 25 to 300 mg a day. May take several weeks to reach full effect.

Comments

- Side effects, including anticholinergic and sedative effects, as well as low-blood pressure upon standing, are less severe than the above-mentioned medications. Otherwise, similar to amitriptyline.

Nortriptyline

Brand Names

Pamelor and Aventyl.

Dose Range

25 to 100 mg per day. May take several weeks to reach full effect.

Comments

- Similar to amitriptyline, but with milder side effects.

Trazodone

Brand Names

Desyrel, Trialodine.

Dose Range

Usually 50 to 600 mg per day. (Lower dose ranges for pain; higher dose ranges for depression.) May take several weeks to reach full effect.

Comments

Trazodone is one of the newer antidepressants, and it causes relatively few side effects—an exception is drowsiness. For this reason, it is often chosen when poor sleep is a problem.

Precautions

- A side effect that men should be aware of is that the drug occasionally causes unexpected or prolonged erections. Should this occur, the patient should discontinue use and contact the physician.
- Trazodone should be taken with food.

ANTICONVULSANTS

Anticonvulsants are particularly useful in treating nerve pain because, like seizures, pain is a sudden electrical phenomenon. By suppressing the spontaneous firing of neurons (nerve cells), anticonvulsants quiet their excitability and interfere with the generation (the start) of the pain message. Thus, although doctors may prescribe an anticonvulsant to help with pain, this has nothing to do seizures. The anticonvulsants are particularly useful for nerve pain that is intermittent, shooting, burning, or stabbing in nature. They are either used with or without a tricyclic antidepressant to treat pain.

Carbamazepine

Brand Names

Tegretol, Epitol.

Dose Range

The starting dose is 100 to 200 mg a day, with increases of 100 mg every three or four days if needed, up to 800 to 1200 mg a day.

How Long It Takes to Reach Peak Effect

Carbamazepine will usually take from two to four weeks for a peak effect.

Comments

- This anticonvulsant is by far the drug of choice for shooting, shocklike nerve pain—it can relieve symptoms in up to 90 percent of cases; it is less likely to be effective for aching, burning nerve pain that is constant.
- It may be recognized as a drug commonly used to treat epilepsy.

Precautions

- This is the most common of the anticonvulsants used to treat pain, because it has been studied the most and seems to be the most effective. Unfortunately, side effects—nausea, vomiting, loss of muscle coordination (ataxia), dizziness, lethargy, and confusion—are more common with this anticonvulsant than others in this drug group. If administered in low doses, and increased only gradually, side effects should not occur very often.
- Very rarely, more major side effects may occur, affecting less than 1 in 20,000 patients. Carbamazepine may be toxic to the liver and the bone marrow, and as a result, if doctors keep the patient on this medication for more than a few weeks, they order regular blood tests of liver and bone marrow function. The bone marrow is where blood cells are made and stored, and its function can be monitored by checking the patient's CBC (complete blood count). Doctors will be looking for thrombocytopenia (a shortage of platelets; platelets help the blood to clot), granulocytopenia (a shortage of white blood cells; white blood cells help fight infection), and anemia (a shortage of red blood cells; red blood cells carry oxygen). Patients with low platelets may bruise or bleed easily, and may have trouble getting a cut to stop oozing. Patients with a low white blood cell count may be prone to developing infections, and those with anemia may fatigue easily. The symptoms of liver problems

are more vague and may include flu-like symptoms, confusion, fatigue, and bleeding problems. Blood tests are carefully checked if carbamazepine is prescribed for patients who have recently undergone chemotherapy or radiation therapy because their bone marrow may already be depressed.

Phenytoin

Brand Names
Dilantin, Diphenylan, Phenytex.

Dose Range
Usually started at 100 mg a day and increased gradually by increments of 25 to 50 mg, with daily doses usually not exceeding 300 to 400 mg.

How Long It Takes to Reach Peak Effect
It normally takes one to three weeks to reach its full effect.

Comments

- Although the most well-studied drug for seizure control, phenytoin has not been studied as thoroughly as carbamazepine for controlling pain. This is true of the other antiseizure drugs discussed here as well. As a result, carbamazepine is usually the first choice when nerve pain needs treatment with an anticonvulsant, but the others have also been found to work well, and are usually prescribed when carbamazepine cannot be given or is ineffective.
- Phenytoin may interract with other medications that are being taken. Check with the doctor or nurse.

Precautions

- Similar to those of carbamazepine, but usually mild and less often a problem.
- Mouth hygiene is very important to prevent gum problems—namely, gingival hyperplasia, which is an overgrowth of gum tissue and which can occur in up to 20 percent of patients; this is usually a problem only in children and adolescents. (See Chapter 11 on side effects and other discomforts.)

Valproic Acid or Valproate

Brand Names
Depakene, Depakote, Depa, Deproic.

Dose Range

Usually started at 250 mg, once or twice per day. This dose can be increased gradually, usually up to 500 mg, three times a day.

How Long It Takes to Reach Peak Effect

It may take from 1 to 4 hours for a peak effect, and may take one to three weeks before pain is relieved.

Comments

- Valproic acid can be used for nerve pain as an alternative to carbamazepine.
- It can be prescribed in a syrup preparation for patients with difficulties swallowing.
- It should not be chewed because it could cause mouth and throat irritation.

Precautions

- Side effects are similar to those described for carbamazepine, including pancreatitis, nausea and vomiting, insomnia, headache, tremor, hair loss, weight gain, and (rarely) liver problems.

Clonazepam

Brand Name

Klonopin.

Dose Range

Usually started at ½ mg twice daily, and may be increased gradually to up to 1 mg four times per day.

How Long It Takes to Reach Peak Effect

1 to 2 hours; may take several weeks to reach full effect.

Comments

- A relatively new antiseizure drug, clonazepam seems to be very effective in controlling pain due to nerve irritation. It is a benzodiazepine (minor tranquilizer), like diazepam (Valium), so in some states it requires a triplicate prescription.

Precautions

- Its most common side effect is drowsiness.
- Dizziness, sedation, and fatigue are also relatively common.
- If used for a long time, withdrawal symptoms may occur if the drug is stopped suddenly.

ORAL LOCAL ANESTHETICS OR SODIUM CHANNEL BLOCKERS

For nerve pain, either continuous or shooting, when tricyclic antidepressants and anticonvulsants have been ineffective, a sodium channel blocker may be recommended to calm unstable nerve membranes and prevent them from firing erratically. These are oral versions of local anesthetics that were developed for heart arrhythmias. Doctors find them particularly useful for unrelieved nerve pain.

Mexiletine

Brand Name
Mexitil.

Dose Range
Usually started at 150 mg, once or twice a day, which can be increased to up to 800 to 1,200 mg day.

How Long It Takes to Reach Peak Effect
1 to 2 hours, but several weeks of treatment may be needed for full effect.

Comments
- Mexiletine works by calming and stabilizing nerve membranes, which may quiet other kinds of pain as well.
- It is usually, prescribed for the burning, tingling, or itching pain that accompanies nerve injury when the antidepressants and anticonvulsants have not been helpful.

Precautions
- Side effects that may occur include drowsiness, stomach problems, nervousness, dizziness, and lightheadedness.

Tocainide

Brand Name
Tonocard.

Dose Range

200 to 400 mg twice a day.

How Long It Takes to Reach Peak Effect

½ to 2 hours; may take several weeks to reach full effect.

Comments

- When mexiletine does not work, this medication may be useful.

Precautions

- Side effects similar to mexiletine, but may be more severe.
- Breathing problems should be reported promptly.

OTHER MISCELLANEOUS DRUGS

Medications called calcium channel blockers (such as nifedipine [Procardia]) and beta blockers may be useful to treat certain types of headaches. Bone pain that persists, despite standard medications, has been treated with various medications such as diphosphonates, calcitonin, and even the amino acid L-dopa, with some success. Another amino acid, L-tryptophan, has been reported to have an additive pain-relieving effect with morphine and to renew the anesthetic effect after a cordotomy (see Chapter 9). It might be particularly useful when the patient can't tolerate antidepressants but has nerve pain.

Other amino acids, such as arginine, have also been reported to help treat herpes sores (herpetic eruptions) and nerve pain from chemotherapy or radiation, but these reports have not been confirmed by research.

Baclofen (Lioresal) is a medication usually prescribed to treat muscle spasms in patients with multiple sclerosis. It may be useful for certain pains, especially nerve pain around the head and neck, that has not responded to other measures. Usually doses are from 20 to 120 mg per day.

To treat burning, itching, tingling, numbing, or nerve pain, the use of an over-the-counter cream called Zostrix has been found helpful for some patients. Made from the substance that makes red peppers hot, Zostrix is usually prescribed for shingles (herpes zoster) but sometimes also for rheumatoid or osteoarthritis. Zostrix is thought to make skin and joints less sensitive by using up a chemical known as substance P, which is thought to be part of the pain-transmission process. By depleting substance P from nerve endings and preventing it from reaccumulating, the area may become less painful. It may also work by being a "counterirritant," in that by exciting some nerves, pain signals from other areas get blocked, much like

TENS (transcutaneous electrical nerve stimulation; see Chapter 9) or skin stimulation that can include vibration, pressure, hot or cold packs (see Chapter 12). When Zostrix is applied, patients sometimes initially feel a burning sensation, which usually stops within three days, although sometimes it can take up to several weeks. Though expensive, Zostrix may prove soothing once the burning sensation stops.

Adjuvant Drugs for Symptoms Other Than Pain

As opposed to the drugs that have been mentioned so far, most of the drugs in this group do not have direct pain-relieving properties. They are useful in patients who are suffering from anxiety and other psychological problems. In low doses, they do not affect mood very much, but are extremely useful in controlling nausea and vomiting. They should not be used as substitutes for painkillers, but may be prescribed along with painkillers when patients are anxious, fidgety, or nauseated. While most of these medications don't have a direct effect on pain, some patients' pain thresholds go down when they are restless, upset, and can't sleep—that is, they can tolerate less pain.

These medications include prochlorperazine (Compazine), chlorpromazine (Thorazine), and Haldol (haloperidol); each is discussed separately below. Two of the medications in the group, however, seem to have pain-relieving properties: a little known medication called methotrimeprazine (Levoprome), which does have pain-relieving properties similar to morphine (but is used only occasionally because it must be given by injection), and fluphenazine.

TRANQUILIZERS THAT HELP RELIEVE PAIN

Methotrimeprazine

Brand Name

Levoprome.

Dose Range

10 to 20 mg by intramuscular (IM) injection, every 6 to 8 hours. Methotrimeprazine has been reportedly used in IVs with no problems. An oral form of this medication is not available.

How Long It Takes to Reach Peak Effect

1½ hours.

Equivalent Pain Relief

15 mg of methotrimeprazine IM is equivalent to the pain-relieving effect of 10 mg of morphine IM.

Comments

- The pain-relieving effect of methotrimeprazine may be as strong as morphine, and is also good for treating nausea.

- Because its mechanism for relieving pain is different from that of morphine, methotrimeprazine may be particularly useful in patients who have become tolerant to high doses of opioids or who can't take opioids. The recommended starting dose is 5 to 10 mg, because it may cause oversedation, unless that is desirable in anxious patients who have not responded to more conventional analgesics or who are unable to take opioids.
- Sedation and sudden low blood pressure upon standing quickly (orthostatic hypotention) tend to diminish after the initial days of taking the drug, and so over time, doses may be increased as needed.
- It is also useful in avoiding severe constipation or respiratory depression due to opioid use.
- It is not available in oral forms.
- Methotrimeprazine is particularly useful in the advanced phase of cancer when the side effects associated with the drug (low blood pressure problems when standing, sedation, and anti-anxiety effects) are not a problem; in fact, they may be desirable.

Precautions

- Side effects include sedation, low blood pressure when patient stands (orthostatic hypotension), and discoordinated motor movement, such as uncontrollable jerky movements (tardive dyskinesia).

Fluphenazine

Brand Names
Prolixin, Permitil.

Dose Range
1 to 3 mg a day, by mouth.

Comments

- This drug helps prevent vomiting.
- It may relieve nerve pain and is usually prescribed in conjunction with a tricyclic antidepressant (such as amitriptyline or imipramine) for pain relief, and with an opioid for its anti-nausea property.

Precautions

- Side effects include sedation, low blood pressure upon standing (orthostatic hypotension), and uncontrollable jerky movements (tardive dyskinesia), similar to Parkinson's disease.

TRANQUILIZERS USED TO PREVENT NAUSEA AND RELIEVE ANXIETY

In general, the following medications are primarily used when patients suffer from nausea, delerium, or anxiety.

Haloperidol

Brand Names

Haldol, Haloperon.

Dose Range

Starting dose is ½ to 2 mg by mouth, every 4 to 12 hours.

If given to treat psychiatric symptoms (agitation), doses may go up to 10 to 15 mg, two or three times a day.

Children's doses are based on weight.

Comments

- This drug is used extensively in the United Kingdom to manage vomiting, nausea, and agitation, in part because it seems to produce less drowsiness than other anti-nausea medications.
- Haloperidol is useful as a morphine-enhancer (also may allow morphine dose to be reduced), especially in cancer patients who are agitated, confused, or psychotic.

Precautions

- This drug may cause drowsiness, dry mouth, urinary retention, and jerky movements.

Chlorpromazine

Brand Names

Promapar, Thorazine, Sonazine.

Dose Range

10 to 25 mg, every 4 to 8 hours, by mouth.

Comments

- Although not a pain reliever, its anti-anxiety and anti-nausea properties are often useful when anxiety is aggravating the pain.

Precautions

- Side effects include low blood pressure, blurred vision, dry mouth, difficulty in urinating, constipation, rapid heart beat (tachycardia), and jerky movements (extrapyramidal effects).

Prochlorperazine

Brand Name

Compazine.

Dose Range

5 to 10 mg, every 4 to 8 hours, by mouth.

Comments

- This drug is useful as an anti-nausea, anti-vomiting medication, but also helps quell anxiety.
- It is available in oral form, IM, and as a suppository.

Precautions

- It can cause dry mouth, drowsiness, dizziness, jerky movements, and blurred vision. May turn urine pink or purple.

Trimethobenzamide

Brand Names

Tigan, Arrestin, Benzacot, Bio-Gan, Stemetic, Tebamide, Tegamide, Ticon, Tigect-20, Triban, Tribenzagan, Trimazide.

Dose Range

Usually 250 mg, three or four times a day.

Usual suppository dose is one suppository (200 mg), three or four times a day.

For children, dose is calculated by weight: for 30 to 90 pound children, usually 100 to 200 mg (oral or rectal) are prescribed, three or four times a day.

Comments

- Trimethobenzamide is helpful to relieving nausea and vomiting.
- It is available in capsules to be taken by mouth, as a suppository, or as an injection.

Precautions

- It can cause drowsiness, dizziness, jerky movements, and blurred vision.
- Tigan and other anti-emetics should not be used in children suspected of having or developing Reye Syndrome.

Thiethylperazine

Brand Names

Torecan, Norzine.

Dose Ranges

Usually 10-mg tablet, one to three times a day.

In children, appropriate doses have not been determined.

Comments

- Thiethylperazine is helpful in relieving nausea and vomiting.
- It is available in tablets, as a suppository, or as an injection.

Precautions

- Medication contains a sulfite that may cause allergic reactions in sulfite-sensitive people, especially those with asthma.
- It may impair mental and physical abilities and so the patient should avoid driving and other potentially dangerous activities.
- Occasionally, this drug may cause jerky movements, convulsions (more common among young adults), dizziness, headache, and drowsiness with the initial dose.

MEDICATIONS FOR TREATING ANXIETY

These anti-anxiety (anxiolytic) medications are called the minor tranquilizers, sedatives, or hypnotics. Anxiety is common among cancer patients and may range all the way from feeling a little nervous to experiencing full-blown panic attacks. When symptoms are minor, the best treatment is simple reassurance and loving contact. When anxiety persists, treatment usually includes some form of psychotherapy (with a psychologist, psychiatrist, or trained social worker) and anti-anxiety medication.

Anti-anxiety medications do not directly relieve pain and should not be used as a substitute for a strong painkiller. However, if the pain is relieved but significant anxiety persists, both the pain and anxiety may need to be treated at the same time. Someone who is nervous and jumpy may have a lower pain threshold and may complain of pain when it is really more a question of them feeling ill at ease or frightened. When complaints of pain seem to be based at least in part on anxiety, treatment with an anti-anxiety medication can be extremely helpful.

Psychological and physical dependency can develop with most of these medications, so doctors are often hesitant to prescribe them, especially on a frequent basis for chronic complaints. Moreover, in some states, a triplicate prescription is required for their use. Nevertheless, they should not be denied to a cancer patient with a genuine need for them. Taken over long periods of time, they may actually increase depression, and if they are stopped suddenly, patients may experience physical withdrawal.

Benzodiazepines

Diazepam (Valium) is the best known of this class of drugs, although many new benzodiazepines have become available and are widely used, both as sleeping pills and to counter anxiety.

Diazepam

Brand Names
Valium, Valrelease, Vazepam, Diazepam Intensol.

Dose Range
This drug is usually started at a dose of 2 to 10 mg, and can be taken once at night for insomnia or several times each day as needed for anxiety.

Comments
- Although not an "all-purpose" pain reliever, diazepam helps treat pain that is caused by muscle spasms because it relaxes the muscles.
- It also is used to relieve anxiety.
- It is available in oral forms, as a rectal suppository, or as an injection.

Precautions
- Most common side effects are drowsiness and disorientation.
- It may increase depression if used on a frequent basis.

Alprazolam

Brand Name
Xanax.

Dose Range

0.25 to 2 mg, three times a day, or 0.125 to 1 mg, every 6 hours.

Comments

- Recently introduced and commonly prescribed, its effects are relatively short-acting and so may be preferred in elderly patients in whom there could be a problem with a buildup of drugs in the body.

New Benzodiazepines

Many new benzodiazepines have become available and are widely used, both as sleeping pills and to counter anxiety. Ones that are usually used once at night to improve sleep include flurazepam (Dalmane; 15 to 30 mg), triazolam (Halcion; 0.125 to 0.5 mg), and temazepam (Restoril; 15 to 30 mg). A popular drug used to quell anxiety (and used during the day or night) is lorazepam (Ativan; 0.5 to 4 mg every 6 hours). Midazolam (Versed), only available as an injection in the United States, is extremely short-acting and may be used to provide sedation for hospitalized patients before stressful procedures and tests.

Nonbenzodiazepine Sedatives

The barbiturates (Seconal, Nembutal) are used less often now because of their potential for abuse and the availability of better drugs. They are still sometimes helpful, however, in a single nighttime dose to enhance sleep. A new drug, buspirone (Buspar), also an antidepressant, seems to avoid the habituating effects of the more traditional medicines mentioned in this section.

A drug in this class that is sometimes used for cancer pain is hydroxyzine (Vistaril), because it is a sedative and has the added benefit of having pain-relieving effects, although these are slight.

Hydroxyzine

Brand Names

Vistaril, Atarax, Anxanil, E-Vista, Hydroxacen, Hyzine-50, Quie SS, Vistaject, Visazine.

Dose Range

10 to 50 mg by mouth or 25 to 50 mg by intramuscular injection, three to six times a day.

Children's doses are based on weight.

Comments

- Also considered an antihistamine, hydroxyzine may dry secretions.
- This drug is particularly useful for the nauseated patient who is also anxious and in pain. It produces an additive pain-relieving effect when prescribed with morphine or another opioid.
- Its role in cancer pain is controversial because it is sometimes used to ease pain when larger doses of strong opioids would be more effective.

Precautions

- Hydroxyzine can cause sedation or hyperexcitability.

STIMULANTS

This class of drugs has traditionally been avoided by doctors because they were highly abused in the 1950s and 1960s to promote weight loss. Also, one of the stimulants, methylphenidate (Ritalin), is used to treat hyperactivity and behavior problems in children, creating another source of controversy. They require a triplicate prescription in many states. The research on their use in cancer patients is still relatively new, so some doctors may not be fully experienced with their important uses in patients with cancer. They are used mainly along with the opioids when the sedative effects of the painkilling drugs are compromising quality of life. Taken during the day, they are often very effective in reducing the sedation produced by the opioids. They may also enhance the effectiveness of stable doses of opioids, improve alertness, and boost mood. All of these drugs have the potential to make people jittery, and occasionally appetite may suffer. They should generally not be prescribed to patients with severe psychiatric problems or brain metastases.

Methylphenidate

Brand Name
Ritalin.

Dose Range
The usual starting dose is 10 mg on awakening and 5 mg with the noontime meal. Tolerance may occur and, as a result, dose increases to 40 mg a day, or more, may be needed to maintain a beneficial effect.

Comments

- This medication should not be given at night.
- It has been shown to help with pain in advanced cancer while minimizing or counteracting sedation. It may improve mood as well.
- It acts quickly
- It poses a low risk for serious problems; occasionally causes agitation.
- Consumers may recognize this drug as being the controversial medication often prescribed to children who are hyperactive (attention deficit disorder).
- It is available in a controlled-release form.

Dextroamphetamine

Brand Names
Dexedrine, Oxydess II, Spancap No. 1.

Dose Range
5 to 20 mg by mouth, twice a day.
  In children, dose is based on weight.

Comments

- Known as "speed" in street language, Dexedrine can offset the drowsiness and sedating effects of the opioids.
- It should not be given in the evening because the patient may have trouble sleeping.
- It may help enhance the pain-relieving effect of morphine and improve mood.
- It is also available in a controlled-release form.

Precautions
An occasional side effect is agitation.

COCAINE

Although used for a long time as part of the Brompton cocktail (a drink described in Chapter 6, which was frequently used for pain relief in the 1970s and before), studies have shown that cocaine, in fact, has no pain-relieving effect. It can, however, help prevent opioid-induced sedation, but other psychostimulants are preferred for safety reasons. It is not recommended as part of a standard regimen for treating cancer pain.

CAFFEINE

Although not usually prescribed by doctors, caffeine may be useful for patients who are drowsy. Caffeine is included in many over-the-counter headache medications, and a strong cup of coffee or tea may help improve alertness.

STEROIDS OR CORTICOSTEROIDS

There are two general types of steroids. One group is called the *anabolic steroids,* which are familiar to us as the drugs that have been abused by some professional athletes; they have little medical use. The corticosteroids, however, are used for many medical conditions, including problems related to breathing, arthritis, and infection. Administered over a period of years, they are likely to cause many side effects, some of which are serious, like weight gain, suppression of the adrenal glands, fractures, and liver failure. But used for short periods of time, their benefits strongly outweigh their risks. They are commonly used in patients with cancer, both as a part of chemotherapy and to control symptoms.

General Use

The steroids have many potentially useful roles in the treatment of patients with cancer. They are very potent in reducing inflammation and its related swelling, and are used in some chemotherapy treatments to shrink tumors and to reduce excessive levels of calcium that are sometimes caused by tumors. They are effective in controlling nausea and vomiting, may improve mood, and may help promote weight gain. One of their most important roles is as a painkiller.

Their traditional role is to relieve pain and other symptoms when a tumor is growing in a small enclosed space, like a brain tumor within the skull, or a spinal cord tumor within the spine. By reducing swelling (edema) and inflammation around the tumor and nerves, they may dramatically relieve headache and backache, although this effect sometimes only lasts a few weeks. They may actually be helpful any time pain is caused by pressure from a nearby tumor, and may be prescribed for pain due to a swollen liver, a tumor near the nerves to the arm, or cancer (carcinoma) of the esophagus or rectum. They are also used when there is swelling in the upper body (superior vena cava syndrome) or lower body (inferior vena cava syndrome).

Until other drugs or treatments can be found, high doses of corticosteroids can sometimes provide quick dramatic short-term relief when severe pain is caused by bone tumors or tumors that have spread to nerves.

These drugs are useful in boosting a patient's mood, stimulating appetite, reducing sweating, increasing strength, and just giving the patient an improved sense of well-being. If a patient has a serious illness with a short expected survival time, these drugs may be used more freely because the side effects from long-term use are less important. Yet, side effects still may occur, especially the longer the drug is used, and include increased susceptibility to infection, diabetes, fluid retention, acne, depression, psychotic episodes, and delirium.

However, the benefits of the corticosteroids often only last several weeks; doctors don't know whether the reason is because the drug's effectiveness diminishes with time, or whether the progress of the disease overrides the drug's benefits.

Nevertheless, the use of corticosteroids is becoming more and more widespread. Studies have shown that half of all patients in some special cancer units are given corticosteroids to relieve their symptoms. Another benefit of these drugs is that they often allow opioid doses to be reduced, thereby alleviating opioid-induced side effects. And finally, these medications may also help relieve the feeling of breathlessness in certain circumstances and may improve breathing.

Thus, steroids can improve the quality of life in some cancer patients. At least one study, conducted in Britain, has shown that selected patients on corticosteroids live longer as well. However, caution must be exercised with these medications. In particular, patients with peptic ulcers or high blood pressure are not good candidates for treatment with steroids.

The first steroid of choice for most doctors seems to be dexamethasone.

Dexamethasone

Brand Names
Decadron, Decaspray, Dexasone, Dexone, Mexadrol, Maxidex.

Dose Range
A common starting dose is 4 mg once or twice a day, by mouth, often dropping after a week or so to a lower maintenance dose.

Higher doses (up to 100 mg a day) are often used for pain, especially when due to the pressure of brain or spinal tumors.

This medication can also be given intravenously.

Comments

- Dexamethasone is particularly useful for shooting or burning nerve pain, pain resulting from skull pressure, pain resulting from nerve compression in the spinal cord, and bone pain.

- This drug may have an antidepressant effect—it has been reported to help patients eat better and enjoy an overall better sense of well-being.
- It is a good choice when large doses of opioids are ineffective and pain is caused by tumors growing in the nerves of the arm or leg (brachial or lumbosacral plexus).

Precautions

- Side effects include infection, weight gain (often a reassuring and comforting effect for the family), GI bleeding (especially when taken with NSAIDs), muscle weakness, insomnia, high blood sugar, and, rarely, hallucinations and other psychotic episodes.
- It should not be taken with NSAIDs.
- This drug should not be withdrawn suddenly but gradually.

Other corticosteroids that are sometimes used with cancer patients include prednisolone (brand name: Prednisolone and Prelone), prednisone (brand name: Deltasone and Sterapred), and methylprednisolone (brand name: Medrol). For a more complete listing of selected corticosteroids used with cancer pain, see the Appendix.

ANTIBIOTICS

Antibiotics help fight infections. Sometimes tumors break through the skin, a process known as *ulceration,* and can get infected. Antibiotics can help relieve the pain from these open sores, particularly the ones from the head and neck. Occasionally, tumors that do not break through the skin can get infected as well.

Infection is usually accompanied by fever and other symptoms, but it has recently been observed that pain from head and neck tumors often improves when antibiotics are given, even when there are no obvious signs of infection. Antibiotics can usually be administered orally, except when an infection is severe, in which case they must be given intravenously, usually in the hospital.

Even when the best of care is given, some ulcerated tumors may produce odors, fluid, and pus. This odor can be a source of tremendous embarrassment for patients, and they may try to isolate themselves from others. Antibiotics, such as metronidazole (Flagyl), either administered orally or placed directly on the open sore, may help control this unpleasant smell. Other treatments to help control odor are described in Chapter 11.

Table 8.2. *Adjuvant Drugs That May Help Particular Types of Conditions*

Bone pain	Aspirin or NSAID, such as flurbiprofen (Ansaid) or naproxen (Naprosyn), among others; corticosteroids, such as dexamethasone (Decadron); biphosphonates
Pain from brain tumor swelling	Corticosteroids, such as dexamethasone; diuretics (to expel fluids); and NSAIDs
Tension headaches	An anti-anxiety drug, calcium channel blocker, or beta blocker
Pain from pressure on nerves	Anticonvulsants, antidepressants, mexiletine, corticosteroids, such as Decadron or prednisone
Pain from nerve damage	Antidepressants, anticonvulsants, corticosteroids, sodium channel blockers, mexiletine
Shingles and other superficial burning nerve pain	Antidepressants, anticonvulsants, mexiletine, Zostrix
Intermittent stabbing pain	Anticonvulsants, such as carbamazepine (Tegretol) or valproate, or antidepressants, mexiletine
Nerve pain after chemotherapy or radiation	Antidepressants, anticonvulsants, or mexiletine
Pain from swollen stomach, hiccups	Metoclopramide or an antigas antacid
Infected skin ulcer	Antibiotics such as metronidazole or clindamycin
Rectal or bladder pain and spasms (tenesmus)	Chlorpromazine, an anti-anxiety drug, or other anti-anxiety drug; an anti-spasmodic drug, such as bethanechol (Urecholine) or oxybutynin (Ditropan); suppositories (belladonna and opium)
Pain from swellings in lymph system and other tissues	Steroids, diuretics
Pain and depression together	Any tricyclic antidepressant, such as amitriptyline, unless anxiety is present; caution with the long-term use of the benzodiazepines because these drugs may aggravate depression over time
Severe pain with anxiety and insomnia	Anti-anxiety drug, such as one of the benzodiazepines
Back pain due to spinal cord injury	Corticosteroid like dexamethasone (Decadron), or a diuretic, or both

Table 8.2. (*Continued*)

Pain due to muscle spasm	Anti-anxiety drug, such as diazepam, sometimes a muscle relaxant, such as baclofen (Lioresal) or dantrolene, may help
Pain and anxiety together	Benzodiazepine or phenothiazine
Depression and insomnia	Antidepressant
Daytime drowsiness	Stimulant, such as an amphetamine

Note: This list presents only a guide to *possible* treatments and should in no way be used as a directive. Complete medical evaluations are necessary to determine the best treatment for a particular patient. Some of the listings in the table are also considered controversial, and should be discussed thoroughly with a physician.

MUSCLE RELAXANTS

The traditional drugs used to treat muscle spasm (cyclobenzaprine or Flexeril, carisoprodol or Soma, methocarbamol or Robaxin), though often prescribed, are not actually very effective, and are best avoided, because their main effect is to produce drowsiness. If muscle spasm is chronic and painful, the best choice may be treatment with diazepam (Valium), which is also an anticonvulsant and a sedative (see discussion above). More recently, baclofen (Lioresal; mentioned earlier in this chapter under miscellaneous pain relievers), a drug used to treat the severe muscle spasm associated with multiple sclerosis, has been used successfully to help treat muscle spasms as well as nerve pain, especially around the head and neck.

9
"High-Tech" Options

In recent years, a number of exciting and important advances in cancer pain management have made great strides in making the cancer patient more comfortable. Although some of these advances are still being tested, others are being used rather routinely by specialists at medical centers around the world. But since the field of medicine changes so rapidly, today's "high-tech" treatment is often tomorrow's routine procedure. This chapter will sort out the various "high-tech" options available to today's cancer patients, help the reader balance the potential benefits and risks of each treatment, and understand which kinds of patients should consider the various options.

THE MOST IMPORTANT ADVANCE:
A NEW VIEW OF OPIOID DRUGS

Even though innovative techniques are now available, the most important advances are actually much more basic. They relate to a new appreciation by physicians that cancer pain is treatable and that standard analgesics, which can be taken by mouth, should be prescribed much more liberally than previously believed. As we've discussed, most cancer pain can be controlled with the careful use of these very simple and readily available medicines.

The cancer patient's physical and mental health is a very fragile and precious commodity. The doctor's main responsibility is to do the most that he or she possibly can with the least invasive form of treatment, since the more invasive procedures involve some risk or may be physically demanding. Patients and doctors alike must be cautious and not to be enticed to try innovative treatments simply to avoid using opioids because of unsubstantiated concerns about addiction or mental impairment. Sticking with oral painkillers is always the preferred route—it is reversible, is associated with very low risks, and can be adjusted when the type of pain changes. With some trial and error, *good comfort levels can usually be obtained by choosing the right dose of the right drug for the right individual at the right time.* This is often a time-consuming process, though, because several types of painkillers may have to be tried in combination with other medications to alleviate side effects. And so doctors will often use *sequential drug trials*, as we have already mentioned—an orderly trial-and-error process that even the most expert specialist adopts. It is only when pain cannot be relieved or side effects from these concerted efforts persist that the "high-tech" methods described in this chapter should be considered to control pain.

STRATEGIES TO RELIEVE PAIN

As described in Chapter 3, once a doctor has performed a complete medical workup to determine the source of pain (not all pain is related to the cancer or treatment), three general strategies are used to relieve cancer pain:

1. *Eliminate the source of the problem* by removing or shrinking the cancer, either with surgery, radiation treatment, or chemotherapy (including hormones). Like all therapy, each of these treatments has some risk. Unfortunately, not everyone is a candidate, and there are limits as to how much radiation and chemotherapy can be administered.

2. *Interfere with the interpretation of the pain message,* which is the most common intervention. Here, pain is controlled by altering the way the brain interprets the messages it receives. By using an analgesic such as morphine, pain is blunted because the drug changes the brain's perception of the pain in a selective and reversible way.

3. *Interfere with the pain signal itself,* which is the least common intervention because it is the most invasive. Here, the pain signal is interrupted somewhere between the tumor and the central nervous system—that is, the spinal cord and brain—by methods that act to short circuit the system; they are not unlike cutting an electrical wire to cause a short circuit. Treatments include neurosurgical procedures that actually cut nerves and certain anesthetic procedures called *nerve blocks* that interrupt the pain transmission by injecting chemicals near the nerves. This chapter will focus on these techniques.

"CUTTING THE WIRES": NERVE BLOCKS AND NEUROSURGERY

Temporary Nerve Blocks

While the term *nerve block* may be unfamiliar to many, most of us have experienced a form of nerve block when the dentist has temporarily dulled tooth pain with a "shot of novocaine." A nerve block involves using a drug, usually injected with a needle, near the path of a nerve, and "putting it to sleep" so that the painful signals are blocked and can't be transmitted to the spinal cord and brain.

Another common example of a nerve block is the epidural anesthesia commonly used to dull the pain of childbirth. An epidural offers more widespread pain relief because the anesthetic (the numbing medicine) is injected through a needle into the epidural space, a compartment that surrounds the spinal cord. Before the needle is removed, a tiny tube or catheter is often placed through it, with its tip placed in the epidural space, so that medication can be reinjected painlessly when the anesthetic eventually wears off.

These kinds of injections or nerve blocks are often called *temporary nerve blocks* because the anesthetics wear off within three to four hours. As a result, they have a limited but still important role for treating cancer pain. When pain is not specifically related to the tumor, it can often be relieved with repeated nerve blocks or injections through a catheter. These temporary or secondary pains may result from muscle spasm, shingles (herpes zoster), or nerve irritation called *reflex sympathetic dystrophy*. Sometimes a steroid will be added to these injections to reduce any associated inflammation. The potential benefits of a local anesthetic in this situation include temporarily breaking a cycle of pain and spasm, and improving movement and local blood flow. This type of nerve block is also called a *therapeutic nerve block*.

Temporary nerve blocks may also be used to help diagnose the source of a pain, much like an X-ray or CAT scan. In the case of some perplexing pains, it is difficult to know which of the body's many nerves is responsible. A skillful anesthesiologist may use a *diagnostic nerve block* to identify the specific nerve that is causing pain by injecting each of the potential "suspects" in turn with a local anesthetic.

Finally, a temporary or local anesthetic nerve block can be used to predict whether long-lasting pain relief may result from cutting the nerve or injecting a stronger substance to destroy the nerve. The temporary block, called a *prognostic nerve block*, is used to mimic the ultimate effect of a more permanent procedure, and hopefully would predict any side effects that might result from a more enduring procedure. Unfortunately, the results of the temporary block are not always completely accurate in predicting the effects of a more permanent block.

"Permanent" Nerve Blocks

The term *permanent nerve block* is actually inaccurate. A more useful name might be *semipermanent block*, because such procedures actually only last, on average, from three to six months. A permanent or semipermanent nerve block usually refers to an injection of medicine that is intended to destroy a portion of a nerve. Called a *destructive* or *neurolytic block*, or more generally, *neuroablation*, these procedures most commonly use 100 percent ethyl alcohol (*absolute alcohol*) or *phenol* near the nerve. Less commonly, instead of giving an injection, the tip of the needle is superheated with electricity (*radiofrequency thermoablation*) or frozen with gas (*cryoablation*) to block the nerve, usually in the head or neck.

Since most cancer pain persists over time, more permanent (destructive) nerve blocks are usually reserved for pain that is very well localized—a pain which the patient can point to reliably. Destructive nerve blocks are usually avoided when the pain covers a wide area (except for abdominal pain) or is located in many areas that are distant from each other. Destructive blocks are also usually performed only when the cancer is not expected to get better.

Destructive blocks require a great deal of skill and training to be safe, and so are performed only at a limited number of centers, usually by anesthesiologists. They can also have side effects since some nerves not only transmit pain, but are also important for transmitting information to the brain about light touch and for sending the commands required for movement to occur. Unfortunately, the effects of injected alcohol and phenol are indiscriminant or *nonselective,* meaning that they will destroy any nerve with which they come into contact.

To avoid injuring healthy nerves, therefore, these procedures must be performed with the utmost accuracy, often with help from X-rays or CAT scans. Even when the most skilled doctor performs the procedure, patients may occasionally experience muscle weakness of an arm or leg, or even bowel or bladder problems, which may persist for months or longer. Obviously, if a patient already urinates through a Foley catheter (bladder tube) or is confined to bed, these are less important considerations. In the relatively healthy patient who gets around well, however, these kinds of problems would present frustrating difficulties. Although these risks are small, they are the main reasons *neurolytic* blocks are not performed more frequently.

Another consideration is that, while successful nerve blocks eliminate or reduce the pain, they numb the area somewhat, making it less sensitive to touch. Most patients gratefully exchange pain for numbness, but occasionally the numb feeling is irritating, a condition called *anesthesia dolorosa* (*dolar* is Latin for pain). For these reasons, a destructive nerve block may be preceded by a temporary prognostic block to assess whether long-lasting effects of the procedure are likely to be satisfying.

Unfortunately, no treatment has a perfect success rate, and even when done properly, pain may be only partially relieved or not relieved at all. Since many doctors would rather limit how much alcohol or phenol is injected to lessen the risk, repeated treatments are often needed. This approach is like covering a fence with several coats of whitewash instead of putting on one thick coat all at once. To alleviate the discomfort of a nerve block, doctors will often numb the area or administer a pain reliever intravenously so discomfort is minimized. The doctor usually cannot "put the patient out" *(general anesthesia)* because he will need the patient's feedback about whether the temporary nerve block relieves the pain or not. Patients should also be prepared for a severe burning pain when a *neurolytic drug* (alcohol or phenol) is injected, which is difficult to blunt, but lasts only about a minute.

TYPES OF NERVE BLOCKS BY ANATOMY

The body's nervous system is complex and consists of hundreds of nerves, both large and small, each with a different function. Any nerve in the body can be blocked, either temporarily or permanently. And with each different nerve, there are different potential benefits and risks, which can vary from patient to patient. There are some general guidelines, however, that apply to everyone.

Peripheral Nerve Blocks

Treatments of this type involve injecting individual nerves or bunches of nerves *(nerve plexus)* that are outside the spinal cord—on the periphery of the body. Many of these nerves are *mixed nerves*, meaning that in addition to sending information about touch and pain, they also send messages necessary for movement and strength. As a result, neurolytic or destructive blocks are performed very cautiously to avoid adding a limb weakness to the other burdens of being sick. Since there is some overlap in the areas covered by each nerve, sometimes more than one nerve must be blocked. And again, there is usually some numbness after a semipermanent block that may be disturbing or even painful in some cases, so a temporary block is often tried first.

For head or neck pain, a *cranial nerve block,* usually some form of a *trigeminal block,* may be recommended. It usually involves placing a needle beneath the skin of the face with its tip near the skull bone. These are technically difficult procedures requiring X-ray guidance and considerable skill. Because problems with swallowing, breathing, or vision occasionally develop, a temporary block is usually performed first.

When pain involves the chest wall, *intercostal blocks* may be considered. In this case, nerves that run just above and below the ribs are injected. Because of the small chance of a collapsed lung *(pneumothorax)* after this procedure, a chest X-ray is usually taken afterward. Obviously, if the lung has already been removed *(thoracotomy),* this is not a concern. A small collapse can usually just be monitored, but more severe cases need to be hospitalized. In serious cases, a chest tube may be inserted.

Pain involving the arm or leg is particularly difficult to treat with an injection because of the risk of weakening the limb. Temporary blocks can be performed quite safely, but neurolytic (destructive) blocks of the nerves to the arm or leg are almost never performed unless the limb is already severely weakened or nonfunctional. Even then, an arm that is weakened and swollen from breast or lung cancer may still be needed for minor but important tasks like buttoning a shirt or pulling on pants. Nerves sometimes blocked for arm pain are the *brachial plexus,* a group of nerves located in the armpit, and the *suprascapular nerve,* near the shoulder. Sometimes the *sacral nerves* (near the tailbone) are blocked for leg pain, but usually a *spinal block* is selected instead.

Spinal and Epidural Nerve Blocks

Also called *central blocks,* these injections are placed between two of the bones of the spine near the *nerve roots,* just before the nerves become peripheral nerves. Temporary central blocks (with local anesthetic) are commonly performed every day in most hospitals for labor pain and minor surgery. Epidural steroids, often used for common low back pain, may also help some cancer patients. Relatively new, spinal morphine, administered continuously, may also be useful (see page 171).

In contrast, though, as we've said, neurolytic blocks with alcohol or phenol are very specialized procedures that require special training. They are relatively safer when performed in the midback (*thoracic spine*) for chest pain, because the nerves to the arms, legs, and bladder are so far away and shouldn't be affected. They are riskier when near the upper (cervical) or lower back (lumbar), so should be used only under special circumstances. For example, this might be a good treatment for leg pain, but only if the patient were so sick that she was confined to bed, and even then, bladder weakness is a concern.

Treatment involves advancing a needle between two of the spinal bones (after anesthesia to the skin) until its tip enters the sac that holds the spinal cord and its surrounding fluid. Only a few drops of medication are needed to make the painful area numb, but the patient must curl up in an uncomfortable position for about fifteen minutes. Which position is necessary depends on whether alcohol (which floats in the spinal fluid) or phenol (which sinks) is used. Most patients say that the position is more uncomfortable than the needle itself.

Sympathetic Nerve Blocks

The *sympathetic nerves* are those that travel to our internal organs, and so when they are injected, patients are not ordinarily bothered with numbness of the skin or risks of muscle weakness. Although a relatively difficult procedure, one of the most common and successful nerve blocks for cancer pain—especially for pancreatic and other cancers that cause abdominal and back pain—is called a *celiac plexus block,* which involves an injection to the *solar plexus,* near where your ribs meet at the bottom of the chest cavity. Since it is located deep in the abdomen, X-ray or CAT-scan guidance must be used. Usually, two needles are placed on each side of the spine, and either a local anesthetic or alcohol is injected. Even though this group of nerves is near many major organs, treatment is relatively safe because of the help provided by the X-rays.

For burning pain in the arm or face, especially in patients with lung or breast cancer, the *stellate ganglion,* located at the base of the neck near the voice box (larynx), is often injected with a local anesthetic. For burning pain in the leg, nerves on the side of the spine (the *lumbar sympathetic ganglia*) can be injected relatively safely under X-ray guidance. Pelvic pain is treated by a relatively new procedure, also performed with X-ray guidance, in which an injection near the tailbone (*superior hypogastric plexus*) is used.

Neurosurgery

With few exceptions, the many complex neurosurgical procedures developed to manage pain have all but been abandoned. Their decline is due in part to high risks, but also to the undesirability of a prolonged recovery from surgery as well as a shortage of specialists.

But when pain is on one side of the body, below the trunk or waist, one procedure that cuts a specific part of the spinal cord to interrupt pain transmission is very useful. In trained hands, it is a relatively simple, safe, and effective procedure, which does not require a prolonged recovery period. In its original form, still occasionally practiced, *open cordotomy* involves major back surgery. The modern procedure is much less invasive; called a *percutaneous* (through the skin) *cordotomy,* it actually resembles a nerve block because a heated needle is placed in a very specific part of the upper spinal cord, where a small spot is burned to interrupt pain. Other forms of neurosurgery are occasionally performed and are mentioned under "Miscellaneous Techniques" later in this chapter.

INTRASPINAL OPIOID THERAPY: ANALGESICS DELIVERED DIRECTLY TO THE SPINAL CORD

This is a new and promising way to relieve pain that has gained popularity because of its high rate of success and relative safety. However, like other "high-tech" approaches, it demands more of patients and their families than treatment with simple oral medications, and so it is reserved for times when these medications don't provide enough relief or cause unpleasant side effects. Many terms are used to describe a similar type of procedure, among them *epidural morphine, intrathecal* or *subarachnoid morphine,* and *spinal implants* or *spinal pumps.*

The Basic Theory: Drug Receptors

As described earlier, morphine is an important painkiller and can be taken either orally, rectally, or directly into a vein or under the skin. In all of these cases, relatively large amounts of morphine must be given so that enough can eventually get to the specific parts of the body where morphine is most effective. Morphine actually works at sites that are called *receptors,* tiny locations on cells primarily in the brain and spinal cord. These receptors can be compared to a "lock" which is only opened or activated by a specific "key," such as morphine and related drugs. Once the receptor is activated or the "door is opened," a complex series of biochemical events occur in the body and pain is relieved.

The main advantage of this type of treatment is that by placing morphine directly where it is most effective, very tiny doses of the drug can bring dramatic relief; the doses are usually so low that very few, if any, side effects ever occur. Patients that may require doses of 100 to 1,000 mg of morphine when they take it by mouth may get the same or better relief with doses of only 1 to 10 mg given near the spinal cord.

Delivering the Drug: Pumps, Implants, and Catheters

The main disadvantage of treatment with spinal opioids is that for consistent, reliable pain relief, the drug must be given continually over time. This usually involves minor surgery to implant a *tiny catheter,* or drug delivery tube, which is placed with its tip near the spine, either outside the sac that holds the spinal cord and its surrounding fluid (in the *epidural space*) or in a location where the medication can mix directly in the spinal fluid (in the *intrathecal* or *subarachnoid space*). A key advantage to treatment with intraspinal morphine is that before having surgery for the placement of a permanent catheter (*implant*), a temporary catheter can be taped to the back for a trial period to determine whether treatment is effective. When placed by a skilled anesthesiologist, the insertion of a temporary catheter is relatively painless and takes only a few minutes. The temporary catheter is usually only used for several days or weeks before placing a permanent catheter. But when a patient is very sick, a temporary catheter can be used for longer periods.

The catheter is only one part of the system that is needed to give intra-spinal morphine. The drug must also be administered through the catheter.

Years ago, patients or their family members were taught how to inject morphine through ports in the catheter in a sterile fashion. This is still an acceptable way of treatment, is relatively simple and inexpensive, but requires a great deal from family members.

Using Pumps Outside the Body

Now that home-care nursing has become more available, rented or purchased portable pumps are usually used (and paid for by most insurers). The simplest device is called an *external pump*—usually battery powered and about the same size as a Sony Walkman. A home-care nurse usually supervises its use and teaches patients and families how to use it, and how to change its batteries and morphine cassettes. For this kind of treatment, a nurse should always be available to handle technical problems, and a doctor should provide backup in case the dose needs to be changed or problems occur.

Using Pumps Inside the Body

An even newer and more sophisticated way of administering drugs to the spine involves actually placing a small pump (about the size of a hockey puck) under the skin of the patient's abdomen during surgery, a procedure much like that used to insert a pacemaker. This device is refilled with morphine every 1 to 2 months, and the drug dose is adjusted in the doctor's office with a laptop computer. One important advantage is that patients are freed from cumbersome equipment and can more readily go about a normal life. Unfortunately, such pumps can cost up to $10,000 and cannot be reused, so doctors are very selective about which patients should receive them.

Regardless of the system that is used, one end of the catheter goes into the epidural or subarachnoid space to deliver the morphine near the spinal receptors. The other end is either left protruding from the patient's abdomen (*externalized catheter*) or, in the computerized system, it is attached to the implanted pump under the skin. Alternatively, it may be connected to a *port*, a small plastic dome the size of a silver dollar, placed under the skin. A portable infusion pump is then either attached to the external catheter or to a tiny needle placed through the port.

Problems and Alternatives

No medical procedure is entirely risk free. Although uncommon, implanted catheters can become plugged, may kink, or may even break. Infection is also a concern, and although it too is unusual, it is a real problem because if an infection spreads near the spine, a serious illness called *meningitis* may result, and hospitalization would be usually required. As with drugs taken by mouth, tolerance to spinal morphine may develop, requiring higher doses. If pain becomes difficult to control, other medications can be administered near the spine. These range from strong opioids, like *fentanyl* (Sublimaze) and *sufentanil* (Sufenta), to weak solutions of anesthetics, like *bupivacaine* (Marcaine). Strong anesthetics are usually not used because they may produce weakness in the legs and bladder, but often a weak solution will produce just enough mild numbness to relieve even severe pain. Newer drugs, like clonidine, a medication used for high blood pressure, are currently being tested to provide relief for pains resistant to treatment. One of the advantages of intraspinal opioid treatment is that, unlike nerve blocks, treatment is reversible (no nerves are destroyed) and can be adjusted as needed.

ELECTRICAL STIMULATION AND THE GATE CONTROL THEORY OF PAIN

The commonly accepted *gate control theory of pain* was suggested by pain specialists Drs. Ronald Melzack and Patrick Wall to explain why certain types of mild electrical shocks can relieve certain pains. They proposed that if many, many nonpainful messages are sent to the spine, there might be enough of a "traffic jam" to block out the painful messages. An example is a burned hand or a finger banged by a hammer; sometimes, the pain is lessened if the hand or finger is held under cold water or sucked on—the nonpainful stimulus closes the "pain gates" in the spinal cord. The use of the cream Zostrix (see Chapter 8) and skin stimulation (vibration, massage, and hot and cold packs; see Chapter 12) are other examples.

In practice, three types of electrical stimulation have been used with some success, although they are not often recommended for cancer pain.

TENS (Transcutaneous Electrical Nerve Stimulation)

TENS uses a mild electrical current on the skin to reduce or eliminate the feeling of pain. Like acupuncture, it may work by triggering the body's natural chemical painkillers, but studies have shown that it may have longer lasting effects than acupuncture. Commonly used for low back pain, it can be used for cancer pain, although it is often not strong enough to block severe pain.

A small battery-powered box, about the size of a beeper, is connected with wires to patches (like EKG stickers) that are placed on the skin of the area that hurts. When the TENS unit is on, a gentle tingling or buzzing sensation is felt that, in about half of patients, may interfere with the pain sensation.

The patient can adjust the unit with its many controls, much like the volume and tone knobs of a portable stereo. The advantages of TENS are that it is extremely safe, has almost no side effects, is portable, easy to use, and can usually be leased inexpensively (it is also covered by most insurers). TENS is usually not effective for severe pain, however, and often, the pain relief wears off, usually within three months. For this reason, many units come with a thirty-day trial.

Spinal Cord Stimulation

This is a more costly and complicated treatment that involves hospitalization and minor surgery to place an electrode near the spine in the epidural space. The electrode is attached to an implanted battery pack (like for a pacemaker). This treatment is mostly used for low back pain, and even then is controversial because most systems cost more than $10,000. It is not very effective for cancer pain.

Brain Stimulation

Though still considered experimental, brain stimulation (also called *deep brain stimulation* and *thalamic stimulation*) has been used for cancer pain, and may be one of tomorrow's answers for the few pains that cannot be treated with standard methods. By activating the brain's opioid receptors, deep brain stimulation seems to release more of the body's natural painkillers (*endogenous opioids* or *endorphins*). Stimulation of the *thalamus*, one of the brain's relay centers, is currently being investigated for help with certain nerve pains, like shingles and phantom-limb pain. Under local anesthesia, a small electrode is guided to the correct spot in the brain through a small hole drilled in the skull; it is then attached to a battery pack. Brain stimulation is performed by neurosurgeons specializing in the procedure and only in a few medical centers. It also may not be covered by insurance.

MISCELLANEOUS TECHNIQUES

Other than cordotomy, most neurosurgical operations for pain are performed only rarely; however, a few specialists have been able to achieve very good results. These kinds of procedures include *neurectomy* (which involves cutting nerves), *myelotomy* or *commissurotomy* (which involves making an incision in the spinal cord to sever certain nerves), and many others that are even more technical.

Pituitary Ablation

This procedure is performed in only a few medical centers, but it can be very helpful for a relatively few patients with many different areas of bone pain, especially when pain is due to breast or prostate cancer. Patients are given a light general anesthetic and a needle is carefully inserted through the nose into the pituitary gland, where, under X-ray guidance, a few drops of alcohol are injected.

Psychosurgery: A Defunct Method

Years ago, severe pain was treated with techniques under a general category called *psychosurgery*. Prefrontal lobotomy, the most well-known example, was also used to treat mental illness before successful drugs were available. These operations "cut the wires" responsible for giving meaning to the sensations, so that, if asked, patients still admitted to having pain, but they were not bothered by it and no longer considered it distressing or unpleasant. Unfortunately, most psychosurgery also results in irreversible personality changes, as depicted so horribly in *One Flew Over the Cuckoo's Nest*. As a result, these procedures have mostly been abandoned. Some more minor, modified procedures (*cingulotomy*) still are occasionally used and have some popularity, probably because personality changes are so rare.

In the next chapter, we'll begin to look at how other problems, such as side effects of treatments and other discomforts, can be relieved.

Part III

OTHER APPROACHES AND CONCERNS

To Cure Sometimes
To Relieve Often
To Comfort Always

—Robert G. Twycross and Sylvia A. Lack

10

Dealing with Constipation, Diarrhea, Nausea, and Vomiting

Pain is not the only factor that can take its toll on a patient's quality of life. Side effects from radiation, surgery, chemotherapy, and other medications, as well as other ailments resulting from cancer, can be the cause of significant discomfort. Just as cancer pain can be well controlled when treated aggressively, many of these other symptoms, such as nausea, vomiting, diarrhea, and constipation, can also be effectively managed.

Just as with pain, families shouldn't ever assume that these other unpleasant symptoms are inevitable and must be put up with. It's rare that a doctor will say, "I give up, there is nothing I can do." Time-tested remedies are available for many of these symptoms, as are new treatments for persistent problems. Effective treatment, may be simple or may be complex—cooperation and communication between the patient and doctor are as important for these symptoms as they are for adequate pain control. To ensure a cancer patient an optimal quality of life, the same attention that is required to control pain must be marshalled to manage other symptoms and discomforts as well.

MOST SIDE EFFECTS CAN BE TREATED

Cancer has been described as a multi-symptomatic disease. In other words, cancer can produce a tremendous variety of problems; though if recognized and treated, many can be brought under control. Problems may arise from substances the cancer produces, from the cancer pressing on normal structures, or from organ failure. Symptoms may also result from the treatment of the cancer—chemotherapy, radiotherapy, and analgesics. A person may suffer from problems that are caused indirectly by the cancer, such as those related to depression or being confined to bed for a long period. Finally, problems may arise that are completely unrelated to the cancer or its treatment. Some of the symptoms that can occur with cancer are listed in Table 10.1, along with their estimated frequency. The frequency of the symptoms vary widely among the four studies from which these data were obtained; for example, one study found that 9 percent of those with advanced cancer

Table 10.1. *Symptoms in Patients with*
Advanced Disease

Common Symptoms
   (*occurring in more than half of patients*)
Pain
Weight loss
Lack of appetite (anorexia)
Constipation
Weakness
Nausea/vomiting
Depression

Less Common Symptoms
   (*occurring in less than half of patients*)
Difficulty breathing (dyspnea)
Coughing
Swelling
Insomnia
Urinary problems
Difficulty swallowing (dysphagia)
Bed sores (debutitus ulcer)
Bleeding (hemorrhage)
Drowsiness
Diarrhea

Occurs More Rarely
   (*occurring in less than 10 percent of patients*)
Paralysis
Jaundice
Colostomy
Dry skin (pruritus)
Mouth sores

had difficulty breathing, while another found that 50 percent did. These symptoms can vary greatly.

It goes almost without saying that if the doctor is not aware of distressing symptoms that are plaguing the patient, he or she cannot help. That is why it is essential that the doctor be informed of any problem that arises, particularly if it is unusual, no matter how small. *Do not assume that these symptoms cannot be controlled.*

Remedies for some of the common symptoms of cancer—especially nausea, vomiting, and constipation—have been well known for years, and most doctors will have recommendations readily available to treat them. Even symptoms that persist or used to be thought of as untreatable are now undergoing extensive research with many promising results. For example, difficult symptoms like weight loss, fatigue, and shortness of breath have responded well to new treatments. Some of these approaches are so new that it is difficult for all doctors to keep up with every recent development; if something in this chapter may be helpful for a loved one, share the information with your doctor. Most of these symptoms can be treated effectively by your family doctor or oncologist. If the condition persists despite aggressive treatment, the doctor may consult with a pain or palliative care specialist (for example, through the service for doctors called the Pain Management Information Center; see the Appendix), or may choose to refer the patient to a specialist.

CONSTIPATION

As Cicely Saunders, one of the first proponents of palliative care, has said, nothing matters more than the bowels when it comes to helping a person who is ill with cancer. Constipation is exceedingly common among cancer patients because many of the drugs used to treat cancer or cancer-related symptoms (including opioids, anticonvulsants, antidepressants, tranquilizers, muscle relaxants, and chemotherapy agents, such as vincristine [Oncovin] and vinblastine [Velban]) can contribute to constipation. Constipation may also be triggered by lengthy stays in bed with no exercise, by tumors in the gastrointestinal region, by changes in the diet, such as reduced food and liquid intake, by low fiber or low vegetable and fruit intake, by dehydration from fever and vomiting, and by anxiety and depression. Patients who are too weak, have difficulty breathing, or are suffering from paralysis or leg weakness—all may have problems with constipation as well.

Sometimes, constipation causes pain that patients do not suspect as being the result of constipation, because the pain can be perceived as being as high up as in the ribs. If allowed to get too bad, constipation can be extremely serious, even life threatening. Patients should not feel embarrassed or ashamed to bring up problems with bowel movements. Nor should they assume that a doctor's help is not needed just because many of the medicines can be bought without a prescription.

Maintain Patient's Own Schedule of Regularity

Probably because it involves a very private bodily function, constipation and bowel habit are not generally discussed fully enough and, as a result, bowel problems may go undertreated. Because many laxatives are available over-the-counter (o.t.c. or without prescription), patients are often left on their own to seek a remedy. This should be highly discouraged—it is important to put embarrassment aside and consult the doctor on how to manage constipation.

One of the problems with regulating bowel habit is that each of us defines regularity differently. Some individuals feel constipated if they do not have a bowel movement daily, while others are accustomed to waiting several days or even a week between normal bowel movements. Treatment should try to reestablish an individual's regular bowel habit as much as possible. Most authorities feel that a bowel movement at least every three days is an appropriate guideline.

Finally, it is most important to discuss constipation with the doctor because:

- If treated before it gets too bad (in other words, prophylactically), constipation can almost always be managed effectively.
- If allowed to become severe, constipation can produce extremely serious health problems, sometimes bad enough to require hospitalization and even surgery.

Be Sure to Get a Recommendation for a Laxative

As with most conditions, prevention is always preferable to having to deal with chronic constipation. Since many of the drugs administered by the doctor, especially the opioids, can produce constipation, each time an opioid is prescribed, it should be accompanied by a recommendation for a laxative. Tolerance to these constipating effects occurs only slowly, if at all, and treatment with laxatives usually is required for as long as these medications are taken. Likewise, as the dose of opioid is increased, the dose or strength of the laxative should be increased as well. Just as more than one type of painkiller may be needed, it is not unusual for more than one type of laxative to be needed.

Fecal Impaction

If constipation persists despite treatment, the doctor will check for a condition called *fecal impaction* by performing a rectal examination. This is occasionally overlooked, because such an examination—even though brief and relatively painless can be unpleasant. In fecal impaction, a small piece, or pieces, of dried stool becomes hard and lodges itself in the rectum, usually near the anus, blocking the passage of other wastes. This is dangerous if unrecognized, because if increasingly strong laxatives are given, they may produce severe cramps and even a rupture or perforation of the bowel. Another reason that fecal obstruction is sometimes missed is that liquid stool (produced by laxatives) may leak around the impaction, giving the illusion of diarrhea.

Treating Fecal Impaction

One way to treat this condition once it has become established is for the doctor or caregiver to place a gloved finger through the anus into the rectum and remove the hardened stool manually. This is painful and may require anesthesia or a sedative. Sometimes, fecal impactions occur higher in the colon and can be relieved with enemas. When combined with enemas (especially with mineral oil) and laxatives, the impaction can usually be relieved, and with continued treatment with laxatives, repeated episodes can often be avoided.

Practical Strategies to Prevent Constipation

- Drink eight to ten glasses of liquids a day. Fruit juice or warm tea upon awakening is often suggested. Prunes (stewed preferably) or warmed prune juice twice a day (morning and evening) can help produce more regular bowel movements.
- Try eating high-fiber foods including bran, fresh raw fruits and vegetables, prunes, dates, whole-grain cereal products (whole wheat bread, grains such as brown rice, barley, couscous, etc.), nuts, corn, raisins, and coconut.
- Avoid foods such as cheese and highly refined grain products, such as cookies, cakes, donuts, and crackers.
- Exercise as much as possible, even if just regular walking, to stimulate intestinal activity.
- Keep a chart of bowel movements; they should occur around every two days. If the patient does not have a bowel movement within three days in spite of stool softeners and stimulant purgatives, a rectal suppository or stronger laxative is usually recommended to prevent severe episodes of constipation and fecal impaction.
- Encourage the patient to defecate as soon as he or she has the urge; a commode close by can often help. A squatting position is ideal for the patient, if possible. A toilet seat may be adapted with a plastic ring, which is often used on toilets for the handicapped, to make the seat higher, but patients will probably need a footstool to support their feet so they can bear down. Bedpans should be avoided as much as possible, since they are difficult to use for defecating; if necessary, however, try to help the patient maintain a crouched position on it, with the feet bearing down on the mattress or over the side of the bed onto a chair or table (avoid leaving the feet dangling).

Medical Management of Constipation

Starting with a Laxative

As stated before, as soon as persons start taking opioid medications, they should also start taking some action to prevent constipation. Although a stool softener (which keeps stools soft by retaining water) is useful, if constipation is already present, a stool softener alone is probably not adequate. These medications produce a soft stool, but it may still be difficult to evacuate, especially if fluid intake is low. That is why most doctors recommend starting treatment with a stool softener and mild stimulant laxative (which enhances bowel activity) combined.

Common softeners include methylcellulose, psyllium (Metamucil), and natural fibers, such as bran. If using Metamucil, drinking eight to ten glasses of liquid a day is very important. Common mild stimulant laxatives include Doxidan, cascara sagrada, senna—a natural product which is available alone (Senokot) or combined with a softener (Senokot-S), bisacodyl (Dulcolax), and docusate (Colace). *Note:* Avoid laxatives with magnesium in patients with kidney disease and laxatives with sodium in patients with heart disease.

These medications are usually taken once in the morning and once in the evening, in increasing doses as needed, to produce a bowel movement of appropriate consistency at regular intervals. (For example, one tablet of laxative will usually counter the constipating effects of 60 mg of codeine or 30 mg of oral morphine; if on 60 mg oral morphine, then 2 tablets may be needed; higher doses of morphine will often require higher doses of laxatives.) Many patients prefer to use laxative medications that they have taken in the past because they have worked well; that's fine, as long as your doctor knows.

Treatment should proceed on what doctors often call a "sliding scale" basis. This means starting with regular (around-the-clock) treatment with a laxative that is strong enough to produce bowel movements regularly. If two to three days have passed without activity, patients should then take a stronger medication; if constipation still persists, their medication should be increased. Other laxatives such as lactulose, magnesium hydroxide (Milk of Magnesia), and especially magnesium citrate may be used as needed. Mineral oil can be used occasionally, but not in patients who are very sick and possibly prone to breathing and swallowing problems (aspiration). A variety of enemas are available, but regular use of enemas should be avoided.

DIARRHEA

Diarrhea is relatively uncommon in cancer patients and may actually result from the overzealous use of laxatives. The presence of diarrhea may require the physician to perform a brief manual rectal examination to be certain there is not a blockage around which liquid stool is leaking. Diarrhea may occur in conjunction with chemotherapy or with radiation treatments to the abdomen or pelvis; and it may persist for up to several weeks after such treatments. Diarrhea also can be caused by anxiety and stress, lactose intolerance (when the body can't digest milk products), and certain dietary supplements.

Practical Strategies

- Eat low-fat and low-fiber foods, such as cottage cheese and other low-fat cheeses, eggs that aren't fried, natural yogurt, broth, baked, broiled, or roasted fish, poultry or ground beef, rice pudding, custard, tapioca made with low-fat milk, gelatin, hot cooked cereals, bananas, applesauce, apples without skins, apple or grape juice, white bread or toast, white crackers, white pasta or rice, potatoes, cooked vegetables such as green beans, carrots, peas, spinach, or squash, or soups from these vegetables. Many nurses and the American Cancer Society suggest using nutmeg as much as possible because it is believed to help slow down the gastrointestinal tract.
- Foods to avoid: all those mentioned above to help constipation, fried or greasy foods, raw fruits and vegetables, pastries, potato chips, pretzels, strong spices (chili powder, licorice, pepper, curry, garlic, horseradish), olives, pickles, gas-producing foods such as beans, broccoli, onions, and cabbage, caffeine-containing drinks, alcoholic drinks, and tobacco products.
- If the patient with diarrhea is fatigued as well, it may be a sign of low potassium. High-potassium foods such as potatoes, bananas, green beans, halibut, and asparagus tips should be eaten or potassium supplements taken. Those with kidney problems should be especially concerned with eating adequate high-potassium foods.
- To prevent dehydration during episodes of diarrhea, at least eight to ten glasses of liquids should be taken daily, especially fruit juice, bouillon or broth, weak warm tea, gelatin, and flat caffeine-free sodas (those in which the carbonation has been allowed to escape).
- If significant weight loss is associated with the diarrhea, or if adequate fluid intake cannot be maintained, contact the doctor at once.
- Eat small but frequent meals, and stick to liquid foods if diarrhea is severe. Extremely hot or cold foods may aggravate the condition, so consume foods that are of moderate or room temperature.

Medications

- For milder cases, over-the-counter medications such as Kaopectate or Pepto-Bismol can help.
- For more severe cases, when diarrhea lasts longer than two or three

days, the doctor may prescribe Lomotil or paregoric. As already mentioned, all of the opioid analgesics work to slow bowel function and should help reverse diarrhea. Discuss this with the doctor if relevant.

Making the Patient More Comfortable

Frequent diarrhea can irritate the bottom. To soothe it:

- Clean up after each bowel movement with warm water, rinse well, and pat the area dry with a soft towel. Don't rub.
- Creams for the anal area that can help soothe irritation include Desitin or Proctodon.
- If very sensitive, a topical local anesthetic prescribed by the doctor or a corticosteroid spray or cream may be applied.
- Warm baths or sitz baths may be soothing to the region.
- Allow the area to be exposed to air. If the patient has difficulty controlling the liquid stool, a disposable brief or pad (such as Depends, which is made for incontinent adults) can be helpful.
- Lay a disposable, plastic-lined bed sheet under the patient.

NAUSEA AND VOMITING

Although many patients may never experience nausea or vomiting, those that do can be miserable. And unfortunately, nausea and vomiting are relatively common—either as occasional problems associated with chemotherapy sessions (usually during administration or within hours afterward) or as a chronic problem. Nausea and vomiting most commonly occur together, but may occur separately. Since the causes and management of both symptoms are usually similar, most of the comments made here about nausea can also be applied to vomiting, and vice versa, unless specifically stated otherwise.

Causes of Nausea and Vomiting

Chronic nausea and vomiting may result from many factors. They may be triggered by tumors partially or even completely obstructing or blocking the gastrointestinal tract, in which case, swelling of the abdomen (distension) may or may not be present. They may be caused by radiation injury to the bowel, scarring (adhesions) from surgery, and even by simple constipation.

Injury to the kidneys or liver can reduce the purifying functions of these organs, and nausea may result from a buildup of the body's toxic waste products. Nausea may be caused by a tumor in the brain, either one that starts there (primary tumor) or has spread from elsewhere (metastatic tumor). Metabolic imbalances—changes in the body's fluid and salt (electrolyte) content—are common causes of nausea as well, especially when there is an excess of calcium, which is particularly common in patients with bone cancer. Nausea can be caused or worsened by mouth problems—such as infection, sores, or tumor growth.

Nausea is also a potential side effect of many medications, including those used to treat pain. The NSAIDs can irritate the stomach lining and produce ulcerlike symptoms, including nausea and vomiting. All of the opioids, including morphine, have the potential to produce nausea and vomiting that are usually transient. In fact, up to one-third of patients will experience nausea after first starting to take an opioid medication, as well as after its dose has been increased. Such nausea can usually be effectively treated with a simple anti-emetic (see later in this chapter), and since it rarely lasts for more than a few days, treatment with the anti-emetic can, in most cases, be tapered and then discontinued with continued use of the opioid.

The fact that the body usually becomes rapidly tolerant to the nausea induced by the opioids (so that treatment with the anti-emetics can usually be tapered off) is a relatively new finding; it doesn't hurt to check with the doctor about whether an anti-nausea medicine needs to be used continually or just for a short time. The opioids, as well as the antidepressants, can cause constipation, as we've said, which also must be managed to minimize the risk of nausea.

Finally, nausea may be psychological in origin (which is not to say that it is less severe or significant or any less real). Doctors have recognized a specific nausea of this type, which they call "anticipatory nausea and vomiting." It usually occurs in patients who have had nausea after chemotherapy, who then go on to become nauseated at the next session, even before treatment is started. This reflex may be so strong that simply driving by the hospital, or seeing one's nurse at the supermarket, can trigger an episode of nausea and vomiting.

Practical Strategies to Counter Nausea and Vomiting

- Encourage the patient to eat plain crackers (Saltines, for example) or to sip on warm, flat cola soda or ginger ale when feeling nauseated.
- Switch, at least temporarily, to a clear liquid diet including foods such as apple juice, cranberry juice, broth, ginger ale, gelatin, tea, Gatorade, frozen fruit pops, cola or lemon-lime drinks, etc.
- If the patient has no mouth sores, sometimes sour foods such as lem-

ons, pickles, or sour hard candy can help ward off nausea. Rinsing with a dilute lemon-water solution may also help.

- Foods to avoid: sugary, high-fat, highly salted, greasy, or spicy foods, or those with strong odors, such as cheese or salami.
- Foods usually well tolerated: bland foods, such as toast, potatoes, applesauce, crackers, and cottage cheese. Eat slowly.
- Avoid smells or sounds that could trigger nausea, such as cooking smells and perfumed body scents.
- When in chemotherapy, some relaxation exercises (see Chapter 12) before the treatment may help. During chemotherapy, sucking on hard or sour candies or mints may counter the distasteful metallic flavor that some patients taste during sessions. If nausea consistently occurs, try switching appointments to a different time of day.
- Experiment with different eating patterns. Some patients do better when they don't eat or drink for several hours before chemotherapy; others do best when they eat heavily three or four hours before a session and then continue throughout the day with light meals or snacks. Others prevent nausea by switching to a liquid diet for the day before and after the chemotherapy session. Still others prevent nausea by eating only light but frequent meals throughout the day. Some doctors recommend avoiding favorite foods on days the patient may become nauseated so the patient will continue enjoying their favorite foods.
- Get plenty of fresh, cool air, either through an open window or with a fan.
- Use the relaxation, distraction, imagery, and breathing techniques described in Chapter 12. Acupressure or acupuncture may also help.
- Other distractions may help, too, such as watching a movie or television, doing a craft, talking with a friend.
- Try to sleep after chemotherapy, when nausea may be expected.
- If the patient vomits, keep a log of the time, amount of vomit, and what it looked like (color, consistency) to report to the doctor or health-care team. Avoid eating solids until vomiting spells pass; sometimes that might be up to 24 hours. Rinse the mouth after each episode with dilute lemon water. Afterward, try sucking ice chips or eating one of the liquids already mentioned as part of the clear liquid diet.

Medical Management of Nausea and Vomiting

Medications, known as *anti-emetics*, can help most people. When nausea and vomiting are the result of chemotherapy, the anti-emetic should be taken 6 to 12 hours before the next chemotherapy session to avoid anticipatory nausea. The doctor will recommend that medication be continued every 4 or 6 hours for at least 12 to 24 hours, or longer if any nausea persists. Since many chemotherapy drugs have the potential to produce nausea, patients are often treated in advance of any problems with a combination of anti-emetics, many of which are given intravenously. Even so, nausea and vomiting may still occur and may occasionally be severe enough to require hospital admission.

Choosing an anti-emetic can be difficult. Nausea may be triggered by several different mechanisms, and since the anti-emetic drugs work by different mechanisms, a trial-and-error approach using different drugs is usually taken. The first medication selected to treat mild nausea, including chemotherapy-induced nausea, most often comes from the group of drugs known as the major tranquilizers. These drugs are usually tried first because they are effective in most cases, can be given orally, are relatively inexpensive, and are unlikely to cause serious side effects. These medications include prochlorperazine (Compazine), trimethobenzamide (Tigan), thiethylperazine (Torecan, Norzine), haloperidol (Haldol), and droperidol (Inapsine which has no oral form), among others. They are usually prescribed in tablet form, but are available as rectal suppositories (and even injections) if the nausea is accompanied by such severe vomiting that oral medications cannot be kept down. Again, they are usually prescribed every 4 to 6 hours, and when nausea is persistent, they should be taken regularly for a period of time, and then tapered off. The main side effect of these medications is drowsiness. Rarely, they trigger a side effect that produces sudden involuntary movements (called extrapyramidal signs) which can be frightening but are not harmful. Extrapyramidal signs are more common in younger individuals and, fortunately, can usually be easily reversed with diphenhydramine (Benadryl).

The medications mentioned so far are the ones used most commonly. If they are not effective, however, the treatment takes a new strategy. If one of the major tranquilizers has been only partially effective, a medication that works by an alternative mechanism can be added, or the old medication can be stopped and a new one started. Although treatment with the major tranquilizers is sufficient in most patients, sometimes several different medications must be tried, often together.

Metoclopramide (Reglan) is frequently used as a "second-line" drug. It has dual effects, working both in the brain (on receptors for dopamine, a neurotransmitter) as well as in the periphery to increase the speed that the stomach empties food. Because of this stomach action, it may be particularly effective in cases when the stomach is slow to empty, because of lack of activity or pressure from a tumor nearby in the abdomen. Some preliminary evidence suggests that metoclopramide also has some pain-relieving effects.

Scopolamine (Transderm Scop, Transdermal Therapeutic System) is another second-line drug that is usually administered in the form of a patch, which after a short time is effective for about 72 hours. Used primarily to treat vertigo and nausea from motion sickness, it may be especially effective for the patient whose nausea worsens when she gets up and moves around and the room seems to spin. Treatment with scopolamine may also produce some degree of drowsiness.

The corticosteroids such as prednisone (Deltasone, Sterapred), prednisolone (Prednisolone, Prelone), and dexamethasone (Decadron, Hexadrol) are used as second- or third-line drugs. Although it is not well understood how they work, they can be extremely effective and may have other beneficial effects as well, such as temporarily improving appetite and mood, and alleviating some types of pain. Over time, they may produce serious side effects, especially when used chronically—over a period of months to years, but they are generally well tolerated for days, weeks, and even months.

Tetrahydrocannabinol (THC), the active ingredient of marijuana, can be an effective second- or third-line drug for both acute nausea due to chemotherapy and chronic nausea. Marijuana itself is not legally available for medical use, but THC can be prescribed in pill form (as dronabinol or Marinol), and doses that are usually sufficient to relieve nausea do not produce a "high." Grogginess or dysphoria (an unpleasant mental state) may, however, occasionally occur, and can usually be managed by reducing the dose. Treatment with dronabinol may also improve appetite.

A new drug, odansetron (Zofran), has been shown to be very effective (helping 60 to 80 percent of patients) in blocking nausea due to chemotherapy and radiotherapy, and is being studied in chronic nausea with promising preliminary results. It seems to work by reducing blood levels of serotonin, another neurotransmitter, and its effectiveness has paved the way for research on other drugs with a similar action.

Another common anti-nausea (or anti-emetic) medication is lorazepam (Ativan), which is used primarily as an anti-anxiety medication. When given intravenously with chemotherapy, it may erase the memory of a vomiting episode. Occasionally, a defoaming agent, usually available over-the-counter (o.t.c. or without prescription), such as simethacone (Mylanta, Riopan Plus, Digestol Tablets, Extra Strength Maalox Plus), is useful to relieve gas pains.

Severe Vomiting Due to Obstruction or Pressure on the Digestive Tract

After swallowing, food is transported along the digestive tract, where it is processed and eventually eliminated as waste. It goes from the mouth to the esophagus (swallowing tube), stomach, small intestine (jejunum and ileum), large intestine (colon), and out from the rectum. When the digestive tube is blocked at any of these points, problems may occur. These kinds of problems may arise with any tumor that grows within the abdomen, especially esophageal and gastric (stomach) cancer, colon and liver cancer, as well as any primary tumor that has metastasized (spread) to the abdomen. Compression from the outside of these organs (somewhat like the blockage that occurs when you step on a garden hose) can result from tumors or adhesions (scars) that stem from previous surgery or radiation treatment.

The symptoms of obstruction depend on whether the blockage is *partial* or *complete,* and whether it is *persistent* or *intermittent* (steady or comes-and-goes). Depending on these factors, there may be loss of appetite, swelling of the abdomen, pain, intermittent or persistent nausea, retching, and vomiting.

Ideally, an obstructing tumor would be shrunk with chemotherapy or radiotherapy, or treated surgically either by removal or a bypass (colostomy). Regrettably, this is often either not possible or advisable, and so in many cases, only symptomatic or palliative treatment can be used.

If the blockage is severe and persists, dehydration and malnutrition follow over time, and patients may become weak. These factors go hand-in-hand with the progressive weakness and failure that is associated with advanced cancer. It is obviously hard to "sit by and watch" while a friend or relative appears to be starving before one's eyes. When intestinal blockage cannot be relieved with surgery, there are two things a doctor can do. The traditional and most common method used by doctors in the United States is to hospitalize the patient and to insert a plastic tube through the nose and into the stomach (nasogastric tube) to drain its contents; at the same time, fluids are given continuously through an intravenous line. This method is costly, uncomfortable to the patient and, because it requires hospitalization, inconvenient.

An alternate method of treatment, practiced quite extensively in the United Kingdom and sometimes in the United States, takes a very different approach and usually allows the patient to stay at home, at least for a while. Anti-emetic medications, which have already been described, are administered very vigorously, often subcutaneously by a portable pump—a method that is much more convenient and comfortable than maintaining an intravenous line. In this manner, nausea can usually be controlled, often for a period of months (if needed), and sometimes the blockage opens a bit, and even vomiting may cease. Patients are allowed to eat what they wish, although most prefer to restrict their intake to liquids only. When a blockage is severe, even though nausea is controlled, patients may continue to vomit, but usually only once or perhaps twice daily. While this sounds unpleasant, patients generally do not mind the occasional episode of vomiting, once the nausea is controlled.

Occasionally, when nausea and vomiting cannot be well controlled with these methods, and patients are otherwise relatively well, a minor surgical procedure called a *venting gastrostomy* is recommended. It involves placing a short plastic tube from the stomach to a small bag that collects its contents; this relieves the pressure and eliminates the need to vomit. This is different from a feeding gastrostomy, which administers nutrition through a feeding tube. Decisions concerning whether a patient would benefit from a feeding tube depend on the nature and stage of the disease. (See Chapters 11 and 15 on nutrition in advanced stages of cancer.)

11
Dealing with Other Side Effects and Discomforts

Patients with cancer, even the same cancer, can have very different experiences, some of them more distressing than others. Many families will find over time that the status of their ill loved one will unexpectedly change. Families frequently feel unprepared and caught off guard about how to help when what feels like an emergency occurs (sudden nausea, difficulty breathing, coughing spells, etc.). Caregivers should not be alarmed that there are so many different symptoms described here; it is unlikely that a given patient will experience many of them. And even when they are experienced, their intensity, frequency, and duration vary greatly among patients.*

BREATHING PROBLEMS

Difficulty breathing is generally referred to as *dyspnea* and may include a variety of altered patterns of breathing. *Hyperventilation* refers to rapid breathing (sometimes also called *tachypnea* or *hyperpnea*). Breathing too fast is a normal response to illness and stress, but is an inefficient form of breathing. When one breathes too fast, there is no time to take a deep breath. Most of these shallow breaths go only in and out of the mouth and throat, without enough getting to the lungs where the actual exchange of oxygen and carbon dioxide occurs—a vicious cycle that only makes the breathlessness worse.

Apnea refers to an absence of breathing, and it is fairly common for brief periods of apnea, lasting from a few seconds to half a minute (periodic breathing), to occur in patients who are weak and very ill. While this can be a sign that the end of life is approaching, this condition can persist, on and off, for days or weeks.

*Many of the practical suggestions offered in this chapter have been adapted from the excellent American Cancer Society booklet, *Coping with Problems Related to Cancer and Cancer Treatment* (1987) by Joyce M. Yasko, R.N., Ph.D., and Patricia Greene, R.N., M.S.N.

Causes of Breathing Problems

Difficulty breathing may arise from many factors and is a symptom that should be followed carefully by a doctor. The most common cause is a tumor growing in the lung, either one which has started there (primary tumor) or has spread from another site (metastatic tumor). If this is the case, breathing problems can often be reduced, at least temporarily, with radiotherapy or chemotherapy.

Sometimes the tumor causes fluid to build up around the lung (pleural effusion) or heart (pericardial effusion). These conditions can usually be detected by a doctor's examination and X-rays. Breathing and fatigue will often improve dramatically when the fluid is removed from around the lung with a needle, a relatively simple procedure called *thoracentesis*. Because fluid usually builds up again, often quite rapidly, thoracentesis is often followed by a *pleurodesis*, a somewhat more complex procedure that involves injecting an irritating substance between the lung's linings (pleura) so they will stick together, which usually prevents fluid from reaccumulating. Pleurodesis usually requires the placement of a chest tube between the ribs to initially drain the fluid and a few days in the hospital. A similar procedure, a *pericardiocentesis*, removes fluid from around the heart to improve breathing and circulation.

A more indirect cause of breathing difficulties is the presence of fluid or a large tumor in the abdomen which compromises the downward movement of the diaphragm, our main breathing muscle. This type of breathing difficulty is more difficult to treat.

Pneumonia is another treatable cause of breathing difficulties, and is usually signaled by the presence of fever, weakness, and productive cough. Once the type of pneumonia has been identified by blood tests or sputum (mucus that is coughed up), unless the patient is very run down, symptoms usually improve with antibiotics, taken by mouth (at home) or, for more severe cases, intravenously (in the hospital).

Breathing difficulties may not be directly related to cancer—they may be due either entirely to problems that predate the cancer, or to basic problems that are worsened. These are more common in smokers and include diseases like chronic obstructive pulmonary disease (C.O.P.D.), emphysema, bronchitis, and asthma. Even when made worse by cancer, they can still be treated with some success using standard measures.

The functions of the heart and lungs are very closely related, and heart failure, from a variety of sources, may produce breathing difficulties. The most common is pulmonary edema, a condition involving fluid buildup in the lungs (rather than around them) because of the heart's diminished strength. It is usually treated with diuretics (pills that remove fluid), which increase the volume of urine, and various heart medications, including digitalis.

Pulmonary embolus, a condition in which the lungs' blood supply is blocked by a blood clot, can cause sudden and severe breathing difficulties. Patients with poor circulation due to spending a great deal of time in bed are at greatest risk. Wearing special support stockings and encouraging regular movement of the legs can sometimes prevent this condition. Medical treatment of pulmonary embolus usually involves prescribing blood thinners, either heparin or coumadin.

Finally, psychological causes are a part of most breathing difficulties. Feeling breathless can be terrifying, and frequently patients panic, causing them to breathe all the more rapidly and inefficiently. An important part of managing breathing problems is to offer reassurance and to try to eliminate the element of panic. Comforting the patient and instructing the patient to practice relaxation techniques can be very beneficial; in some cases, as we'll see, anti-anxiety medications can also help a great deal.

Practical Strategies

Although patients with lung cancer most commonly experience trouble with breathing, other patients too may experience trouble breathing as the cancer progresses. Specific techniques not only help keep the lungs clear, but also promote circulation, since the blood carries oxygen to the lungs.

- Breathing properly can help shortness of breath. If possible, inhale through the nose from the stomach, not the chest—the abdomen should enlarge when you inhale. Exhale about twice as slowly as you inhale, and breathe out through pursed lips, as if you are blowing out a candle.
- When short of breath, be sure the head and chest are elevated on pillows if in bed. When possible, sit up and lean shoulders forward, with arms either spread out on either side, or leaning forward on a support, such as a table. If sitting up, feet supports are more helpful than allowing feet to dangle from the bed or chair. While in bed, patients should frequently change sides to keep lungs clear.
- When possible, improve circulation by standing, or even walking. Take it slowly if it is difficult to breathe.
- Patients should not stay in any one position too long because this will inhibit circulation. When sitting, they should try not to cross their legs. Special pressure stockings can be worn to prevent blood clots, especially if the patient is on steroids.
- Keeping a patient moving, even if bedridden, can be helpful. Nurses often help patients do a range of motion exercises with the arms and

legs, and families may, if they wish, ask the nurses how best to help with the exercises.

- If possible, the patient should drink as much as ten glasses of water a day to help mucus membranes clear lung secretions.
- Ask a nurse, physical therapist, or respiratory therapist about proper coughing techniques to clear the lungs. One technique involves breathing deeply twice, and on the third breath, bracing the feet on the floor or other support to hold for three seconds. While braced, cough as deeply as possible, three times.
- Keep air moist with a vaporizer (cold water), humidifier, tea kettle, or even pans of water near a heat source.
- Since breathlessness can be severely aggravated by anxiety, patients may be trained and coached in relaxation techniques, as described in Chapter 12. These exercises include:

  - Progressive muscle relaxation in which every muscle in the body is tensed, one at a time, and then relaxed. The patient learns how to recognize the state of tension, as experienced by the muscles, and to compare it with the state of relaxation.
  - Meditation in which the patient closes her eyes and listens to her own slow and steady breathing, all the while thinking of a calming word, such as "calm," "relax," or "peace."
  - Autogenic techniques which involve a person thinking about how heavy, warm, or relaxed her body and body parts are, working on one part at a time. The goal is to induce relaxation through these thoughts.
  - Imagery and visualization which involve the patient imagining he is somewhere that calms him—on a sailboat in the Caribbean, on a beach, in the forest. The person imagines all the details of the spot, using imagery in his mind and trying to visualize what it would be like to be there.

Medications for Breathing Difficulties

- Although needed in only a few cases, oxygen therapy involves keeping an oxygen tank handy or even in continual use, if needed. Despite its relatively high cost, which is not always reimbursed by insurance, simply having oxygen available often has a reassuring, psychological value that can be quite important. Be certain that no one smokes, lights a match, or even has a pilot light going nearby because any of these could trigger an explosion of the tank. Be sure the tubes are untwisted at all times.
- Opioids have a variety of complex effects on breathing, which are beneficial overall in the cancer patient. Because opioids slow breathing,

doctors are cautious about prescribing morphine to patients with both breathing and pain problems. There is a growing positive experience with the use of opioids, in low doses, specifically to ease distress and breathing problems in cancer patients. They reduce the sensitivity of the brain's breathing center, while also relieving the sensation, pain, and anxiety of having trouble breathing. The overall result is that the distress is lessened and patients are able to take slower, deeper breaths.

- The anxiety related to dyspnea, which aggravates the condition, is also sometimes treated with tranquilizers such as diazepam (Valium); these medications can reduce anxiety and are muscle relaxants as well.
- Other medications which may help, depending on the cause of the problem, include steroids, bronchodilators, antibiotics, diuretics (which help expel extra fluid), heart medications, and blood thinners.
- When a patient is very sick and near death, they may not be strong enough to cough up accumulated secretions in the back of the throat. The drug scopolamine (administered by injection or patch, which is marketed as Transderm Scop; hyoscine is used in the United Kingdom) may be used to dry up these secretions, and may have the effect of sedating the patient as well.

COUGHING

Coughing occurs in about 30 percent of patients with advanced cancer and in about 80 percent of patients with cancers involving the lung or bronchial tubes. It may also be caused by irritation to the lower throat or lungs or from factors unrelated to cancer, such as a postnasal drip, asthma, cigarette use, or heart failure. Some simple measures can help alleviate coughing:

- Keep air moist with a vaporizer or humidifier.
- Avoid lying directly on the back, since this position makes coughing difficult.
- If cigarettes seem to be part of the cause, realize that if the decision is made to give up smoking, it will still take two to four weeks for coughing to gradually diminish. Families and patients need to consider how much gratification is obtained from the cigarettes, how difficult it would be to quit, and whether the attempt is worth it.

Medications for Problems with Coughing

- If the patient has difficulty coughing up secretions that make him nauseated or cause vomiting, a medication can be given by mouth to help break up the secretion.

- Although over-the-counter cough medicines are sometimes effective, if coughing persists, or is disturbing, painful, or dry, the doctor may recommend a medication containing codeine or a related compound. When the patient has a tumor involving the lung area, which is responsible for the coughing, an opioid such as hydrocodone or morphine may be needed.
- Corticosteroids may also be prescribed for persistent coughs.

MOUTH OR THROAT SORES

Chemotherapy, radiation, reduced intake of liquids or food, altered hygiene, and infection can all contribute to mouth sores or inflammation in the mouth. The sores may be like canker sores or they can be open ulcers, both of which may bleed or get infected. They may make eating painful and difficult, but are often overlooked.

The need for mouth care may present an opportunity, rather than be viewed as just a problem, according to some authorities. Sometimes, when patients are very sick, loving caregivers feel frustrated that they cannot do more to help. Learning the basics of mouth care and applying them regularly can be an excellent way for family members or other caregivers to spend time with the patient in a loving, meaningful, and helpful way.

The best strategy for these conditions, known as *stomatitis* and *mucositis*, is prevention. Simple daily routines should be undertaken twice a day, or even every 4 hours if the patient is undergoing chemotherapy treatments. Physicians more accustomed to managing acute medical problems may forget to advise how to prevent mouth problems, and an oncology nurse may be a valuable resource in providing instructions.

Mouth Hygiene to Prevent Problems

- Brush the teeth with a soft nylon bristle toothbrush only. To soften the bristles even more, use hot water on the bristles before and after use. If toothpaste is irritating, try a paste composed of baking soda and water. If brushing hurts too much, clean teeth with cotton swabs or commercial sponge-tipped sticks called Toothettes.
- Floss with unwaxed dental floss; avoid flossing if there are bleeding problems or if platelet count is low. Using a Water-Pik can help keep the mouth clean, too.
- A mouthwash should be used as often as every 2 hours, such as one composed of half-strength hydrogen peroxide (one part 3 percent hydrogen peroxide to one part water) or baking soda. Avoid lemon, glycerin (which will make the mouth drier), or commercial mouthwashes

containing alcohol (alcohol is a common ingredient in these and may irritate or dry the mouth). A very effective commercial preparation is a chlorhexidine mouthrinse.

- Keep dentures clean and only use them if they fit properly; if they don't fit, they may injure the mouth during eating. If weight loss has occurred, dentures may need to be refitted.
- Keep gums stimulated by encouraging the patient to chew foods or by gently rubbing a finger over the gums.
- If patient is on long-term chemotherapy, ask about using a fluoride preparation on the teeth to prevent cavity formation, which is common during chemotherapy.
- Radiation therapy in the region of the mouth greatly increases the risk of dental cavities. To prevent them, frequent fluoride applications are often recommended—consult with the doctor or a dentist. Avoid sugary foods. To avoid complications later, many physicians and dentists will recommend pulling high-risk teeth before radiation is administered.

When the Mouth Is Irritated

- Keep lips moist with vaseline, cocoa butter, or other water-based lubricant.
- Avoid hot, cold, acidic, rough, or salty foods. These may include spicy foods, vinegar, citrus foods, toast, and pretzels, crackers, and other snacks.
- Avoid alcoholic drinks and tobacco products.
- Rinse frequently with mouthwash, as described above. Do not floss. If brushing is too painful, teeth and gums should be wiped regularly with moist paper towels or cotton.
- Warm tea or a paste made from an antacid such as Maalox, diluted Milk of Magnesia, Mylanta, or Gelusic may help healing; place antacid into a warm liquid, and once settled, pour off excess liquid and apply the paste with a cotton-tipped stick or gauze. Rinse 15 minutes later with water.
- Offer a high-protein, high-calorie diet served at room temperature.
- If pain is severe, mouthwashes should be used every two hours, but brushing and flossing may be discontinued.

Medications for Mouth and Throat Sores

- When irritated, mouth sores can be treated with a topical anesthetic, such as lidocaine, Xylocaine, or Hurricaine, to reduce the pain and promote healing; these are effective not only for mouth sores but for sores in the throat too (some sprays are available).

- To reduce pain, Benadryl liquid or lozenges may help.
- When mouth infections (usually yeast infections such as candidosis or thrush) occur, mouth rinses with hydrogen peroxide and a saline or sterile water solution, with the addition of flavored nystatin (an antifungal medication), or an antifungal pill may be prescribed by the doctor. The nystatin should be applied four times a day to each side of the mouth, kept there three minutes, and then swallowed.
- The doctor may prescribe another antifungal medication (such as ketoconazole) for certain infections.
- Expect medications to take several days to become initially beneficial and about two weeks to be fully effective.

DRY MOUTH

Radiation to the head and neck area can cause dry mouth, known as *xerostomia*. The reduction of saliva production may last from six months to a year and, in some cases, may be a permanent side effect of radiation therapy. But the most common cause of dry mouth in cancer patients is from the side effects of certain medications, especially tricyclic antidepressants, antihistamines, opioids (narcotics), some chemotherapeutic agents, and major tranquilizers (phenothiazines). Reviewing the medication list with the doctor may make it possible to delete problematic medications and substitute others. Dry mouth can also be caused by a tumor near the salivary glands, mouth infections, and tobacco and alcohol use. Sometimes, a patient's general dehydration, lack of eating, or breathing through the mouth can cause dry mouth as well.

Dry mouth causes food to taste differently and sometimes contributes to loss of appetite. This condition can cause the patient a number of problems: it may make it more difficult to digest starches, promote mouth irritation and sores, inhibit taste, make it difficult to chew solid foods, promote cavities and mouth infections, and can even make it difficult to form words.

Practical Strategies

- Avoid spicy, very hot, or very cold foods, citrus products, and carbonated beverages, as well as foods hard to chew. Serve foods well-moistened with gravies, sauces, or mayonnaise.
- As much water or other liquids that aren't irritating should be consumed as possible—at least several times an hour. Small frequent sips of water and rinsing the mouth with cold water also helps.

- Keep a thermos or pitcher near the patient with a straw or spout, if necessary.
- Keep lips lightly lubricated with lip balm, cocoa butter, Vaseline, or similar product.
- Sucking on smooth and sour hard candies, lozenges, popsicles, and pineapple chunks as well as chewing gum may also help promote saliva production.
- Keep something in the mouth, such as a pipe or lollypop.
- Keep air humid with a vaporizer (cold water), humidifier, tea kettle, or pans of water near a heat source.
- Maintain mouth hygiene as described above (see under mouth and throat sores). That means brushing the mouth with a soft toothbrush after eating anything. Every two hours, a mouthwash should be used, such as one that produces an effervescent wash: a mixture of one part Cepacol, one part saline solution, and one part hydrogen peroxide (3 percent solution); or glycerine and citric acid washes, which may help stimulate salivation. Ask the doctor or oncology nurse for a recommendation.

Medication for Dry Mouth

When dry mouth is severe, artificial saliva products such as Moistir or Mouthkot are available by prescription.

DROOLING

Tumors in the mouth can cause excessive drooling (*sialorrhea*), which may be upsetting to the patient and family. There are few practical measures, other than wiping the mouth as necessary.

Medication the Doctor May Recommend

- Atropine drops can provide temporary relief; for longer term relief, atropine tablets can be used, although they can cause dry mouth and, occasionally, irritability.
- The antidepressant amitryptyline (Elavil) can work for some patients. The anti-emetic, Transderm Scop, can also dry secretions.
- When very troublesome in selected circumstances, radiotherapy can be used to modify salivary gland function.

DIFFICULTY SWALLOWING

Chemotherapy and radiation may interfere with the function of the esophagus (swallowing tube), which can make it difficult to swallow (*dysphagia*). Tumor growth into muscles or nerves involving the pharynx (the area around and including the esophagus) may also be a cause of this condition.

Practical Strategies

- Avoid tobacco and alcoholic drinks, as well as spicy, acidic, hot or cold, hard, crunchy, or coarse foods.
- Serve a high-protein but well-balanced diet.
- Use milk and dairy products, such as yogurt, sour cream, or cottage cheese, to coat the throat.
- Keep foods well-moistened with liquids, gravies, sauces, etc.
- Keep bites small; when severe, foods may be mixed in a blender or food processor and served as a "shake."

Medications for Handling Difficulties in Swallowing

- If swallowing is painful, liquid aspirin or acetaminophen may be helpful, as well as anesthetics applied directly in the mouth. For more severe pain, other non-steroidal anti-inflammatory medications in liquid form or morphine can be used.
- If tumors are involved, corticosteroids (such as dexamethasone) can temporarily shrink a tumor and improve swallowing. In some cases, radiation may also be able to shrink the tumor.
- If cancer in the esophagus is involved, and radiotherapy doesn't help, a feeding tube may be considered.

PROBLEMS WITH TASTE

Cancer can alter taste perceptions in a variety of ways, a problem that affects about half of all cancer patients, regardless of the type of cancer they have. Doctors believe several causes may contribute to the problem. The taste buds themselves may lose their sensitivity because of chemicals produced by the cancer or poor dental hygiene may lead to loss of taste. Usually, food tastes bland or tastes slightly "off," having a metallic or medicinal flavor, or has no taste at all. Some people find they either want no sweets or want more sweets; many lose their desire for meat and bitter foods.

When taste problems occur, an extra effort should be made to prevent or treat sores and dry mouth (see preceding sections on Mouth and Throat Sores and Dry Mouth).

Practical Strategies

- Brush teeth often; use a mouth rinse such as a mixture of water and baking soda.
- Assuming the patient doesn't experience nausea, the aroma of foods cooking may stimulate the desire for food.
- Flavoring food with mild spices such as salt, vanilla, cinnamon, or lemon may enhance flavors.
- When all foods taste bitter, good selections may include white meat, eggs, and dairy products. Some suggest adding honey, Nutrasweet, or sweet fruits to foods that taste bitter. Adding beer or wine to soups, marinades, sauces, and seasonings may also help. Marinate meats and fish; use strong seasonings; and avoid hot foods—wait until they are room temperature or even cold.
- Unpleasant aftertastes can be masked with mints, chewing gum, or mildly sweet or pleasant desserts.
- Tart food may be enjoyed more, such as pickles or foods flavored with lemon or vinegar.
- Try starchy foods such as potatoes, rice, pasta, and bread without any butter or margarine.

LOSS OF APPETITE

Cancer patients may lose their desire to eat *(anorexia)* either temporarily or chronically at various stages of the disease; it may, in fact, be one of the first symptoms of cancer, and is also common in advanced cancer. Foods may taste different; have metallic or medicinal "off" flavors, or be downright unappealing. It is often disorienting to patients when they find that foods they have enjoyed for a lifetime no longer hold much pleasure, and that they can suddenly tolerate foods they never cared for. They should be reassured that this is a common side effect of cancer and its treatment, and patients should be encouraged to experiment with different foods.

Failure to eat is one of the most distressing aspects of cancer for patients and their families. The degree of concern that this symptom should raise depends very much on the specific case, the prognosis, and stage of the disease.

Practical Strategies

When a patient has a chance for a cure, or is in the early or middle stages of cancer, aggressive methods to counter malnutrition should be undertaken. These may include:

- Providing small but frequent meals.
- Selecting favorite foods of the patient.
- Offering a milkshake-like dietary supplement if solid food can't be taken. Ask the physician to recommend one of the highly nutritious food supplements available as "shakes." They may range from common products like Carnation Instant Breakfast to others usually recommended by doctors (for example, Ensure). Patients frequently find these most palatable when served chilled over ice; the manufacturer may also be able to provide information on how to prepare these foods in interesting ways.

Medication for Loss of Appetite

Preliminary research suggests that treatment with medications may stimulate appetite, with a relatively low risk of serious side effects.

- Corticosteroids (dexamethasone, prednisone) administered in relatively high doses may be successful for a short time. The administration of high doses of megestrol (Megace), a hormone, may be effective for longer periods with fewer side effects. Taken at night, the antidepressant amitriptyline or the tranquilizer chlorpromazine may boost appetite and general attitude as well.
- The active ingredient in marijuana, THC, currently only legally available in pill form as dronabinol (Marinol), may also be effective in some patients.
- In some cases, aggressive treatment that includes tube feeding (gastrostomy) or intravenous feeding (total parenteral hyperalimentation) will be recommended. These methods, however, are appropriate in only a small proportion of cases.

Lack of Appetite in Advanced Stages of Cancer

When patients do not have a good chance of long survival and are in the advanced stages of cancer, lack of appetite is relatively common. Yet, patients and families may not admit to themselves that the patient's prognosis is poor. Doctors often find it difficult to discuss a poor prognosis, either because they do not have specific training in discussing such difficult topics with patients, because they are not comfortable admitting that some cancers are beyond cure, or because they simply do not want to upset their patients. But, even experts in palliative and hospice care cannot always predict life expectancy with certainty, and so many experts will be hesitant about conveying that death is imminent. Finally, patients and their families are often naturally reluctant to receive unpleasant news and may discourage doctors from engaging in such conversation.

Nevertheless, patients with progressive cancer commonly lose their appetite and families often feel helpless when this occurs. Many families equate preparing and offering food with providing love. Some view their central role or job as providing food and feeding the patient; when the patient won't eat, they feel like failures. Families in this situation should not be discouraged: they are witnessing an unavoidable but natural part of the disease process. Patients with advanced cancer usually don't want to eat and may try to do so simply to make their families feel better. Most experts concur, however, that dehydration and missed meals are not particularly uncomfortable for a very ill person with cancer. Forcing the person to eat or drink may not help them and can make the very ill patient feel even more uncomfortable. Although it may be difficult to witness a loved one lose their appetite, it is unkind to pressure patients to eat when they are unable to do so. It is a challenge for the family to find more direct, verbal ways to show that they care.

LOSS OF WEIGHT

Many cancer patients will lose weight and, over time, may appear emaciated. Weight loss can be caused by a variety of factors, such as loss of appetite, diarrhea, vomiting, hemorrhaging, ulcers, poor absorption in the gastrointestinal tract, a failing metabolic or digestive system, and even the chemical by-products of a tumor.

Patients who lose a great deal of weight (a condition known as *cachexia*) may look ill, feel weak, look pale, and feel full when they have only eaten a little. Their changed appearance can cause distress, fear, and feelings of being isolated as friends and family members note the marked change in appearance. Clothes will no longer fit well; dentures may become loose and may not only cause problems with eating but can be painful.

Unfortunately, cachexia is common and can't be avoided or treated in many cases. Although the medications mentioned under the section "Loss of Appetite" can be tried, attention should really be focused on relieving the social implications associated with the changed appearance, dealing with more practical matters, such as obtaining clothing that fits better, and using coping strategies to ward off depression and other potential psychological problems. Dentures may be refit (even at bedside) and can help the patient chew and look better. Caring for the skin and mouth is important during this time, as described in this chapter (under Skin Problems).

Do not force foods aggressively. The person will have a fickle appetite and will feel full with a small amount of food.

FATIGUE AND WEAKNESS

For a variety of reasons, cancer patients often suffer from fatigue. Fatigue is said to be "multifactorial," meaning that it is usually caused by many factors. As a result, it is often difficult to determine which is the main culprit. Reasons for fatigue include side effects of chemotherapy or radiotherapy, poor nutrition, infection, the effects of chemicals made by the tumors, the effects of other medications used by the patient, liver or kidney failure, imbalance of the body's salts and electrolytes (calcium, potassium, and sodium), depression, fever, and anemia. Even so, the doctor may recommend some simple tests to find correctable causes. Although medications prescribed to treat pain may contribute to fatigue, reducing them to heighten alertness does not usually make sense, because patients will suffer more from untreated pain, and they will become tired out from "fighting the pain."

Practical Strategies

Sometimes, fatigue or weakness will be a temporary side effect of treatment. To help relieve it during treatments:

- Be sure the patient rests often. She should stay relaxed, and go to bed earlier and sleep later.
- Try to maintain a normal routine, but slow it down a bit for the patient. Step it up gradually.
- Encourage the patient to keep drinking plenty of liquids—ideally, eight to ten glasses a day.
- Offer the patient foods that are complex carbohydrates (rice, beans, grains, vegetables) which provide more energy than highly processed foods or sweets.
- Encourage the patient to accept help with simple chores they can't easily do, such as cooking and cleaning.
- In more advanced stages of the disease, weakness and fatigue can be expected, and distraction, such as conversation, music, television, and so on, will continue to bring pleasure to the patient who is weak.

- A careful regimen of fresh air, exercise, and physical therapy may be helpful for some patients. However, these remedies are situation-specific ones: rest instead of exercise may be the best thing for many patients who are weak.
- When fatigue is a sign of depression (see Chapter 14), it will sometimes get better when the depression lifts. Simple measures are often sufficient—such as conversation, companionship, reassurance, hugs, and encouragement with small activities. When depression persists, professional counseling or treatment with one of the antidepressants should be considered. Patients need to be reassured that depression is common in patients with cancer. If the fatigue is attributed to a major depression, then antidepressants may help.
- If pain or anxiety is preventing normal sleep, it should be treated aggressively (see Chapter 12).
- Ensuring that sleep and rest are maintained is a key factor in minimizing fatigue. Pay attention to the "sleep-wake" cycle, which often gets reversed in ill patients. It is very common that, for one reason or another, patients are unable to sleep well at night. As a result they are drowsy during the day, nap at odd times, and then are even less likely to sleep well at night, perpetuating a vicious cycle that is hard to reverse. If this seems to be occurring, minimize or eliminate daytime sleeping so that patients are more tired at night, and talk to the doctor about adding either a nighttime sleeping pill or daytime stimulant.
- Consider renting a hospital bed, a bedside commode, wheelchair, ramps, raised toilet seat, walker, and stool for the bath or shower. These simple measures will help conserve the patient's strength.

Medications and Other Treatments for Fatigue

- Review the patient's medication list with the doctor periodically. Sometimes patients continue to take medications that are no longer essential which, if eliminated, may give them more strength.
- Blood tests may indicate an abnormality, such as anemia, potassium that is too low, or calcium that is too high. A transfusion or other treatment may be recommended. Keep in mind that not all abnormalities should be treated—for example, a blood transfusion does not make sense if it will only correct the problem for a few days, or is unlikely to promote well-being.
- To boost a sense of well-being, prednisolone is very commonly used for patients with advanced cancer and usually helps them feel stronger and hungrier.
- The stimulants, methylphenidate and dextroamphetamine, may be use-

ful to reduce sleepiness and fatigue, especially when they are caused in part by the treatment of pain with the opioids.

HAIR LOSS

Hair loss, known as *alopecia,* is a fairly common side effect of chemotherapy or radiation to the scalp. Severity may range from hair thinning to complete loss of hair. Strangely, when hair grows back, it may be softer, thicker, or of a different texture than before. Sometimes, grey hair that falls out is replaced with hair of the patient's original color. Occasionally, patients may also lose hair in other area of the body, such as from the eyebrows, arms, groin, and so on.

Although much less disturbing to the body's functioning than nausea or other side effects, patients arc often devastated psychologically by hair loss because it is often such an integral part of the patient's body image.

To minimize hair loss and protect new hair that's growing in:

- Though unproven, some patients wear an "ice turban" or keep cold compresses on the head during chemotherapy treatments to inhibit the drugs from reaching the hair follicles.
- Before treatments, cut hair into a manageable style that won't require a lot of brushing or combing.
- Use mild products on the head, and keep shampooing to a minimum. Pat hair to dry.
- Avoid hair dryers, curling irons, clips, elastic bands, hair spray, and all other hair products, including brushes and combs.
- Satin pillowcases may help prevent hair tangles.
- If hair loss is expected, choose a wig before treatment. Synthetic wigs are more comfortable and less expensive that real-hair wigs.
- Consider obtaining a wig through the American Cancer Society, the hospital, or support groups. Check with insurance about reimbursement.
- Use a hat, scarf, or turban if hair loss has occurred. A hairnet at home can help contain hair and minimize shedding.
- In summer, keep head covered to avoid sunburn; in winter, keep head covered to prevent heat loss.

BLEEDING EPISODES

While it is relatively rare, bleeding can be a side effect of chemotherapy or radiation, may be a result of the cancer itself, may be the result of an allergic reaction to some medications (especially quinidine, quinine, digitalis, sulfonamides, or thiazides), or may even be caused by stress and anxiety. Bleeding may occur directly on the skin, or may emanate from the mouth, nose, groin, or elsewhere.

To Prevent Bleeding, Be Sure the Patient

- Avoids activities that might be too physically strenuous which may cause even minor trauma.
- Avoids hand razors, cuticle scissors, tight-fitting clothes that could irritate the skin, tourniquets, and aspirin.
- Avoids strenuous activities, such as lifting, bending over from the waist, or pushing during a bowel movement.
- Drinks plenty of liquids to keep mucous membranes moist.
- Follows hygienic precautions listed under the section Mouth and Throat Sores, earlier in this chapter, to avoid mouth bleeding.
- Keeps stools soft and avoids using anything in the rectum (thermometers, enemas) to avoid bleeding from the anus.
- If on steroids, takes an antacid or milk with the medication to prevent irritating the stomach. Women may want to use a lubricant before sexual intercourse to prevent friction and bleeding; they should avoid douches and vaginal suppositories.
- Blows nose very gently through both nostrils and keeps air humid with a vaporizer or humidifier to avoid bleeding from the lungs or nose.

If Bleeding Occurs

- Apply pressure to the area for five to ten minutes, and if a limb is involved, elevate it. Call the doctor if bleeding continues for more than five minutes.
- If nose bleeds (*epistaxis*) occur, squeeze nostrils gently shut below bridge of the nose; tilt head forward to prevent blood from backing up. If it persists, place an ice pack on the bridge of the nose. Contact the doctor if bleeding doesn't stop after five minutes.

SEXUAL PROBLEMS

In many ways, cancer interferes with sexuality—the patient may be tired, nauseated, anxious, or fearful; he or she may lose sexual desire or be unable to function normally. Cancer reminds us of our mortality and vulnerability. Just the psychological impact of being diagnosed with cancer, let alone the body changes that might occur, can affect our body image and make us feel less sexy and less lovable. Couples need to communicate during this stressful time about their needs, fears, and anxieties. When intercourse is not possible, physical intimacy (hugging, holding, caressing) can go a long way in keeping the couple close. Sexual partners may be fearful to initiate intimacy out of concern that they will hurt their mate. This concern can easily be overcome with communication.

During chemotherapy, women are more prone to bleed heavily during their periods, and many doctors advise that women of child-bearing age take birth control pills to stop menstruation during this time. During radiation of the genital area, women may be advised to have regular intercourse or even to use a "dildo"-like device to retain the vagina's natural shape. If these matters are not discussed, patients and their families should make a special effort to discuss them with a nurse or doctor.

SKIN PROBLEMS

Itching and Dry Skin

Chemicals from the tumor, side effects of treatment, dehydration, and even anxiety or boredom may cause or aggravate dry, itchy skin, a condition known as *pruritus*. To relieve it, patients may:

- Use water-based moisturizers and avoid oil-based ones. Use these moisturizers after bathing and every night.
- Drink plenty of fluids (eight to ten glasses a day).
- Protect skin from wind, heat, hot sun, and cold.
- Avoid hot baths and soap. Soothing bath solutions include cornstarch, baking soda, Aveeno, or soybean powder. Pat the skin dry rather than rubbing it.
- Keep cool wet packs on the itchy area for 20-minute intervals.
- Don't exercise excessively.
- Keep clothes loose and light; avoid heavy fabrics such as wool and corduroy.
- Avoid scratching by using ice packs, by practicing distraction or another relaxation technique (see Chapter 12), or by applying a vibrator or extra pressure to the area. Cut nails if necessary and encourage rubbing instead of scratching.
- For dry patchy areas, try placing a wet cloth over the area for 15 minutes and then apply cream before allowing it to dry.

Medications for Dry, Itchy Skin

Physicians may prescribe an antihistamine if the patient feels itchy all over; for local patches of itching, a corticosteroid cream or local anesthetic may be used. Small doses of naloxone can relieve itching when it is severe and is due to treatment with a narcotic.

Tumors That Break Through the Skin

Tumors that ulcerate, or break through the skin, are distressing for any patient and family, and although not very common, such sores can be unpleasant, devastating a patient's body image and escalating a sense of helplessness. Such tumors may also leak fluid.

Caring for these problems requires plenty of support from health-care professionals, such as a visiting nurse. Wounds should be kept dry and cleaned twice a day. Certain creams should be used to clean and dress the wound. To control any odor, special charcoal dressings may used; an effective home remedy is yogurt gently spread over the wound. When such a tumor constantly bleeds, the wound can be dressed in gauze that has been lined with a gelatin sponge material. Protect the surrounding area with petroleum jelly or zinc oxide. An air freshener may also help minimize the odor. When a large wound is involved and massive bleeding is feared, an entire blood vessel can be closed with minor surgery.

Medications for Problem Tumors

When a tumor has an odor, an infection is probably involved and should be treated. Antibiotic treatment often helps reduce pain.

The antibiotic clindamycin or the antibacterial medication metronidazole (Protostat) can be effective. Metronidazole can cause nausea and nerve damage and is dangerous if taken with alcohol; clindamycin can severely irritate the gastrointestinal tract. Powdered and cream preparations of metronidazole, however, hold promise for topical treatment and are now available.

URINATION PROBLEMS

The urinary tract is particularly sensitive in the cancer patient; problems such as burning during urination or feeling the urge to urinate often are fairly common. Symptoms of an infection include dark urine, fever or chills, and low back pain.

When a bladder infection is diagnosed:

- Try to get the patient to drink up to three quarts of fluid a day, avoiding coffee, tea, and other caffeine products, as well as alcoholic beverages.
- Avoid foods that could be irritating to the bladder lining, such as alcohol, coffee, tea, and spicy foods.

- Vitamin C or large quantities of cranberry juice (up to three quarts) may help acidify the urine.

When too much uric acid (hyperuricemia) is the problem after some chemotherapies:

- Drink at least three quarts of fluid a day, but avoiding tea and wine, which are high in substances known as purines.
- Avoid lentils, dried beans, liver, sardines, or anchovies which can make the condition worse.

Other guidelines:

- When incontinence (leakage) is a problem, sometimes a medication to increase the sensation of having to urinate (an anticholinergic drug) or a catheter may be used.
- Urinary retention, an uncommon side effect of opioids and a few other drugs, is most common in elderly men. Tolerance to the drug often eventually develops. If it is not particularly uncomfortable or severe, it may be left untreated.
- Occasionally, the outflow of urine becomes completely blocked, either due to medications, swelling, or pressure from a tumor. This is usually accompanied by swelling of the lower abdomen, feelings of pressure, and discomfort. If simple measures to help the urine flow do not work, the doctor should be informed, or if he is unavailable, the patient may need to go to an emergency room to have a catheter passed to empty the bladder. Usually, bladder catheterization is not uncomfortable, especially for women.
- A catheter is often left in place when patients chronically leak urine or are bedridden and do not have the strength to get to the bathroom. The use of a catheter may increase the risk of a bladder infection, but can make life much easier for patients who are fatigued by frequent trips to the bathroom.

SLEEPING PROBLEMS

If the patient can't sleep, try to determine whether it's because of pain, anxiety, night sweats, fear of urinating, or other reasons. To help monitor a sleep problem, try to keep track of how long it takes for the patient to fall asleep, how long he sleeps, how many times he wakes up, why he wakes up, and how rested he feels afterward. Counseling and certain medications may treat the insomnia if anxiety or fear is its cause (See Chapter 14). If night sweats persist, a suppository of a non-steroidal anti-inflammatory drug, such as indomethacin, often helps.

Practical Strategies

- If anxiety is the root of the problem, any of the relaxation and distraction exercises in Chapter 12 (breathing, progressive muscle relaxation, music therapy, guided imagery) can be used to soothe patients, allowing them to more easily drift off to sleep.
- Opioids used for pain will help induce sleep; families should not be overly concerned if the patient seems oversedated at the beginning of an opioid regimen. Most patients build a tolerance to the opioids within a week or two (see Chapter 7 on morphine and the other strong opioids).
- A soothing back rub or massage can often reduce anxiety and relax the person, helping him to fall asleep.
- Pay attention to whether the "sleep-wake" cycle has gotten reversed. It is very common that, for one reason or another, patients are unable to sleep well at night. They then become drowsy during the day, nap at odd times, and then are even less likely to sleep well at night, perpetuating a vicious cycle that is hard to interrupt. If this seems to be occurring, minimize or eliminate daytime sleeping so that patients are more tired at night, and talk to the doctor about adding either a nighttime sleeping pill or a daytime stimulant.

Medications for Sleeping Problems

- Traditional sleeping pills (such as Dalmane, Halcion, Amitol, Nembutal, and Seconal) are commonly prescribed but may be habit forming or cause daytime drowsiness. Tricyclic antidepressants may be used to treat insomnia in cancer patients because they help induce sleep and enhance the pain-relieving effects of opioids. However, they should not be taken as needed; instead, they are usually prescribed to be taken regularly so that they can help relieve pain as well.

CONFUSION AND DELIRIUM

Many conditions can trigger confusion in the cancer patient. Unlike delirium, a confused patient will from time to time be mixed up, but behavior remains normal. The patient is not agitated, and even if she occasionally hallucinates or seems to be "losing" her mind, she becomes aware of these episodes. If this condition becomes more profound or the patient becomes agitated, then the patient may be described as delirious. Delirium, by definition, is marked by passing episodes of disorganized thinking or incoherence, in which the patient is disoriented as to the time of day and displays impaired attention. Patients with delirium can hurt themselves and often do. Delirium tends to be worse at night.

The terms confusion and delirium represent a continuum, are not sharply defined, and need to be distinguished from dementia, a gradual intellectual decline over months or years. Patients with dementia may be unaware of commonly known facts, but are usually more alert and aware of their surroundings than those with delirium.

Delirium and confusion can stem from infection or the side effects of some drugs, such as diuretics, which help the body rid itself of excess fluids. Confusion may also occur from too much insulin, especially if a patient has suffered great weight loss and persistently shows a lack of appetite. Many medications, including benzodiazepines, narcotics, steroids, and anticholinergic drugs, and even nonprescription drugs like aspirin or antihistimine, if taken often, can trigger confusion. Other causes include poor pain control, lack of sleep, fecal impaction, urinary retention, and brain tumors. In most cases, the cause is a result of the disease and not a form of any kind of mental illness. Families should be prepared, however, for incidents of confusion or delirium because some 85 percent of terminally ill cancer patients will experience such episodes. Almost all patients will experience some degree of confusion or delirium at least intermittently in the last few days of life.

It is important not to panic if patients experience confusion. Most spells pass quickly, but may return. If persistent, the doctor should certainly be consulted. Keep in mind that patients may be very embarrassed by such episodes. They should be reassured that these are normal for patients in their condition.

When possible, drug substitutions can be tried. Those that have much lower risks for delirium as a side effect include sucralfate (Carafate), which can be substituted for cimetidine (Tagamet), and nortriptyline (Pamelor) which can be substituted for amitriptyline (Elavil).

Symptoms and Management of Delirium

Delirium, usually associated with agitation, is a confusional state in which the autonomic nervous system is overactive. Symptoms include flushed face, dilated pupils, sweating, and rapid heartbeat. It may be caused by a physical problem, such as by a tumor which is affecting the central nervous system, organ failure, infection, or other complication. It may also be caused by an indirect effect on the central nervous system which stems from medications (including chemotherapy).

Some 15 to 50 percent of cancer patients that are hospitalized show episodes of delirium. Often just the change of scenery and the absence of familiar surroundings are disorienting. When sudden episodes of agitation, cognitive impairment, change in attention span, or levels of consciousness occur, chances are these changes are from the cancer or side effects rather than a new psychological problem. If there is severe agitation or hallucinations, an antipsychotic medication that helps sedate the patient may be called for. Haloperidol (Haldol) is commonly used because it is sedating and has fewer side effects than other antipsychotic medications. It can be given orally, intravenously, or intramuscularly.

Yet, caring for a confused or delirious patient can be difficult because patients may become unintentionally violent and disruptive. The following strategies may be appropriate for either confusion or delirium.

Practical Strategies

- Frequently reassure the patient, keep familiar objects near him, and speak simply and clearly. Don't be frightened. Acknowledge the abnormal behavior, stressing that it will probably be temporary, is likely to be the result of needed medications, and is harmless. Sometimes it may even be appropriate to joke about it together.
- Keep the patient's room quiet and well lit at night with a nightlight.
- Try not to awaken the patient during the night.

Medications for Delirium

Families and physicians usually prefer to make the patient less restless and aggressive with an antidepressant, haloperidol (Haldol), or the antipsychotic medication chlorpromazine (Thorazine, Promapar) if needed. For more on sedation in patients who are very ill, see Chapter 15.

HICCOUGHS

In cancers affecting the stomach, diaphragm, and sometimes the brain, hiccoughs are not uncommon. They may also be triggered by kidney failure (*uremia*) or infection. Many of us don't realize how exhausting and demoralizing hiccoughs can be when they last a long time.

Practical Strategies

- Hiccoughs can sometimes be managed with simple physical maneuvers like holding the breath or breathing in and out of a paper bag (by boosting the amount of carbon dioxide in the bag).

There are a number of folk remedies, mostly scientifically unproven, but which cannot hurt to try. They include:

- Sipping water from the "wrong" side of a glass.
- Drinking water with two heaping teaspoons of sugar.
- Drinking two glasses of liquor.
- Running a cold key down the back of the person hiccoughing.
- Drinking peppermint water which can relax the sphincter to the swallowing tube, or esophagus, when the hiccoughs are due to pressure on the stomach.

Medications for Hiccoughing

- When the hiccoughs are due to pressure on the stomach and peppermint water doesn't work, an anti-flatulent might (such as Maalox after eating), as might metoclopramide.
- When the hiccough reflex is stimulated (when the tumor presses on the diaphragm), chlorpromazine can sometimes help; possible side effects include drowsiness, lightheadedness, and heart palpitations.
- When hiccoughs are caused by a brain tumor, phenytoin or carbamazepine may help.
- Other medications that are occasionally used to suppress hiccoughs include quinidine, benzonatate, atropine, and methylphenidate.
- If hiccoughs persist despite all these efforts and are troubling to the patient, a phrenic nerve block (see Chapter 9) or surgery to the phrenic nerve may even be considered.

MUSCLE JERKING

No one knows what causes muscle jerking, which can be much like twitching, or why high doses of opioids can have this effect. The movement is not sustained, but sudden and uncontrollable. Muscle jerks may make drinking a cup of water unpredictably difficult but, otherwise, muscle jerks are not particularly bothersome to the patient. Although they may disturb the family members, they should be reassured that these involuntary movements are an expected side effect of the medication and would stop if the medication were stopped. Sometimes, jerking causes pain. If so, the doctor may consider a benzodiazepine or steroid for this side effect, or the pain medication may need to be changed.

MUSCLE CRAMPS

Muscle cramping may be totally unrelated to cancer, or can be a symptom of a systemwide problem such as uremia (a buildup of toxic substances in the blood due to poor kidney function), cirrhosis, or other metabolic conditions. In cancer patients, muscle cramps may also be caused by the tumor exerting pressure on certain nerves, dehydration (from sweating or diarrhea), or be a side effect of medication (such as diuretics), radiation, chemotherapy (when vinca alkaloids or cisplatin are used), hormone therapy (such as those used for breast cancer), or surgery, which may cause nerve damage.

Practical and Medication Strategies

- In cases where the cramping is caused by dehydration or medications that aren't vital, withdrawing suspect drugs, if possible, might help.
- When the culprit medication can't be withdrawn, other medications may help so the patient can more comfortably continue with chemotherapy or hormone therapy. Quinine taken at bedtime can prevent cramps that typically occur during the night. Doses are kept low.
- For bothersome cramping during the day, the anticonvulsants phenytoin (Dilantin) and carbamazepine (Tegretol) are considered most useful and have been well studied. Other substances that have been reported to help cramping, but whose studies have been scant, include diazepam (Valium), dantrolene, procainamide, diphenhydramine, fluoride, riboflavin (vitamin B), vitamin E, verapamil, and nifedipine.

12

Mind-Body Approaches
to Easing Pain

Mind and body are inextricably linked, and their second-by-second inter-
action exerts a profound influence upon health and illness, life and death.
Attitudes, beliefs, and emotional states ranging from love and compassion
to fear and anger can trigger chain reactions that affect blood chemistry,
heart rate, and the activity of every cell and organ system in the body—
from the stomach and gastrointestinal tract to the immune system.

All of that is now indisputable fact.

Kenneth R. Pelletier, Ph.D., M.D.
Stanford Center for Research in Disease Prevention at the
Stanford University School of Medicine

So far, we've been discussing how doctors ease the pain and discomfort of
cancer by drawing from an arsenal of drug therapies and medical treatments. But just focusing on the treatment of the body is neglecting the very
powerful influence the mind has on the body. In recent years, more and
more Western physicians in almost all fields of medicine are recognizing
that the mind and body are not two separate entities, but integral parts of
the whole body system. Physical illness, the immune system, and the mind
are all, in fact, intimately connected, and, as we'll see, many studies are
showing how feelings, thoughts, attitudes, and behavior can all have powerful and pivotal influences on well-being, health, illness, and pain.

Though not a miracle cure, mind-body approaches can help us harness
the power of the mind to better control thoughts and emotions such as
worries, pessimism, negativity, hostility, and depression and to promote
relaxation, hope, control, and optimism. Some evidence even suggests that
such techniques may help arrest or perhaps even reverse the disease process
and promote longevity. Whether these benefits will be substantiated by further research, most doctors nevertheless acknowledge that these techniques
can greatly improve the quality of life for cancer patients and others by
helping them better cope with the fear and anxiety of having cancer and
with the treatments for cancer which may have very unpleasant side effects.
By helping patients improve their spirits, mind-body techniques can go a

long way in reducing the severity and frequency of medical problems, including pain. As we'll see, a growing body of evidence is showing that these mind-body approaches can relieve nausea, for example, a common side effect of chemotherapy, reduce the amount of pain medication that cancer and surgical patients need, and even speed up recovery.

These mind-body techniques include relaxation, meditation, mindfulness, yoga, coping strategies, hypnosis, self-hypnosis, support groups, biofeedback, and music therapy, among others. Most of these alternative therapies were considered totally unconventional and "on the fringe" just 20 years ago. Today, they are becoming more widespread and accepted in hospitals and clinics throughout the country as effective, no-risk strategies that can ease distress, muscle tension, anxiety, depression—all of which can improve quality of life and enhance the medical treatment of pain and other discomforts associated with cancer.

Although none of these techniques are meant to substitute for medical treatment and although none can actually "cure" pain, they can usually help enhance the patient's relief while allowing him to regain some control and mastery over his life.

HOW DISTRESS AGGRAVATES PAIN AND ILLNESS

First, let's look at how the stress of cancer can make pain and illness worse. Obviously, having cancer is enormously stressful. The disease turns a person's life, and the family's, upside down and, in many ways, the individual feels out of control. Stress bombards the cancer patient on all fronts, from worry and anxiety about the disease, its progression, its treatments, potential disabilities and perhaps disfigurements, to concerns about its negative role on the family's emotional, financial, and even physical well-being and anxiety over losing control of one's life and independence. At one time or another, the typical cancer patient is plagued by feelings of despair, depression, hopelessness, and helplessness. And a cancer patient will be fearful about pain and dying. (See Chapter 14 for more about psychological aspects of cancer and cancer pain.)

There is little doubt that emotional distress can lower a person's pain threshold and increase pain. Stress also takes a serious physical toll: many studies have shown that a person's stress causes muscles to tighten up, disturbs appetite and sleep habits, and triggers the production of "stress hormones." These hormones, such as adrenaline and cortisol, increase heart rate, blood pressure, muscle tension, and blood sugar and, over time, can wear down one's pain threshold and weaken the immune response.

Another way that stress may influence health is through the chemistry of the emotions. Researchers have discovered that emotions can influence the production or activity of chemical messengers called neuropeptides which travel through the body and influence the nervous, immune, and endocrine systems. Thoughts and feelings may also influence levels of brain chemicals such as endorphins, the body's natural painkillers that are chemically similar to morphine.

Whatever the exact mechanisms between the brain, nervous system, and immune system, growing evidence is showing their intimate connections. Studies at Ohio State University have shown, for example, that people under stress—those taking important exams, family members caring for loved ones with Alzheimer's disease, and women who have recently endured a difficult divorce—had lower levels of immune-cell activity. Other studies have shown that people who had undergone significant levels of stress were much more likely to become ill. Similarly, studies at Duke University have shown that people with "angry" personalities or those who are easily upset by life's stressors are more prone to heart disease.

Well, if psychological states such as stress and anger can wear down or inhibit the immune system, making one more vulnerable to illness and infection, can the mind work to promote health? The answer appears to be a resounding yes. The evidence that reducing stress, loneliness, and depression and boosting control, relaxation, hope, and optimism may bolster the immune system has been gaining such momentum in recent years that a new medical subspecialty—called *psychoneuroimmunology*—has been born. Psychoneuroimmunology is the study of the relationships among the mind, the brain, and the immune and endocrine (hormonal) systems. Although the evidence is far from conclusive, findings so far have been so provocative that the National Institutes of Health established a new Office of Alternative Medicine in early 1993. It will take many more studies to validate the effectiveness of many of these treatments; yet many researchers now agree that mind-body techniques have merit and can play a definite role in pain management. For example, Dr. Steven Locke, a psychiatrist at Harvard Medical School and a researcher in mind-body medicine, reviewed the medical literature and reported to *Consumer Reports* (February 1993) his findings: "More than 40 published studies have looked at the ability of human beings to alter some aspect of immunity using some mental strategy—biofeedback, guided imagery, meditation, hypnosis, and so on. Most of them report some positive outcome." Although, Locke says, some studies were excellent, others have been inconclusive.

These positive results, however, should not be interpreted to mean that negative emotions can cause an illness or that positive emotions can cure it. What researchers are growing more convinced of is the positive effect of the emotions on an individual's overall well-being. Even if these mind-body approaches prove to be ineffective in actually influencing the course of disease or indirectly relieving pain, patients can benefit from these strategies by reducing stress, improving outlook and coping strategies, and regaining some control over their thoughts and feelings—all of which can help reduce the intensity of perceived pain.

FIND OUT WHAT TO EXPECT

Having accurate and detailed information is a fundamental key for many patients in helping them to cope, because such knowledge helps restore autonomy and a sense of some control over one's life. Before any procedure, for example, be sure that the anesthesiologist, surgeon, radiation technician, and so on, reviews what to expect—details about what will happen before, during, and after the procedure. The patient should understand beforehand what sensations might be felt—pulling, bloating, stinging, and so on. Some studies, though not all, have even found that such information can raise pain tolerance, diminish the use of painkillers, and is linked to faster recovery rates and shorter hospital stays. In patients who tend to repress their anxiety and avoid seeking information, training in coping skills may be helpful (explained later in this chapter).

HOW COUNSELING OR SUPPORTIVE THERAPY CAN HELP

Once a patient is given clear and straightforward information about his or her disease, simple supportive therapy may be very useful in allaying fears, anxieties, and emotional conflicts. Many doctors do this automatically; in other cases, the patient could benefit from talking instead to a nurse on the staff, a social worker, or other type of medical or mental health professional who specializes in working with cancer patients and families. The professional listens carefully to the patient's concerns and responds with understanding and empathy, providing knowledgeable reassurance, support, and advice about the concerns. Supportive counseling should also focus on helping the patient communicate openly and on enhancing her coping skills.

Group Support and Support Groups

Participating in groups with other cancer patients can also help; a professional may or may not lead the group. Participants benefit from talking with others who have similar problems, which make them feel less isolated, different, alienated, and alone. The support provided in settings like this may help promote communication among the family as well. In fact, doctors are finding that cancer patients who participate in a support group with other patients like themselves not only feel better but may live longer. David Spiegel, a Stanford psychiatrist, for example, compared two groups of women with breast cancer, all receiving conventional therapies. One group of 50 women participated in a weekly discussion group, sharing their feelings and practicing stress reduction and pain control techniques (as explained later in this chapter); the other group, comprised of 36 women, did not participate in a group. He found that, after a year, the women in the support group were less depressed, experienced 50 percent less pain, and had a brighter outlook. Even more intriguing, however, he found that the women who attended support groups ended up surviving almost *twice* as long as those in the control group! Similarly, research at the University of California at Los Angeles found significantly more active and greater numbers of immune cells in patients with skin cancer (malignant melanoma) who participated in groups compared to those who did not.

Likewise, other kinds of studies, known as epidemiological studies (which examine correlations between illness and other factors, in this case psychological factors, in large groups of people), have found similar findings—that people with few social supports had higher death rates from all diseases (including cancer) than people who were the same age but had more social support. A long-term study by the California Department of Health Sciences, for example, showed that older people who lacked social support were more likely to get cancer and die from it than others.

Experts suspect that the benefits of groups come from their ability to reduce stress and isolation and to improve the person's outlook on life; both of these factors help the patient regain control and mastery over life. Unfortunately, many patients are initially reluctant to join such groups and share their feelings with "strangers." Many people are more inclined to suffer in silence, especially if they are depressed or scared. Many individuals are not used to asking for help or admitting fear, particularly to people they don't know. Caregivers may seek the help of a professional mental health worker to initiate discussions or to encourage the patient to just try attending a group, without having to say anything.

HOW COPING AND RELAXATION SKILLS CAN REDUCE PAIN

To help cancer patients cope and improve their psychological state, families and loved ones can help by providing information and support, and by exposing the patient to certain techniques that break the vicious cycle of anxiety—which intensifies pain and, in turn, causes more anxiety. Coping and relaxation skills are among the most studied and recognized of these techniques. A 1987 study at the University of Southern California, School of Medicine, for example, compared how 56 children coped with bone marrow procedures, a traumatic and often painful treatment. At different procedures several weeks apart, the children received one of three protocols: (1) Valium (a tranquilizer); (2) training in breathing exercises, imagery lessons (imagining they were at Disneyland or on the beach), and distraction techniques (imagining scenarios in which the children help Superman or Wonderwoman) with a small reward at the end; or (3) cartoon viewing during their procedures. When the children used the cognitive-behavioral techniques (breathing, imagery, and distraction), they had significantly lower distress, pain ratings, and pulse rates than when they took a tranquilizer or were distracted by cartoons alone.

Although studies like this one abound, some patients are still reluctant or skeptical about trying them. Some resent being asked to try these kinds of techniques, believing they are mere "mental tricks," and that being asked to use them minimizes the legitimacy of their pain and suffering. Others feel silly or have no faith that they can help. One way to help convince these "skeptics" might be to get them to acknowledge how their pain escalates when they're upset. Then, ask them to consider how the opposite could be true—how their pain could be soothed if they were relaxed. Also, they can be reassured that these techniques are safe, noninvasive, and have no risk of side effects. In other words, trying them can't hurt in any way.

A few cautionary notes, however, are in order. These exercises are skills and, as such, they must be learned, practiced, and mastered. Don't be easily discouraged—it may take up to two weeks to feel comfortable with these skills and to experience any effect. They cannot just be adopted passively.

Furthermore, these methods will not *cure* pain—but they do have the ability to help change the perception and experience of the pain and our response to it. For example, if a pain is sharp and stabbing, a patient may try to think about it as dull and spreading. If the pain is burning, the sensation can be countered with thoughts of cold pain. By changing the perception of pain, cancer patients can regain some control over their thoughts and feelings, and hopefully over their pain and discomfort, and over life in general. They may also benefit physically when physiological factors aggravated by stress are improved; they may experience reduced muscle tension, increased blood flow, reduced heart rate, among other benefits.

Moreover, these techniques are most appropriate for patients in mild or moderate pain. Those with mild pain, however, may not be very motivated to practice new skills if simple analgesics are doing the job of relieving their discomfort. Patients in severe pain, on the other hand, may have a hard time concentrating and may not find these techniques particularly beneficial. Patients with lung problems should check with their doctor regarding any deep breathing exercises.

ENHANCING COPING SKILLS

"When you change your mind, you change your life."

An important skill for any patient (and any person, for that matter) is to learn how to notice and change negative attitudes, pessimism, and automatic, self-defeating thoughts. By monitoring thoughts, feelings, and behaviors, ones that are self-defeating, negative, or unproductive can be identified and modified. These would include statements that patients say to themselves that may blow a situation out of proportion or that always seem to imagine the worse. For example, a patient may experience an unfamiliar stomach pain and immediately jump to the conclusion that it means that the cancer has invaded the stomach. When a patient finds himself automatically interpreting a flareup as a sign of worse things to come, it not only escalates feelings of anxiety, depression, and helplessness, but also makes it difficult to concentrate on productive ways of dealing with the problem.

When ill, it is common to have good days and bad days, as well as to experience new feelings and symptoms that sometimes include pain. If there is pain, since it can't be wished away, it might as well be acknowledged. This is a good first step in dealing effectively with a tough situation. Know, too, that it is natural for negative feelings and fears to well up inside; they need to be dealt with head on, which can sometimes be a harder job than managing the pain. Although anyone with cancer has good cause to be concerned, fretting and worrying will not make things better. Worrying can only make it worse. In fact, numerous studies have shown that people who chronically think about the down side to life, its negative aspects—in other words, pessimists—fare worse than optimists in terms of the inability to ward off illness and depression and to gain control over their life (see Chapter 14, section "Sustaining Hope").

Whenever possible, take a positive and action-oriented approach—one that confirms that you are in charge and not a helpless, passive victim. Review and use the techniques and medications available. If the pain persists, the doctor and team should be informed so they can reevaluate the case and prescribe new doses or new medications. If the negative feelings persist and seem overwhelming, it is important to communicate them. Identifying and sharing the problem is the first step to resolving what is troubling the patient. A good heart-to-heart conversation with a close family member, friend, member of the clergy, or professional counselor may help, as might a new medication. These strategies are action-oriented: a problem arises (for example, a new side effect or symptom) and the individual communicates, discusses it with a doctor, and works through the problem without imagining the worst every step of the way.

It may sound like a worthless exercise, but focusing on the positive, rather than the negative, is a powerful means of bringing life's circumstances into perspective. More and more studies, such as the long-term study of 268 men who graduated from Harvard between 1942 and 1944 and have been followed ever since, have shown that optimists, people who "look on the bright side" and who explain adversity to themselves as temporary specific problems, are healthier and live longer. Another study by University of

---

Exercise in Coping Skills

Instead of this negative thought which can feel like a mental catastrophe: "This pain must mean that the tumor has grown and the pain will probably get worse and worse until I can't take it."

Try this type of positive, conscious thinking: "This new pain is unpleasant, but I can deal with it. I will practice deep breathing and consider taking more pain relievers. I will write down what I'm feeling as best as I can, so my family and doctors can know what I am experiencing. It will help them take care of me."

Instead of this negative thought: "This pain only gets worse—it's never going to go away."

Try this type of positive thinking: "This is a bad pain. I know my doctor is committed to my well-being. I must let him and the nurse know that the pain treatment needs to be stepped up. In the meantime, I will take my medication and practice relaxation techniques."

Instead of this negative thinking: "I'm all alone—everyone's given up on me. The doctor and my family haven't come to visit."

Try: "Just because I've been alone all afternoon, I can't jump to the conclusion that everyone's giving up on me. The doctor has always shown up before, and so has my family. I should take this time to focus on what's good in my life. Perhaps I will listen to that new tape I received, or write my niece a letter."

Instead of this negative thinking: "This pain is killing me. I can't take it."

Try this type of positive thinking: "It is a bad pain but I must not panic. Relaxing will make it better. Remember to breathe deeply, in and out. Relax. The more I relax, the faster the pain will subside."

This kind of approach attempts to shift the patient's point of view from one of pessimism, helplessness, and hopelessness to one of resourcefulness, control, and optimism. Learning to replace automatic, selfdefeating assumptions and interpretations with more positive ones is an important coping strategy. By acknowledging, communicating, and dealing honestly with their fears, feelings, and thoughts, people can ultimately gain a greater sense of mastery over their lives.

Miami and Carnegie-Mellon researchers found similar results: graduating students with a pessimistic outlook ended up experiencing more physical problems than optimistic graduates who started out with the same level of health. These researchers also found, for example, that optimistic men recovered from bypass surgery much more quickly than pessimistic men.

In sickness, we may naturally dwell on negative thoughts, so we have to make a conscious effort to look for the life-affirming, meaningful, and positive aspects of life, even in the face of serious illness. A statement that does nobody any good might be one like this: "I can't go shopping anymore, I can't drive anymore, and I can't even clean the house anymore. I am useless and helpless."

On the other hand, a more helpful thought or statement might be: "I've started to read novels again after all these years, and to listen to all the works of Mozart, something I've always wanted to do. Also, spending so much time with my daughter has really strengthened our relationship." Such statements not only highlight what personal goals have been attained, but empower persons, allowing them to feel a greater sense of control over their lives, and to acknowledge some good changes that have come out of misfortune and illness.

Gaining Control and Relief by Changing the Meaning of Pain

How persons think about their pain can have a direct impact on their ability to cope. Consider the different meanings people can have about their pain: one person might believe the pain is a punishment for something done in the past; another sees it as an enemy; another views it as weakness; and another as an overwhelming loss. All of these persons will find it harder to maintain a sense of control and power over their lives, since all of them maintain a negative view of their pain. Also, the stress from these self-defeating thoughts can exacerbate pain by contributing to muscle tension and anxiety, and can keep the mind focused on the pain and its negative meanings.

On the other hand, persons who view their pain as, perhaps, a relief from other demands, as a challenge or a vehicle for growth, retain a sense of mastery and control over life. A study by researchers from Ohio University and University of West Florida, for example, found that tension headache patients who learned to use their thoughts to think about their pain differently experienced at least 43 percent improvement in pain relief, with some experiencing as much as 100 percent improvement; the control group who received no counseling in such skills showed no improvement.

Cancer patients who can view their pain as a challenge may be more apt to view their situation as one that they can exert some control over and try to master. Those who view pain as "punishment," on the other hand, have a more resigned, helpless, and hopeless outlook. By using cognitive techniques to reframe reactions and thoughts about pain, the patient may be able to transform the experience from a threat to a challenge, which in itself, is linked to lower pain levels.

Another way to work on this skill is by using a pain diary (see Chapter 3). Chart when pain is at its worst and what was going on at that time—What were you thinking or feeling? What was the situation? How did you try to reduce the pain? What worked? In looking for patterns, try to figure out what might have aggravated the pain episode—Certain emotions? Particular problems? Thoughts about the meaning behind the pain?

Desensitizing the Patient Who Is Fearful

When patients have uncontrollable fears about a treatment or avoid doing things because of unjustified concerns, which will in the long run make themselves worse, an approach of using very small steps to overcome fears can help. This method is called *desensitization*. First, the patient should be taught one of the relaxation techniques in this chapter (see next section). While deeply relaxed, the patient can be guided to imagine a pared-down version of the fearful stimulus (such as a very thin needle for fear of injections) and then may actually be shown a thin needle. With success at this level, a slightly larger needle can be tried. Likewise, if a patient is afraid of moving or performing some activity, he can be encouraged to master it in very small steps, in which the process or procedure is broken down into manageable chunks. By systematically exposing the patient to feared thoughts or realities in a gradual way, the feared object or idea is rendered significantly more approachable and less threatening. Personal control and mastery are thus gained. This process of desensitization is usually best carried out under the supervision of a mental health professional, like a psychologist or psychiatric social worker.

METHODS TO PROMOTE RELAXATION

Because stress, muscular tension and spasms, distress, and the body's responses to them (perhaps sweating, increased blood pressure, changes in brain chemicals and blood flow, or heart rate) can make pain worse and harder to deal with, techniques to reduce these negative feelings may help alleviate pain. Some conditions—such as irritable bowel, headache, and muscle spasms—may be a direct result of tension states. But even when the pain is unrelated to tension, relaxing muscles can prevent or alleviate increased pain due to tension. Although relaxation and self-hypnotic techniques have been used in Eastern cultures for centuries to produce physiological changes, Western science has only recently acknowledged the powerful effects of these techniques. A robust body of studies has shown relaxation to be very effective in producing physiological reductions in heart rate, blood pressure, respiratory rate, oxygen consumption, and more, with increases in brain waves associated with peace and tranquility (low-frequency alpha, theta, and delta waves)—all of which reduce anxiety and ease muscle tension, thereby calming one's mental condition.

Studies have also shown that relaxation can be directly responsible for reducing pain. Studies at Duke University have shown that relaxation techniques are effective for low back pain, while studies at the State University of New York at Albany have had success with relaxation and chronic headache. Relaxation techniques have also been shown effective for reducing the nausea and vomiting that commonly occur before chemotherapy treatments.

Intriguing studies suggest that the beneficial effects of relaxation—meditation specifically was studied—may come from reducing the secretion of the stress hormone cortisol. Cortisol helps the body muster more energy needed to cope with stress, but at the expense of the immune system and tissue repair. When neurochemists at the Maharishi International University in Fairfield, Iowa, measured cortisol levels in people before and after they practiced meditation for four months, they found a 15 percent drop in cortisol. Another study indicated that meditators experienced up to a 25 percent drop in cortisol levels.

A number of techniques are used to achieve deep relaxation, or what has been called the "relaxation response," or self-hypnosis—including relaxation exercises, meditation, hypnosis, and biofeedback. Whatever works for a particular patient, to enable her to quickly and easily regain a calm inner sense of peace, should be used. Patients who are most willing to use their imagination and have the confidence to do so tend to benefit the most. Patients in severe pain or those who are on higher doses of opioid medications may find it harder to focus on these exercises.

All the techniques should be tried in a quiet place, in a comfortable position, and with the eyes closed. Soothing music in the background may help produce a calming environment.

Progressive Muscle Relaxation or Progressive Relaxation Training (PRT)

This technique involves tensing a body part for ten seconds, and then releasing the body part from the tension. Each body part is squeezed separately, from the forehead, eyes, and mouth, right down to the arms and fingers, down to the feet and toes. At the end of the session (which may be from 5 to 20 minutes), the entire body is tensed up together and then all pressure and tension is allowed to flow from the body, leaving the patient in a more relaxed state and perhaps ready for a mental relaxation exercise.

The reason why PRT is important is because so many of us don't realize we are tense and are exhibiting that tenseness in our body, such as in the lower back, face muscles, or jaw. This procedure actually forces us to tense a body part and then relax it, so we can recognize the state of relaxation. At least two studies have shown that PRT can significantly reduce the frequency with which cancer patients experience nausea before chemotherapy (anticipatory nausea) because they associate nausea with previous treatments. PRT can also markedly reduce how long such nausea lasts and its intensity, says Jimmie C. Holland, M.D., Chief of the Psychiatry Service at Memorial Sloan-Kettering Cancer Center in New York City.

Controlled Breathing

As part of PRT, a patient can learn controlled breathing. The patient progressively relaxes his muscles and then focuses all his attention on his breathing, slowly and rhythmically breathing in and out. Breaths should preferably be through the nose, deep in the back of the throat where breaths become more audible. Inhalations should be held for several seconds, and exhalations should be slow and complete. Progressive relaxation and controlled breathing can be combined by tensing different muscles when inhaling, and relaxing others when exhaling. Upon exhaling, some trainers suggest that a calming word be said in the mind (such as peace, beauty, or love).

Autogenic Training

Patients using PRT may also want to add autogenic training to their relaxation sessions. Autogenic training is a relatively simple technique in which the patient repeats self-affirming statements involving warmth, heaviness, and calmness. The repetitions work to lull and calm the patient into a state of tranquility, and elicit the "relaxation response."

Although it sounds so simple, this technique has been shown to have dramatic effects on the body, much like the other techniques that prompt the relaxation response—including increased blood flow to the mentioned body parts, which relieves pain, and promotes a sense of well-being. In fact, electronic skin-temperature monitors can be used to provide physiological feedback to the patient, showing what works and what doesn't. This process of monitoring a person's ability to change physiological measures is called *biofeedback*. An electronic monitor tells patients when their body is

---

Exercise for Autogenic Training

In a darkened, private space, lie on the floor or a sofa with eyes shut and body comfortably relaxed. Repeat the same thought in 4 or 5 different ways. For example:

"My arms are heavy and warm, very heavy and warm.
My arms are getting even heavier and warmer.
My arms are sinking, sinking down into the floor."

While repeating these statements, the patient should try to visualize a warm bath, bright sunshine, a warm fireplace, or other things that bring warmth and pleasure. Repeat with every body part (substituting legs, neck, feet, back, and so on, in place of arms in the example) for as long as possible, breathing deeply and slowly. The object is to put the mind and body into a relaxed, trance-like state.

---

really responding to some procedure they are trying to learn and sharpen. Biofeedback is discussed in more detail later in the chapter.

Visualization, Imagery, and Distraction

Patients can add visualization, imagery, and distraction exercises to any of these relaxation techniques. Their purpose is to not only distract the mind from focusing on the pain, but to promote relaxation. According to studies at the Pain Evaluation and Treatment Institute of the University of Pittsburgh School of Medicine, which reviewed types of distraction and visualization exercises, all proved to be effective for mild to moderate pain.

The distraction may be as simple as singing, watching television, counting the ceiling tiles, or making conversation. In fact, a study at the University of Alabama Medical Center found that patients in semi-private rooms in hospitals required less medication overall than patients in private rooms because the distractions were greater.

Other kinds of visualization techniques involve conjuring up pleasant images in the imagination—of being on a sailboat, on a beach, on the top of a mountain. Any relaxed or peaceful scene the patient imagines or remembers will do.

As in a daydream, patients can follow any train of relaxing thoughts, perhaps capturing the image of a beloved one or reliving a wonderful experience from the past, walking through a childhood home, imagining a magical holiday moment, fantasizing about a romantic interlude, or spinning a fictional tale of themselves from a favorite novel—all with a pain-free body. The key is to concentrate on the scene as much as possible and imagine as vividly as possible all the possible details, using all the senses, includ-

---

Sample Imagery/Relaxation Exercise

Get in a comfortable position, and close your eyes.

Imagine you are on a raft at a tropical beach. A warm gentle breeze is blowing over you. The sun is beating down on your lightly-clad body. Your raft is gently bobbing up and down.

Feel the warmth in your fingertips, your arms, your toes, up your legs.

Enjoy the gentle rocking motion, lulling you into a gentle, weightless state.

Breathe slowly, deeply. Each breath brings in warmth; each exhalation pushes out poisons.

Imagine that you begin to float. Soon you're on a large, billowy cloud, floating through the sky.

Let yourself be calmed by the rhythms, the warmth, the peace.

---

ing smell, taste, touch, sound, and so on. Scientists have in fact found that the parts of the brain that are stimulated during the visualization are the same as those that would be stimulated when actually experiencing the tranquil scene.

The patient can also use imagery to soothe the painful area in a more direct way, imagining, for example, that a sparkling wand of healing energy, vitality, or colors are coursing through the body and bathing the problem area and that pain. By adding breathing to the imagery, the patient can picture the tension, and poisons exiting the body with the exhales. Try holding the incoming breath for as long as possible, and during that time, imagine that painful joints are easing into their sockets, that tense muscles are softer, even that tumors are shrinking.

Many people benefit from being guided by audiotapes which are readily available through bookstores and several health magazines. Bernie Siegal, author of *Love, Medicine and Miracles*, for example, has produced audiotapes intended specifically for the cancer patient. In them, he leads the listener through meditations and thoughts that can induce relaxation. Although not for everybody, such tapes, with their soothing background music or "white" noises (a seashore or sounds from a night forest, for example), may help the patient drift into a trance-like state and transport him far from the cancer bed. Some report emerging from the experience relaxed, refreshed, calm, and peaceful. Other people like to use tapes they have produced themselves, with or without the help of a professional. On their own tapes, individuals may choose music and imagery that they know suits and soothes them.

The reason that they work is because they help the patient elicit the relaxation response, which, as we've discussed, can create beneficial physiological changes. Later in the chapter we'll discuss the use of imagery for purposes other than relaxation.

Meditation and Repetitive Prayer

According to Herbert Benson, M.D. of the Mind/Body Medical Institute, who is Associate Professor of Medicine at the Harvard Medical School and who coined the phrase "the relaxation response," meditation and prayer may also elicit a relaxation response. By emptying the mind of all intruding thoughts, and therefore tensions, and by repetitively repeating a "mantra," or simple word, in one's mind to minimize distractions, Benson found the same physiological changes that occurred with other methods of relaxation already described in this chapter. This form of meditation is called transcendental meditation (or TM). Benson's group also tested the responses of persons of different religions while praying—he included a *davening*-prayer from Judaism, a rosary-type prayer from Catholicism, and a "centering" prayer from Protestantism—and again found the same physiological responses. Like the deep breathing exercise and TM, repetitive prayer helped to draw attention away from distress and pain and to induce relaxation by emptying the mind of all distracting thoughts.

USING YOGA AND MINDFULNESS MEDITATION

Another type of meditation, known as mindfulness meditation, induces relaxation and well-being as well, but instead of tuning out all thoughts, mindfulness focuses on them. As with other techniques, it is not used instead of medical treatment and has not been shown to slow or reverse disease, but can help people cope more effectively with their illness. The process involves facing, even "welcoming," stress, pain, fear, and other negative feelings, because acknowledging these negative states or emotions is the first step in transforming them. First, the practitioner begins with a deep breathing or standard meditation exercise. Yoga, particularly *hatha yoga*, is often used, because it promotes physical strength and flexibility while focusing on breathing and calmness.

Once relaxed, if the mind wanders, instead of bringing it back to the breathing or the mantra right away, mindfulness involves observing where the mind goes—watching as if from outside what the feelings or thoughts are—without making any judgments or analysis. By observing the thoughts and feelings, the premise of mindfulness is that you become more aware of what is *really* bothering you, or what your true fears or dislikes or preferences are. The object is to be *aware* of what you are feeling by simply observing. As a result, the practitioner is said to be more in touch with herself and her life, and more accepting of it.

According to Jon Kabat-Zinn, Ph.D., Director of the Stress Reduction Clinic at the University of Massachusetts Medical Center in Worcester, where he is an Associate Professor of Medicine, patients who have participated in mindfulness training for eight weeks experience a "sharp" drop in their medical problems, as well as significantly less anxiety, depression, and hostility. They also feel more in control, more self-confidence, and can better view life's stressors as challenges rather than threats. He says the practice (it's not really a technique) works because it reduces the suffering associated with problems such as chronic pain. Through practice, patients can separate their physical discomforts from negative emotions and thoughts, and thereby seem more in control.

"Mindfulness helps patients understand that the depth of pain may come from the fear that it will continue unabated and uncontrolled, rather than from the bare physical sensation itself," says Kabat-Zinn. "This knowledge is usually enough to help people go on to develop effective practical strategies for living with significant chronic pain and the limitations it imposes, so that the pain need not totally dominate their existence and erode the quality of their lives."

USING IMAGERY TO FIGHT THE CANCER

Another technique is to imagine transforming the pain into another sensation. Imagine that, instead of pain, the sensation is an ice cube, a trickle of sand, the tickle of a feather, or a piercing light.

Imagery can also be used in an effort to fight the cancer rather than to just induce relaxation. During chemotherapy sessions, some patients like to visualize that the drugs being injected are like little angels or white knights, coursing through the bloodstream and annihilating each and every cancer cell. Other people picture their tumors being bombarded by an army of white cells. Although some researchers believe that such imagery can actually bolster the immune system, studies have not yet confirmed this. Nevertheless, using this kind of imagery may help the patient feel more in control and can help one regain a sense of mastery.

One way to determine whether this (or other techniques) is working is to keep a log of when such techniques are used, and how the pain or use of pain medication changes. Over a week or two, if positive changes are noticed, then the technique may be helping.

MUSIC THERAPY

Music therapists, employed at some clinics, know how music can capture the patient's mind and mood like nothing else, distracting the patient from the pain. Music therapy involves using music of the patient's own choosing that is intended to improve psychological, mental, and physical health, and to promote a sense of well-being.

Over the past two decades, studies have revealed a link between music therapy and diminished pain reactions in patients after surgery, in patients attending cancer centers, and in those with benign chronic pain. Research has shown that music can affect mood, and since mood can affect pain, changing mood may influence pain. In fact, researchers have found that when patients can choose the soothing music, it can reduce blood pressure, heart rate, pain, and the amount of anesthesia needed for surgery and dental work, says music therapist Barbara Hesser at New York University. Although studies on music's effect on cancer pain are very limited, music therapists are part of the pain teams in some of the leading cancer pain clinics in the country, including Memorial Sloan-Kettering Cancer Institute in Manhattan.

In choosing selections of music that will appeal to a patient, music therapists take into account a patient's mood—a depressed patient, for example, may respond well to music in minor keys; a lonely patient to a solo instrument or a song expressing the need for contact; an emotionally fragile patient to a soft and comforting piece. The music therapist next attempts to progress from a piece that matches mood to one that may transform it. Thus, a solo instrument for the lonely patient would change to a full orchestral piece. The music for the emotionally fragile patient might progress to something more upbeat and dramatic.

At Memorial Sloan-Kettering, patients report that after a music therapy session they generally feel less pain, experience a better mood (with less anxiety, depression, or anger), and are more communicative—that is, they talk more and feel less lonely and isolated. Professional music therapists are not necessarily needed; family members can choose music, provide the patient with headphones, and arrange even to have live presentations. Shared music sessions may be helpful to family members who can reminisce together with the patient and communicate closeness, support, or whatever else is on their minds.

BIOFEEDBACK TECHNIQUES

Biofeedback uses painless electrodes (which are like stickers) that are placed on certain muscles and parts of the body to monitor various functions electronically, such as breathing rate, temperature, muscle tension, blood pressure, brain activity, and pulse. While being monitored, patients practice relaxation, imagery, meditation, or any of the other techniques already mentioned, and can actually see the physiological changes they are producing. By using any or all of the techniques mentioned, patients can thus tangibly monitor their progress with this electronic feedback and hone their skills. Once patients learn how to master the relaxation skills effectively and reliably produce desirable physiological changes, the equipment is usually no longer needed.

Most pain clinics and hospitals have biofeedback equipment; however, sessions may be costly. For more information and referrals, see the Appendix at the end of the book.

HYPNOSIS

Hypnosis is used by some 5,000 physicians in the United States who incorporate it into their conventional medical practice. It has been shown to be useful for some pain patients, such as burn victims and other acute pain cases. When researchers at Case Western Reserve University School of Medicine reviewed clinical trials using hypnotherapy, they found that hypnotherapy could reduce hospital stays, decrease nausea and pain, and promote healing in cases involving hysterectomy, coronary bypass surgery, hemorrhoid surgery, abdominal surgery, among other cases. Its use with chronic cancer pain, however, has been found to be less effective. Experts suggest that only 10 to 15 percent of patients obtain direct pain relief. Nevertheless, it may benefit the cancer patient by reducing distress and tension, and inducing relaxation, all of which may help relieve pain and boost one's sense of control.

Similar to relaxation, deep breathing, and imagery techniques, hypnosis usually involves deep breathing to harness one's attention, closing or fixating the eyes, deep relaxation, and imagery to transform the pain sensations. A person in a hypnotic state, which is somewhat like the floating, drifting feeling we get just before we fall asleep, becomes very receptive to the directions of the therapist, which might be something along these lines: "You are feeling totally relaxed. You are more and more comfortable with each breath you take."

With hypnotism, time can seem compressed or can be made to seem limitless, much like the feeling we have when we lose all sense of time, such as when we're immersed in a riveting movie or when playing a favorite instrument. In these situations, time seems endless. In a setting that is unpleasant, such as a boring meeting or a particularly painful episode, time seems interminable. Hypnotism can help by changing our perceptions, especially that of time.

Of course, not everyone is responsive to hypnosis. Only about one-third of the general population can be induced into a deep hypnotic state; about 10 percent seem completely resistant; and the remainder fall in the middle with varying responses. Nevertheless, that means that up to 90 percent of people may derive some benefit from it. Those who respond the most strongly may find relief in concentrating on changing the temperature of the pain, or even its sensation, or by using their harnessed concentration to focus on an area of the body that feels no pain.

Self-Hypnosis

Some patients also respond well to self-hypnosis, or auto-suggestion, which can be reached by the patient herself through meditation, breathing, imagery-based relaxation exercises, visualization exercises, or progressive muscle relaxation techniques. The physiological and psychological effect is very similar to the relaxation response.

Although very much like a relaxation or autogenic session, experts say that if deep relaxation can truly be attained through hypnosis, then patients may be able to achieve the same state at different times merely by counting backward from 20, relaxing with each number, remembering how it felt when they first achieved a deep hypnotic state. With each count, they feel themselves going deeper and deeper into a relaxed and restful state.

As with any alternative therapy, consumers need to beware of quacks and price tags. (For more information and referrals, ask your doctor or medical center; see the Appendix for specific information.)

ACUPUNCTURE

Practiced for some 5,000 years, this ancient Chinese treatment came to the attention of the West just decades ago when Westerners were allowed back

---

Exercise for Self-Hypnosis

Get in a comfortable position, and close your eyes.

Let all the muscles in the body relax, one at a time if necessary. Each part of the body should feel limp, loose.

Start at your feet. They should feel heavy. Let go of all the tension in them.

Feel your legs; they should feel heavier and heavier. Let go of all the tension in them. Let go of everything, let yourself relax . . . completely.

Continue to move through the body, repeating these phrases for each part. Constantly repeating to yourself that you need to let go completely, to relax, to feel limp and loose. Every muscle is relaxed.

You feel sleepy, and more relaxed. Go deeper, sleepier, more and more relaxed.

At the end of any session, open your eyes and sit up slowly if arising.

into China. Acupuncture bases its success on reestablishing a balance between the body's "Yin and Yang" which, according to Eastern thought, are two forces at work in the human body and the cosmos. They are like opposite sides of a coin, and together make up the body's primal energy. Although scientists don't know how acupuncture really works, they think that the 500 acupuncture points are related to nerve receptors and, when stimulated, somehow muffle pain, perhaps by triggering nerve cells to produce endorphins, the body's natural painkillers. At least one study at the University of Texas Health Sciences Center has supported this theory with its work on rats.

The acupuncturist inserts any number of hair-thin stainless steel needles into selected groups of the hundreds of specific points on the body's "meridians"—energy pathways, the functions of which are believed to be the key to health. Some acupuncturists twirl the needles, stimulate them with mild electricity, or heat them to enhance the effectiveness of treatment.

Although well accepted in some cultures, this ancient practice still is not well understood by Western science, nor is it endorsed by many traditional Western physicians. Yet, many doctors assert that there is little harm in being treated by a reputable (and in some states licensed) acupuncturist. In fact, the American Academy of Medical Acupuncture reports that some 2,000 American physicians use acupuncture in their practices.

Further research, however, is needed to determine the exact role acupuncture might play in the management of pain. In the meantime, even supporters recognize some of its limitations. When improvement does occur, it tends to be short term, up to several days or weeks, with repeated treatments often needed several times a week. In one large study of 183 cancer patients, researchers found acupuncture most useful for pain involving veins or arteries, muscle spasms, bone cancer, and hypersensitivity to ordinary stimuli (dysesthetic conditions). Acupuncture should be avoided, however, in patients getting chemotherapy because the needles heighten the risk of bleeding.

Since most insurers won't pay for acupuncture, it's a good idea to inquire about how many treatments would be needed before relief may be expected, since sessions may be costly. As with any "nontraditional" health care, it is important to inform the primary physician of all treatments being pursued. (For more information and referrals, ask your doctor or medical center; see the Appendix for specific details.)

USING THERAPIES ON THE SKIN

Families should not forget the simplest of pleasures—the bliss of a warm bath, or the soothing relief of a firm but gentle massage on the back, arms, face, legs, or feet. A bath can be revitalizing and may promote a sense of well-being. Here are some simple tips that loved ones can follow to provide soothing care.

If getting out of bed is not too much effort, a warm, not hot, bath can be relaxing. It may be helpful to line the tub with towels so the patient can lean back and rest comfortably; others find a bath chair helpful. If the patient is particularly weak, a caregiver may want to wear a bathing suit, and sit in the tub with the patient. Another helper might be needed in getting the patient in and out of the tub.

When considering a massage, avoid alcohol-based lotions, which might dry the skin, and deep muscle massage unless specifically requested. Choose the scent of the lotion or cream or oil with the patient, or use an unscented one; patients can be very sensitive to scent when they are ill. Sometimes slow circular motions feel the best; other people may prefer light stroking or brushing. For the patient who can't be massaged, or who doesn't want to be touched, try bathing just the feet. With a warm bowl of water near or under the foot, lift the leg and drip a water-soaked washcloth over the foot. Massage with cream afterward if desired. Avoid massaging any areas that are being exposed to radiation treatment.

A similar method to massage, called acupressure, involves applying pressure for from ten seconds up to a minute to areas such as the heel of the hand, the ball or heel of the foot, fingers or fingertips, or around an arm or leg. Try pressing near and around a painful area, looking for particularly sensitive "trigger points" under the skin. Experiment with the patient by asking what feels good, and what doesn't.

Hot or cold compresses can be used to change the pain threshold, relieve muscle spasms, and reduce congestion in a painful area. Cold can minimize the response of the tissues when injured, while heat may help flush out toxins and fluids that have accumulated. Patients are sometimes not sure which to use. Try both to see which is more successful. For warm compresses, either warm, moist heating pads (use only those that are specifically made to be wet), hot-water bottles, or even a washcloth dipped in hot water can be used. Simply wrapping a painful joint in an empty plastic bag, taped around the joint, can elevate heat around the joint by trapping the body's own heat. For cold compresses, either cold gel packs wrapped in a towel, ice bags wrapped in a towel, or wet washcloths from the freezer or refrigerator can be used. Be sure to always cover the skin with a towel or sheet to protect it from the source of heat or cold.

Vibration, friction, or even rubbing with a menthol cream is sometimes used to stimulate the skin and activate the same nerve pathways that are used to transmit pain. By rubbing a cream on an arm, for example, the nerves not transmitting pain may become so excited that they block the painful nerve transmissions from a painful area. This mechanism is known as the gate control theory of pain—when one nerve pathway is excited, other pathways may close off their transmission from other parts of the body, thereby blocking painful transmissions.

Menthol preparations include such creams as Ben Gay, Heet, Icy Hot, or Mineral Ice. Rubbing them on the skin can feel warm and soothing. But be sure to avoid sensitive areas, such as the mouth, eyes, and genitals, and avoid any broken skin areas or rashes.

Similarly, using a vibrator near a painful area may ease the pain temporarily. For headache, for example, the scalp or neck may be vibrated gently. Other areas may also be particularly responsive and can be very soothing—the lower back, the bottom of the feet, or the buttocks.

Experimenting with these simple activities can bring soothing relief and enhance the patient's sense of well-being, as well as affirm a loved one's importance and humanity. Moreover, these activities will communicate love between patient and caregiver.

A few precautions: Avoid areas that are being treated by radiation therapy or that are irritated already; check with a doctor or nurse if unsure. Do not use hot or cold on areas that have poor circulation or poor sensation. Keep treatments to 5 or 10 minutes. Do not use heat on any new injuries, and if a cold compress causes pain or shivering, stop.

OCCUPATIONAL THERAPY

Although not usually a part of the cancer pain team, occupational therapists may be included to assess how the patient wants to spend his time and to facilitate the patient in achieving goals. Occupational therapists can help patients assess what tasks they may need help with to enhance a patient's quality of life. They can use creative means to modify the environment, helping patients adapt to their illness. They may be knowledgeable about the cognitive-behavioral techniques described earlier in this chapter and about support groups that may be available to patients, which include people coping with similar disabilities.

MAKING THE PATIENT COMFORTABLE: SPLINTS, PILLOWS, CUSHIONS, COMMODES, AND BEDS

If the patient is at home and having trouble getting around, some very simple measures may go a long way to conserving energy. These may be useful in the rehabilitation of someone recovering from cancer or surgery, as well as the patient whose reserves are weakening. The family should try to be attentive to the changing condition and needs of the patient, and should try to be realistic. Many families rent a hospital bed and table, although others think the large electric bed is too intrusive.

Others make do by adding extra pillows—a regular pillow or a foam roll under the knees, one at the lower back, one under the head, or an extra "hug" pillow for the patient to manipulate.

If frequent trips to the bathroom become too painful or tiring, consider renting or purchasing a commode. These portable toilets not only allow the patient to relieve himself right next to the bed, but also have arm supports which many patients use to sit up during the day. The idea that using a hospital bed or portable commode is symbolic of "giving in to the cancer" may need to be overcome, especially if the patient's best interests are served by their use. Remember, these items can always be returned.

Many types of splints or supports for joints and the spine are available that can help prevent movement-related pain. If moving an arm or leg or even the back is very painful, talk to the doctor about whether splinting would reduce the pain. When joints or muscles are weak or paralyzed, certain splints (orthoses) can provide support and reduce pain. Pain in the spine is common in patients with prostate cancer, breast cancer, or in tumors that have spread to the spine and weakened the vertebrae. Doctors who specialize in bones and joints—orthopedists—may be consulted. Even if a commercial splint isn't available, consider a hospital's orthotics lab which may be able to fashion a custom device. Ask a nurse or doctor for advice.

If a patient takes to spending most of her time in bed and can't easily turn, try to prevent bedsores by purchasing an inflatable mattress pad or "egg-crate" pad to prevent bedsores. These items are usually covered by insurance. Be sure that the patient turns frequently or is turned, and skin is prevented from rubbing against other areas of skin; in other words, put a pillow between the patient's thighs, a towel between the trunk and arm, and spread the patient's fingers apart. Families can recognize red areas on the skin that indicate places where bedsores may soon appear. These areas may be rubbed gently or massaged, and cushioned to reduce pressure on them. Special bandages are now available (such as Opsite) to protect vulnerable areas; they allow air in but protect the area. Inquire about these and other products from a home health-care nurse or a drugstore that specializes in home-care products.

Prostheses (artificial body parts) can sometimes be used to ease the pain due to cancer, such as leg prostheses to help control amputation pain.

MOVEMENT, EXERCISE, AND PHYSICAL THERAPY

If a patient is bedridden, ask a nurse about gentle exercises to prevent stiffness in the joints. If it's not too painful, moving the arms and legs several times a day to obtain a full range of motion will probably be recommended. Sometimes, an extra ("bolus") dose of analgesic may be recommended before such exercise, or even before a strenuous activity such as going to the bathroom or bath, to prevent the pain triggered by the movement.

If a physical therapist is available through the pain or home-care team, it may be useful to consult him or her about physical therapy after surgery, or about what to do when a patient is unable to get around. Physical therapists can be helpful in suggesting a range exercises to maintain strength. They are knowledgeable about whether to elevate an extremity, how to gently pump the limb or apply a special type of pump called a compression pump for swollen limbs, how to massage, how to use breathing exercises, coughing, and posture techniques, and whether to use a compression garment that applies pressure to a limb to help relieve pain.

NUTRITIONAL AND OTHER ALTERNATIVE TREATMENTS

For years, Western science minimized the role of diet and nutrition in preventing and treating cancer. Today, however, scientists and nutritionists around the world are acknowledging the intimate link between diet and health. Unfortunately, using nutritional practices, such as macrobiotics and other special diets, to modify an established illness has not yet been systematically examined and tested under scientifically controlled conditions. That doesn't mean these diets are ineffective or are quackery. Nor does it mean that they work.

Other alternative cancer therapies include spiritual or faith-healing treatments, megavitamin therapies, herbal and detoxification treatments, among several dozen others. Patients should probably be wary of treatments that seem too good to be true. When interested in pursuing an alternative treatment, patients should gather all the information, pro and con, that is available, including costs and potential risks. Will the new treatment require modifications in the current traditional treatments? If after such investigations, a patient is still interested, consult the primary physician to determine if there is any potential harm, or if such a treatment could interfere with current medications and therapies.

As mentioned earlier, the therapies, techniques, and exercises discussed in this chapter don't "cure" pain. With relaxation and other mind-body techniques, however, we do know that the states achieved have beneficial effects on the body that do seem to last longer than the few moments it takes to perform these exercises. They not only help the patient break the vicious cycle of anxiety and pain, but promote an overall and enhanced sense of well-being by boosting self-esteem, a sense of control, and confidence, because the patient has taken an active role in the treatment that has helped him or her to cope.

Table 12.1. *Strategies for Cancer Pain That Do Not Involve Drugs or Surgery*

To relieve muscle spasms	Massage
	Ice or heat packs
	Exercises
	Repositioning chair, bed, and pillow
To disrupt nerve pathways to interfere with the transmission of pain to the brain (counterirritants)	Menthol cream rubs
	Heat or ice packs
	Vibration, pressure, rubbing, or massage
	Transcutaneous electrical nerve stimulation (TENS)
To relieve tension and stress which aggravate pain	Relaxation techniques
	Deep breathing
	Distraction and imagery exercises
	Progressive muscle relaxation
	Autogenic exercises
	Music therapy
	Mindfulness and yoga
	Meditation and prayer
	Hypnosis and self-hypnosis
To cope more effectively	Group support
	Cognitive coping strategies
To relieve movement-related pain	Splints and other orthopedic supports (collars, corsets, slings)
To promote movement	Strengthening exercises
	Compression cuff for swelling
	Walking aids (cane, crutches, walkers)

13

Special Cases: Children, the Elderly, and Patients with Special Needs

So far, we've discussed techniques that are generally effective for controlling cancer pain. These techniques take into account the variability among individuals, recognizing that each person is unique, and that many of the techniques need to be applied differently for each individual. This is what doctors call "interindividual variability"—an important feature of cancer pain and its management. Yet, certain groups of individuals have special needs—namely, the very young and very old, as well as those with a history of substance abuse.

CANCER IN CHILDREN

People do not usually think much about cancer—until they, or someone they know well, is diagnosed with it. When they find themselves confronting a diagnosis of cancer, most people often reflect on the injustice of the situation. Whether spoken or not, people often think, "It isn't fair . . . I've led a good life, I don't deserve this . . . How could God do this? . . . I must be being punished for something . . ."

Childhood cancer is perhaps the most vivid proof that cancer strikes with neither rhyme nor reason—and that while it follows certain known rules, fairness is not one of them. It is sad whenever a disease like cancer is diagnosed, but it is especially tragic when this occurs in an innocent child.

Unfortunately, the younger the child, the more often his pain and suffering is overlooked or undermedicated. Just recently, doctors have become increasingly convinced that youngsters experience pain as acutely as adults, and need to be treated just as aggressively.

Most Common Types of Cancer Pain in Children

Although all types of cancers may occur in almost anyone—young and old alike—some are much more common in children or adults. In general, adults often get solid tumors, while children tend to get blood-borne cancers. Solid tumors occupy space and grow locally in an organ; if untreated, they would eventually metastasize (spread) through the bloodstream and lymph nodes. If the tumor grows or extends into pain-sensitive tissues, the pain experienced is usually due directly to the tumor.

Cancers in children, on the other hand, are more likely to be a leukemia (cancer of the blood cells) or lymphoma (cancer of the lymph cells). These types of tumors spread through the bloodstream first, and if not stopped, eventually would invade the bone marrow where blood cells are produced and stored. Only later, if at all, would the leukemic cancer cells spread to distant organs.

As a result, children experience pain from the extension of a tumor much less often. Most of their pain problems, which should be treated vigorously, come from the treatment of the cancer itself, not from the tumor. Because of the way most childhood tumors spread, children's most common problems with cancer are with infection, bleeding, and blood clots rather than pain. Pain, whether from the tumor or treatment, should be treated aggressively.

Pain from Treatments—"Procedural Pain"

For problems like mouth sores, bone pain, and nerve pain which can result from radiotherapy and chemotherapy, children receive similar pain treatments to adults. But unique to children—and by far the most common and challenging problem with children—is *procedural pain*.

It is easy to forget, even for doctors, that the small tribulations that arise during a hospital stay and that are usually relatively insignificant to an adult, can be both painful and terrifying to a child inexperienced with hospitals and their routines and staff. Depending on the type of cancer, various diagnostic tests may have to be done. In adults, most of these tests are different forms of X-ray studies which, although sometimes frightening (especially for those with claustrophobia), are rarely painful. In addition to these X-ray studies, children, because of the kinds of cancers that afflict them, are often given other more painful tests, sometimes daily.

Blood Tests, Spinal Taps, and Bone Marrow Biopsies

Blood tests, spinal taps (also called lumbar punctures, which involves inserting a needle near the spine to remove spinal fluid), and bone marrow biopsies (procedures that remove some bone marrow through the insertion of a needle) are tests that are performed frequently in children with cancer, especially when the child has leukemia, to monitor the effectiveness of treatment.

Blood tests, or venipuncture, may be simple procedures for an adult but not necessarily for a child. That's because youngsters have much smaller and more fragile veins than adults. They also tend to be fearful, may be less cooperative, and may require more attempts to obtain satisfactory test samples. Usually, as treatment continues, more and more venipunctures are required, and the easily accessible veins can collapse. This may result both in more needle "sticks" as well as efforts to obtain blood from less conventional areas, such as the ankle, thigh, wrist, chest, or neck—sites that can generate both more pain and more fear. These same problems may occur with lumbar punctures and bone marrow biopsies.

Communication Problems

As we've discussed previously, pain is a personal experience—it cannot be measured or detected with a machine, blood test, or X-ray, so doctors need to rely very heavily on their patient's report of pain. When dealing with children, though, difficult problems arise in trying to assess and treat pain.

Most adults communicate in a sophisticated way. They can discriminate among various types of unpleasantness and can describe, often calmly, how these episodes differ, even when they are in severe pain. Children, on the other hand, generally communicate at a very different level, and depending on their age, in very different ways.

Newborns, Infants, and Toddlers

The newborn is completely helpless and unable to communicate its feelings. The only way the newborn can communicate its distress is by crying. But unlike the older child, there really is little more an infant can do to help a parent, nurse, or doctor determine what might be wrong. With their very limited repertoire, newborns use what seems like the same cry to convey a wet diaper, feeling cold, or feeling pain.

Up until a few decades ago, it was assumed that newborns did not even feel pain; scientists simply thought that their nervous systems were not developed enough. As a result, many procedures, even surgery, were performed with little or no anesthesia. There is good evidence now that, even though they cannot tell us about it, newborns are sensitive to pain. Most doctors now treat infants to prevent and minimize pain, but this has been slow to catch on everywhere. If a procedure has been proposed for a baby— even one as simple as circumcision—it is reasonable to ask the doctor what will be done to prevent pain.

While an infant may experience distress when separated from a parent, he is more easily comforted than an older child might be. Most infants are not sufficiently mature to make fine distinctions among stimuli, which is why a pacifier may often be substituted for a mother's breast, or one warm, comforting body for another—in other words, being held or comforted is more important than who does the holding or comforting.

Toddlers, on the other hand, are very attached to their parents, and separation from a parent is usually much more difficult. Toddlers are unlikely to understand the particulars of what is going on around them, except to recognize an unfamiliar setting as being threatening. As a result, unless special care is taken to reassure the toddler and even, when indicated, to treat him with a sedative or analgesic medication, he is likely to react intensely to events which, though not painful, are strange to him.

School-age Children and Adolescents

Obviously, as children mature and can better communicate and understand what's going on, they can more easily learn to cope. Yet, even without pain, children may suffer intensely from the experience of being sick, from having their lives disrupted, and from facing each new hospital "routine," which may feel like a shocking and terrifying invasion of their self. Children will need constant understanding and support, and as a result, "rooming in" with the child when hospitalization is required may be the most comforting strategy parents can try. This practice is becoming increasingly accepted by the health-care community, especially in children's hospitals. Decorating the room with familiar toys and even providing video games can be reassuring and distracting.

As children mature into adolescents, they become more like "little adults" than their younger counterparts, and can often communicate important information effectively, such as where and how much it hurts, what kind of a hurt it is, whether the medicine is helping, and so on. Parents should not be too surprised (or angry), however, when the "little adult" becomes more "little" than "adult." When stressed by illness and separated from their families, adolescents may revert to their childhood ways and become harder to communicate with; as a result, their problems may become harder to manage.

Usually, though, when given love and support, adolescents can deal effectively with the stress of illness. Such support should come not only from family and friends, but also from doctors and nurses. Newly independent, adolescents may even pride themselves on their ability to "handle" things, and at times may even discourage attention from their family, a phenomenon that may be hard for parents to understand.

Pain Versus Distress

We have already talked about the differences between nociception and suffering: *nociception* refers to the electrical, chemical, and physiologic changes that are triggered when there is an injury, while *suffering* is the person's reaction to the injury. When added together, we have pain. But children commonly react to many different kinds of unpleasant events similarly, making it hard to distinguish whether the resulting distress is due to actual pain or just fear. A child who has stepped on a nail looks very much like a child who has been told he is going to get a needle—and since their reactions are the same, they both need attention.

Preventing Pain

In the last few years, experts have begun to pay attention to undetected and untreated pain in children. Probably, the most important advance has been in recognizing that pain in children exists. Even when they can't tell us, kids may be hurting. This change in attitude has resulted in the view that if it looks as if a child may be in pain, even when parents and doctors aren't sure, the suspected pain should be treated as if it is present.

Because doctors can't differentiate between a young child's response of fear or anticipation and a response to physical trauma or pain, more and more doctors favor treating children's distress preventively, rather than using a "wait and see if it hurts" attitude. Children are learning all the time from the actions of adults around them, and once they "learn" that something the doctor does hurts, chances are the procedure will continue to hurt them. Once this pattern of memory and anticipation of pain is established, it is hard to break, in children as well as in adults. On the other hand, if the children can get through a procedure once without too much discomfort, the child gains confidence and repeat procedures are likely to go more smoothly.

Pain Assessment Tools for Children

There are three basic methods used to assess or measure pain—using the patient's report, making assessments by observing the patient's behavior, and assessing pain based on physiological changes. Ongoing research is focusing on how these methods can be best used in young people.

When children are old enough to report on their pain, most doctors agree that this is by far the preferable way to assess the discomfort. As discussed in Chapter 3, adult cancer patients are often given sophisticated questionnaires to fill out about their pain; these tests, however, are not very useful in young children. Instead, special pain assessment tools for children have been developed that use colors, poker chips, a thermometer, or faces.

As mentioned in Chapter 3, "face scales" are often used with children as young as three. They are shown a group of cartoon or photographed faces that range from a baby crying to one who is smiling, and are asked to point to the one that best corresponds to how they feel. With the poker chip method, youngsters are given chips, each of which is a "piece of hurt," and then they are asked to show how many pieces of hurt they have at a given time. They may also point to where their hurt is on a pain thermometer, or show which colors best describe their hurt.

When children are too young to report pain reliably using one of these or other methods, doctors must rely on less perfect measures of pain—their own subjective observation (does the child look like he is hurting?) as well as physical changes. The physical changes are not always that useful—even though blood pressure and pulse usually change when pain is present, these changes are not very specific. In other words, although the child's pulse may go up during pain, it may go up for many other reasons too. Still, this is used as one indicator, among other observations. The main problem with the observation method is that the results depend a great deal on who's watching (parent, doctor, etc.), but useful information can still be gathered. Researchers interested in perfecting the art of observation are at work analyzing how the quality of an infant's cry, specific facial expressions, and movement change with pain.

Treating Chronic and Acute Pain in Children

As doctors have recognized the problem of pain in children, they have gained more experience with using adult medications to alleviate it. Fortunately, chronic pain can usually be controlled with oral pain medication, usually avoiding the need for additional sticks of the needle. The adult pain medications used are primarily the NSAIDs and oral morphine (or a similar opioid), but in child-size doses and calibrated to the child's weight. Aspirin is usually not given to children anymore because of its risk of triggering an illness called Reye Syndrome—a serious condition that occurs in children, which may cause sudden changes in mental status, such as agitation or mild amnesia, and severe vomiting, possibly even seizures, respiratory arrest, and coma. Acetaminophen and other NSAIDs such as ibuprofen are therefore used instead. Of the NSAIDs, tolmetin and naproxen are the ones that have been approved for children, and are particularly useful for mild to moderate pain caused by inflammation or bone tumors.

As with adults, since children tend not to ask for pain medication until their pain is severe, pain medications should be given on schedule, around the clock, and *not* as needed. Around-the-clock dosing prevents bad bouts of pain as well as provides better relief.

Whereas doctors used to think children metabolized opioids more slowly than adults—and therefore were given fewer doses—today, doctors believe that children from age 30 days old and on process morphine and related drugs the same way that adults do. Newborns, on the other hand, are more sensitive to the respiratory depressant effects of opioids, and should be monitored closely for apnea (when breathing stops) if younger than three months, just to be on the safe side. For special kinds of pain, like nerve pain, the adjuvants (antidepressants, anticonvulsants, and others—see Chapter 8) may also be useful, but again, in lower doses than that prescribed for adults.

When oral medications are ineffective or cannot be taken because of nausea, doctors have other options, and parents can help by making procedures as pleasant as possible, to minimize a child's fear and apprehension. Since children hate needles, for example, injections should be avoided. Older children may be embarrassed by the use of suppositories; if they appear to be, try to substitute another form of medication. Subcutaneous infusions (by pump) require a needle, but need to be changed only about once a week, and are less likely than intravenous lines to become dislodged. If it appears that the child will need medication by injection over a long time, or if many blood tests are planned, it may be best to have an *indwelling catheter* placed surgically. This is a durable plastic intravenous line that is placed (under anesthesia) in a large vein, usually in the chest, but sometimes in the neck or thigh. Although there is a risk of infection, it is low. While not specifically approved for children, a "pain patch" is another good option. Using a bandaid-like skin patch that is changed every three days, a strong opioid (fentanyl) is administered through the skin. A lollipop form of the same strong painkiller (fentanyl) may soon be available. Only rarely are nerve blocks or spinal morphine required in youngsters, but when they are, they have been used successfully even in babies.

Although the risk of addiction in children treated with opioids is *extremely* rare, many doctors—some 40 percent according to a 1986 survey—have erroneous concerns about prescribing them to young children. In most cases, such concerns should not inhibit the use of these very effective painkillers for moderate to severe pain.

Acute pain related to procedures can be controlled by a combination of reassurance, medications, and psychological approaches. As opposed to chronic pain, the problem here is more often fear and apprehension. A good treatment, therefore, is the administration of a sedative medication (like midazolam, a benzodiazepine), either with or without a painkiller, by mouth whenever possible. Youngsters will often then sleep lightly through the procedure and will not even remember it later. If the child should get even more distressed after such premedication, it is probably an indication that the child prefers to know what is going on and feels as though he is losing too much control when sedated. If this is the case, using relaxation or cognitive techniques, which are described in the next section, and in more detail in Chapter 12, can help relax and soothe the child.

Parents as Coaches

As with adults, the many cognitive and behavioral strategies discussed in Chapter 12—such as hypnosis, visual imagery, distraction, among others— can help reduce anxiety and pain in children. Some pediatric oncology centers are focusing on the use of parents as coaches to help youngsters master these techniques. A main goal is to be sure that the parent is calm and relaxed first, speaks quietly and calmly, and knows how to coach the child through a relaxation technique. According to pediatric psychologist Dan Armstrong at the University of Miami Medical School, parents should not necessarily try to reassure the child directly, since his research has found that such behavior is actually linked to more distress in the child. Rather than telling the child what to do (such as hold out your arm) or trying to reassure her (such as telling her it is going to be okay, or it'll be over in a minute), parents are most helpful when they stick to providing facts (such as "The little sting you are going to feel will make your arm numb so you can't feel anything else.") or use statements of reinforcement in a calm voice (such as "That was very good—good job.").

Parents need to be as fully involved in treatments as possible, so that the anxieties and fears they communicate to the child are minimized. Parents can be particularly helpful by incorporating and modifying the behavioral and relaxation strategies described in Chapter 12, which can ease their own stresses as well as their child's. Breathing techniques, for example, may be modified for children by encouraging them to think about their bodies as balloons or bike tires. The goal is to fill the balloon up with air, and to gently empty it. Taking the image further, the parent may ask the child to pretend he is a hot-air balloon or is on a magic carpet. Once relaxed with the breathing exercise, the child can imagine she is floating high above the bed in the balloon or on the magic carpet visiting distant lands. Imagery or distraction techniques may be particularly useful during a painful procedure. Parents can use their imaginations and bring with them party blowers, blow bubbles, video games, or pop-up books to help youngsters imagine pleasanter thoughts than those that overwhelm them in their hospital beds. Helping them pretend they are visiting Disneyland, or are Superman or Superwoman soaring into space, or a character they know from the movies or a favorite book, can ease the pain and pass the time. Parents can help prompt the child to imagine they are somewhere else, doing other things, or can help the child spin a story in which a hero or heroine has the same fears as the child but triumphs over them.

Experts in hypnosis and pain control, such as Karen Olness, M.D., Director of the Division of General Academic Pediatrics at Rainbow Babies and Children's Hospital in Cleveland, point out that children are particularly responsive to hypnosis and self-hypnotic techniques because they are used to harnessing their imagination in pretend play. With a few practice sessions, children can quickly learn effective self-hypnotic techniques to induce a tranquil and distracted state.

Doctors have found that the more control a child (or adult) can exert— such as influencing the timing of procedures, the order of procedures, and placement of injections the more feelings of helplessness associated with a chronic disease can be relieved. Another tactic that some hospitals use to prevent anxiety in children when a nurse comes close is to require that nurses who take blood wear a red apron, so that the child need not become distressed when other nurses approach.

If anesthesia is required for a procedure, talk to the anesthesiologist ahead of time about staying with the child until he or she is anesthetized. Talk with the child about all the interesting things going on around her; calmly explain to her what's going on, allowing her to play with devices as permissible, such as a face mask. By remaining calm, the child will feel secure and follow her parents' lead in viewing the experience as a challenge or adventure rather than a worrisome and fretful experience.

CANCER PAIN IN THE ELDERLY

The management of cancer pain in individuals of advanced age follows the same basic principles that have been described for mature adults:

- The mainstay of treatment for moderate to severe pain is still with potent opioids, like morphine, administered around the clock, supplemented with "rescue doses" of short-acting opioids for "breakthrough pain."
- Pain that is slight or moderate may be treated primarily with the weak opioids, such as oxycodone.
- Depending on the type of pain, treatment may be supplemented with other drugs, such as the non-steroidal anti-inflammatory drugs (NSAIDs) and adjuvant analgesics (antidepressants, steroids, etc.).
- Occasionally treatment with the adjuvant drugs alone is sufficient.
- Individualizing and readjusting therapy to take into account the unique needs of each patient are essential.

Elderly persons do, however, differ in several important ways from younger patients, and knowing these differences can help guide treatment. First of all, older people tend to minimize the pain they experience; they may not mention it or show it, and may have to be asked actively about it. Also, as people age, independent of cancer, various organs and systems (kidneys, liver, brain, etc.) tend to function less efficiently, becoming impaired or more vulnerable to change. As a result, the elderly patient may have a lower tolerance to analgesic drugs, which allows pain to be controlled with lower doses than those usually prescribed. Some doctors also recommend the use of short-acting painkillers rather than the use of long-acting ones, such as methadone (Dolophine) or levorphanol (Levo-Dromoran). Moreover, starting doses may not need to be increased as rapidly as in younger patients. To avoid serious side effects, the doctor usually starts medications at lower doses, being prepared to quickly raise or lower the dose depending on the patient's response.

Just as elderly patients may be more susceptible to the analgesic effects of painkillers, they may also be more susceptible to their side effects. The principles for managing side effects in elderly patients is the same as that for mature adults, and can be summarized as follows:

- Begin treatment with low doses to prevent side effects; if pain persists and there are no serious side effects, be ready to raise the dose quickly.
- As soon as treatment with an opioid is started, a laxative should be administered regularly to prevent constipation. Be prepared for mild grogginess or sedation soon after treatment with an opioid is started, but don't be too concerned—these effects usually disappear after a few days. Be alert for the onset of nausea and vomiting, and if they occur, alert the doctor so that treatment with an anti-emetic (an anti-nausea drug) can be initiated. Nausea also tends to resolves itself quickly, so treatment with an anti-emetic can usually be withdrawn after a few days.
- If grogginess persists, the doctor may want to consider treatment with a psychostimulant, such as methylphenidate (Ritalin) or dextroamphetamine.
- Keep records of the intensity of pain and the presence and severity of any side effects. Maintain regular contact with the physician so that medications can be adjusted upward or downward as needed.

CANCER PAIN IN THOSE WITH HISTORIES OF SUBSTANCE ABUSE

Special attention needs be paid to patients who are either active or recovered substance abusers (alcohol or drugs). It is essential that the doctor be informed, honestly and thoroughly, of any history with drugs or alcohol. If he is not, it could mean potential agony for a patient who is an active abuser of alcohol, narcotics, benzodiazepines (such as Valium), or other street drugs. That's because these patients often have higher levels of tolerance— that is, they may need higher doses of painkillers at the outset to quell their discomfort. If a doctor is unaware of a substance abuse problem, he is likely to unknowingly underprescribe appropriate medications. These patients also may have more problems getting their pain under control than other patients because they or their physicians may be concerned about worsening an addiction or rekindling an old one. On the other hand, these patients will be at higher risk for being undertreated because doctors may be reluctant to prescribe potentially addictive medications such as opioids. As we have emphasized throughout this book, the risk of addiction from cancer pain treatment in the general population (those without any history of abuse) is extremely low. When a patient has a history of abuse, however, that risk is substantially higher. This is not to say that the pain shouldn't be treated or that medications, even strong ones, should not be prescribed; it just means that these risks need to be considered in making a treatment plan.

Discuss with the physician any fears about whether the pain will be treated effectively and whether readdiction might occur. The risk of readdiction should be discussed frankly and balanced against the risks of undertreated pain. With certain precautions, the risks of starting a drug habit can be minimized. The physician may try to treat the pain with nonhabit-forming medications (such as non-steroidal anti-inflammatories, antidepressants, and anticonvulsants) for as long as possible. Many of the pain syndromes associated with HIV, for example, are due to nerve injury and will not require treatment with opioids. Maintain open and regular communication with the doctor, informing him if medications are not effective enough and stronger pain medications are needed.

Expect that the doctor at this point may want to establish some ground rules—to protect both himself and the patient. Most doctors will insist that pain medications be taken exactly as ordered. Some may suggest that a pain medication diary be maintained to reflect the patient's responsible use of the drugs. The doctor will become uncomfortable and may lose some trust in the patient if told that the prescriptions have been lost, the medication accidentally damaged or flushed down the toilet, or given other excuses that appear concocted. If the medication is used as directed, there should be no need to ask for early refills or to call the doctor on nights or weekends for medication. Maintaining a trusting relationship with the doctor is essential, and the patient needs to continue being honest with the doctor.

If stronger medications are needed, the doctor will probably want to prescribe long-acting ones (such as MS Contin or Oramorph), transdermal fentanyl (the skin patch, Duragesic), or methadone, administered around the clock (a-t-c) rather than as needed (prn; see Chapter 7), since these medications relieve pain most consistently and are less likely to produce a euphoric feeling or "high." If the pain is treated with an inappropriately weak analgesic (such as codeine or propoxyphene [Darvon]) or with a stronger painkiller prescribed on an inappropriately infrequent schedule, the patient may become what is called "pseudo-addicted"—that is, the patient may ask for more medication in a manner that appears to resemble the drug-seeking behavior of an addict, because the pain is inadequately relieved due to undertreatment, not necessarily because of a drug craving per se. Around-the-clock dosing is important for pain control and avoids alternating peaks and troughs in the concentration of medication in the blood; such peaks are much more likely to be associated with a sensation of being "high" and may promote more erratic use of the medication. It is important, therefore, that medications be prescribed as they are for cancer patients in general—with adequate doses, around the clock. If the doctor is concerned about whether the medications are being used properly, you may mutually decide to obtain prescriptions for opioids in small quantities—say, on a weekly basis.

Another problem that may occur with patients who are recovered addicts is a reluctance to take the medications as prescribed. Patients may also be pressured by families or peers, especially if in a 12-step program such as Alcoholics Anonymous or Narcotics Anonymous, to back off the needed painkillers. The patient or family may need to reassure the group that it is appropriate to take such medication for medical reasons.

Patients and families need be aware that physical dependence and tolerance will probably occur, as they would with patients with no history of substance abuse. As we have discussed earlier in the book, however, these reactions to opioids are not the same as addiction. (See Chapters 1 and 7 for fuller discussions on these topics.)

As patient-controlled pumps become increasingly common (see Chapter 7), in which the patient pushes a button for an extra dose of painkiller as he needs it (within certain limits set by the doctor on the computerized pump), concern may arise as to whether an active or recovered substance abuser should use one. In fact, the risk of a recovered addict abusing such a medication pump is lower than doctors had previously thought. Again, the risk of addiction needs to be balanced against the need to treat the cancer pain. If the patient is expected to have a temporary pain problem, as opposed to a patient with advanced cancer, the risks and balances will obviously shift.

If a substance abuser is involved with Alcoholics Anonymous or another support group or with counseling, it is important to maintain these supports and to share freely with peers any problems or experiences the patient is encountering with his use of habit-forming medications. Sharing freely with others who can empathize and provide support may go a long way in helping the patient resist abusive behavior.

14
Dealing with Feelings

Finding out you or a loved one has cancer is a shock and usually a major crisis. For most people, the biggest terror is that the diagnosis is a death sentence, which of course, it is not. But it is a vivid reminder of our mortality, and is a very real threat to our security and all we take for granted.

Understandably, a diagnosis of cancer will throw most people into a psychological tailspin as they begin the process of coping with the news. Most of us regard ourselves as fit, healthy, and whole persons with a past and a future. Even if we have had some chronic illness, once we adjust to it, we still tend to maintain a healthy self-image. Unexpected news of cancer causes doubt and uncertainty, and suddenly threatens all of the things we relied on as being dependable and certain.

This aspect of threat is all pervasive—the reliable and predictable things of everyday life are suddenly subject to change. The potential threats are many and include threats:

- To the image of ourselves as being healthy
- To our professional life and goals
- To our role in the family and household
- To our financial security
- To our dreams, hopes, and aspirations

In short, every aspect of our well-being is suddenly called into question. Concerns can pop up almost automatically and cloud everything we think and do. We become victims of a merry-go-round of reactions, including disbelief, shock, fear, anxiety, panic, sadness, depression, feelings of helplessness, despondence, and anger.

However painful, these reactions are common and "normal." In fact, there's more cause for alarm when a person diagnosed with cancer doesn't express such feelings. Keeping strong negative emotions bottled up or denying the illness to oneself and to others can be psychologically and physically harmful. Mates need to catch themselves if they feel the need to overprotect their loved ones, and are fearful of bringing up the cancer. Talking about feelings and fears is healthy, and to some extent, necessary, and family members may need to encourage each other to keep talking.

Yet about half of us adjust "normally" to the news of cancer after learning of a diagnosis or starting treatment. Obviously, no two persons' "normal" adjustment will be the same. Many experience sudden changes in eating or sleeping patterns, or in how they relate to other people, including their loved ones. It's called "an adjustment disorder," and is viewed as a reasonable, "normal" reaction to a crisis, especially to a potentially life-threatening one like cancer. But by and large, with time and support, most patients manage to mobilize their psychological resources and support networks and adapt relatively well.

But when these changes persist for more than several weeks, they may be a warning sign that major problems are brewing. If left alone, they could seriously impair the patient's functioning and well-being and could even interfere with medical treatment. Counseling, specifically short-term supportive psychotherapy, often works quickly—in as little as four to ten sessions. By helping the patient express his bottled-up feelings and fears, sort out the rational from the irrational fears, and learn how to cope with the rational ones, many of the psychological symptoms mentioned above will often subside.

Almost all patients will be fearful and anxious as they cope with the news of their diagnosis, tests, treatments, and symptoms of cancer. How distressing those emotions are for a particular patient depends a great deal on specific personality traits and the coping strategies that have been learned over a lifetime, as well as the support that is available to the patient from family, friends, and the medical team.

A new science called *psycho-oncology*—the study of the psychological and psychiatric aspects of cancer—is identifying what kinds of psychological issues may arise with cancer and how to help by enhancing the patient's supports and coping skills. This chapter will discuss how family members can be supportive and help the patient (and each other) distinguish between realistic and irrational fears, and how to cope with their crisis while minimizing distress. The reason these issues are being discussed in a book about cancer pain is because emotional distress can lead to anxiety and depression, which often increases physical tension and therefore the intensity of pain. Likewise, pain is much more difficult to manage when people are depressed or anxious. Moreover, pain itself can cause psychological changes that may seriously impair physical, psychological, and spiritual well-being, or may make problems seem worse.

HOW PEOPLE RESPOND PSYCHOLOGICALLY TO CANCER

As we've said, about half of cancer patients adjust "normally" to being ill with cancer, according to a U.S. study by the Psychosocial Collaborative

Oncology Group (PSYCOG)—a society of mental health professionals that study cancer patients—of 215 cancer patients from three cancer centers. That leaves about half whose psychological problems may become debilitating. Of those, about two-thirds suffer from reactive anxiety and depression—that is, anxiety and depression that are a direct response to the illness. Symptoms of depression include insomnia, loss of appetite, agitation, and feeling tired and down much of the time, and lack of interest or pleasure in everyday things. Symptoms of anxiety include restlessness, jumpiness, sweating, upset stomach, heart pounding, worry, fear, irritability, difficulty concentrating, and similar symptoms that persist. Thirteen percent of patients in this study suffered from major depression. Not surprisingly, the patients with pain had twice the rate (40 percent compared to 20 percent) of psychiatric disturbances, especially anxiety and depression.

The duration of chemotherapy may be a particularly emotional time—often more so than during radiation or surgery treatments, because of concerns about unpleasant side effects. Of course, if it is the first chemotherapy treatment, or one that is associated with very high chances of success, the primary feelings are upbeat and hopeful. If the cancer advances, the frequency of psychiatric problems among cancer patients increases, as might be expected. Whereas about one in four cancer patients experience severe symptoms of depression, the rate soars to three out of four for those with advanced cancer.

It is, of course, always difficult to know whether some of these symptoms (poor appetite and sleep, etc.) are due to depression, medication, or are direct effects of the tumor. Regardless of the cause, the effort to clear up these symptoms is well worth it, enabling the patient to be as strong as possible during these tough times. You may be surprised at how much a consultation with the doctor, psychiatric or oncology nurse, or social worker can help.

THE TYPICAL DISTRESS OF CANCER PATIENTS

As patients try to cope with their illness and its repercussions, they may experience a rollercoaster of changes. We will first discuss the most common ones, and later suggest how family members and other primary caregivers can help.

Anxiety

From the moment a lump is spotted, a mysterious insistent pain nags, or sudden weight loss is noticed, almost every one feels anxious. First, there is a nagging, usually unspoken fear that it could be cancer. If a doctor confirms it, that gives way to new fears of what is to come, including concerns about treatment, disfigurement, even death. The anxiety—which may range from simple jitteriness, restlessness, and being easily startled, to sweating, heart pounding, clammy hands, upset stomach, poor concentration, insomnia and edginess, among other symptoms—can mushroom into panic (episodes of chest pains, choking, feelings of dizziness, feelings of unreality, hot or cold flashes, trembling, faintness, fear of going crazy, in combination) or chronic anxiety, potentially threatening the patient's ability to cope and comply with a doctor's treatment recommendations.

Denial

Although a person may notice a distressing sign, some ignore it, denying to themselves that something might be wrong. Although denial can sometimes be a useful coping mechanism, if it is severe or persists, it can fester until a crisis develops later on.

Fear

Fear is pervasive in these circumstances: fear of the unknown, of pain, of mental and physical loss, of rejection by the family, and of lingering illness and death. Every time a new pain or symptom surfaces, a fresh wave of fear may sweep over the patient. This is to be expected, and must be expressed so it does not get out of control. Being afraid is bad enough—but handling it alone (perhaps to avoid "burdening" loved ones) makes it especially hard.

Isolation and Detachment

Some people react to cancer by detaching themselves from the whole issue of medical treatment, discussions about their illness, and in the advanced stages of cancer, thoughts of death and dying. This detachment is another form of denial and serves as a buffer for the patient. Sometimes the patient does it as a way to protect family members. Like the other negative emotions discussed here, it is normal up to a point. This form of denial may be just another step in coming to terms with a very unpleasant situation, but if it persists, professional counseling may be needed.

Guilt

Sometimes patients blame themselves for having caused the cancer in the first place or believe that they are sick or in pain as punishment for something they've done. Smokers, for example, may feel shame and guilt for smoking despite warnings of increased risks of cancer. Whether justified or not, this self-punishment does no one any good. Commonly, such guilt can lead to a major depressive disorder.

Worry

In addition to pain and other physical problems linked to cancer, such as nausea or vomiting, difficulty in breathing, or weakness, patients worry about losing control over their daily lives, losing their independence and personal freedom, and having to become more dependent on others. They also worry about whether they can continue working or not, the financial toll their illness takes, and being a burden to their families. All these factors contribute to the patient's overall suffering. These are legitimate concerns that need to be dealt with in a productive way, but worry doesn't help. Instead, constant fretting needs to be talked about with a loved one or mental health professional. The timeless wisdom of taking one day at a time can also help enormously here.

Loss

Cancer patients suffer many losses on different levels, and each one needs to be dealt with directly and, when appropriate, grieved for separately. Loss of esteem, self-control, future dreams, and body image, of sexuality and reproductive abilities, are just a few of the highly important attributes upon which we base our well-being, self-esteem, and quality of life. Again, such concerns need to be faced up front and discussed with a supportive person.

Withdrawal

Disfiguring surgery or side effects from treatment (such as hair loss) may trigger despair and depression, causing the patient to withdraw from seeing or even speaking to friends and acquaintances. Those who lose a breast or have had colostomies, for example, may feel physically mutilated and withdrawn, even from partners and friends.

Self-pity

Patients who are terminally ill and debilitated may pity themselves, and although a certain amount of grumbling and anger may be therapeutic, it can be destructive if sustained. The patient may feel justified in being demanding, in complaining, and in being short-tempered. These behaviors, however, can end up being manipulative and exploitive, turning the patient's powerlessness into a negative form of power. As a result, caregivers and family members may start resenting the patient (and feel guilty as a result) as he alienates them. Then the patient can accuse them of not caring, or of abandoning him. This cycle breeds emotional distance.

Defiance

An opposite tack to self-pity is the decision to fight the disease and its pain at all costs. But by fighting the pain without seeking medical advice to control it, patients end up hurting themselves only more. By waiting and holding out, they're going to end up requiring more medication to relieve the intensified pain when much smaller amounts could have been used for the earlier, milder pain. The defiant, fighting spirit, however, if channeled properly, can be a very positive and powerful response. Remember, every good fighter needs a coach.

Information-seeking Behaviors

Some patients act exactly the opposite of those who deny or avoid; they try to read everything they can about their condition and may panic when the slightest little thing goes wrong or doesn't fit their mental pictures. These patients need to be active members of the medical team so they can feel they have some input and control in the decision-making process.

Irritability and Anger

Many cancer patients become irritable if things don't go as predicted (sometimes it seems like everything goes wrong). They may feel they don't deserve this, that life isn't fair, that God has deserted them, just at a time when faith can be a powerful ally. They seek a sense of meaning for their suffering, and yet there appears to be none. Their expectation of equity and fairness in life is shattered. Cancer has no favorites. Typically, cancer patients may lash out at family members and loved ones, the most convenient and forgiving targets with whom patients feel the safest. Though stressful for everyone, fits of anger, even screaming, crying, throwing dishes, or whatever it takes (without becoming a threat or danger) to get the anger out are therapeutic. After acknowledging the anger, they can harness that energy to fight the cancer.

Resignation

Some patients reject offers of help, choosing instead to suffer in silence and to just be left alone. It is sometimes hard to distinguish between a defeatist attitude and an approach that is realistic, especially since feelings change from day to day. Although it is hard to listen to the expression of negative or pessimistic thoughts—especially when trying to keep one's own attitude positive—they must be talked out so they can be dealt with. Maintaining a positive attitude can help immeasurably during a crisis. With these and other changes, loved ones must be attentive to whether pessimism is a passing phase or a serious problem that needs professional attention. No matter what the situation is—even when it appears bleak—there are *always* things to be hopeful about.

Hopelessness and Helplessness

Since many patients feel that they have little or no control over the outcome of their illness, they feel helpless. When medical help seems inadequate, feelings of helplessness can evolve into feelings of hopelessness. Both of these feelings can contribute to depression and may make other mental and physical illnesses seem worse.

Hopefulness, as long as it is realistic, can be a very positive response that needs to be encouraged. To counteract feelings of hopelessness, patients need to set realistic goals and feel that their lives have meaning and value. Families can reassure their loved ones that time together is valuable. If cancer has rendered the future uncertain, the patient needs to be encouraged to take one day at a time and to work toward having a good morning, a good night's sleep, or a pain-free day. The more control the patient can have over his life—such as the timing of treatments, baths, or other activities, or being asked about everyday decisions (what to eat, who to call, where to go, etc.)—the less negative and hopeless he may feel. Priorities and goals need to continually be reframed and addressed, especially if the disease is advancing.

CANCER AS A POST-TRAUMATIC STRESS DISORDER

When persons believe the diagnosis of cancer is a life-threatening event, they may be thrown into a series of psychological changes that are similar to those triggered by combat, rape, physical or sexual abuse, or other traumatic events that are outside the range of everyday experience. These psychological changes are collectively called *Post-Traumatic Stress Disorder* (PTSD), and in the cancer patient may include attempts to avoid all thoughts or feelings associated with the illness; forgetfulness about what the doctor has said; a sudden loss of interest in things that used to be meaningful, such as young children or a job one loved; feeling and acting estranged from others; inability to have or express loving feelings; and a sense of a suddenly foreshortened future.

The person also may have trouble falling asleep or staying asleep, may find it difficult to concentrate, may be irritable or quick to burst out in anger, have an exaggerated "startle response," or may suddenly break out in a sweat or hyperventilate if exposed to something that reminds him of the trauma (of being told about the illness). These changes don't indicate that a person has suddenly gone "crazy." Instead, he is responding to a deeply disturbing and frightening event in his life.

HOW TO HELP

As a rule, cancer patients are extremely vulnerable. They have important, often relatively simple, needs which, if fulfilled, can make them feel immeasurably safer and, therefore, more physically comfortable. Most can benefit by being well informed about the nature of the cancer and its treatment, and by being reassured that physical discomforts will always be aggressively treated. Family members can help by reassuring them about what the doctor really said and helping the patient see when he may be focusing on something irrational or something beyond his control.

In most cases, though, family members themselves are under enormous stress, often feel physically and emotionally drained and distressed, and need help and support themselves. Naturally, loved ones try to always put the needs of the patient first. A son or daughter, for example, may see the cancer illness as an opportunity to return the love and support they experienced as a child. There are always limits, though, and relatives sometimes need to be reminded to take care of their own needs.

If the family members' basic needs are ignored, they may get too "burned out" to really be there when they're needed. Families should be sure that they have at least one professional they feel comfortable confiding in who is connected with the doctor's team or the home health-care program (a nurse, pharmacist, social worker, or other mental health professional). They may want to take advantage of his or her availability, experience, support, and empathy to talk over their own concerns and emotions.

TYPICAL PSYCHOLOGICAL NEEDS OF CANCER PATIENTS

In general, family members and caregivers can help satisfy the basic psychological needs of patients. Typically, cancer patients need to feel:

Safe

Feeling secure where they are and confident in the hands of caregivers is important and must be established as a foundation for working out other problems associated with the disease.

Needed

Many patients, as they become weaker, may feel like they are a burden. They will need reassurance that they are still needed and loved. In fact, some patients may actually *be* a burden, in which case it needs to be talked out. More likely, the illness can be an opportunity for family members to "give back." The patient can be helped to recognize that relatives and loved ones will need to be given a chance to do what they can, as they also feel helpless in so many ways in the face of the illness.

Love and Warmth

All people benefit from expressions of love and affection; touching the patient, holding his hand, and massaging him are all important. Behaving warmly and touching are common ways for love to be communicated.

Understanding, Knowledge, and Empathy

Family members and other loving caregivers can't make the illness go away, but they can express empathy for the patient's distress. Patients need their family to acknowledge the severity of their ills, but at the same time, they may need to be reminded not to worry too much and that they should take one day at a time.

Patients may benefit from having their symptoms explained—why they're occurring, what can be done about them—as well as from information about the process and nature of the disease. Caregivers should try not to deny or minimize the patient's feelings, especially if the patient is gravely ill. Rather than saying something like "Don't be ridiculous, you're going to beat this and be fine," if it's obvious the patient is terminal; it would be more helpful to say something like "I know you're very sick, and you might die. Are you feeling scared? How can I help?" Acknowledge the patient's feelings and try to get him to talk about them. Don't push—keep communication lines open and be available to listen and offer input when asked.

Acceptance

Patients must feel secure and accepted, regardless of their condition, appearance, mood, and demands. They need to be reminded that just because they may look dramatically different, they are no less the person who was dearly loved before the cancer. Their personhood, essence, and self are just as vital and important to others as ever.

Self-esteem

Many cancer patients feel devastated by the disease because, as mentioned above, they are haunted by thoughts that somehow they are responsible for their illness—that the disease is a punishment of some sort, that if they only had been a better person, hadn't been unfaithful, hadn't had that abortion, or whatever, they may not have gotten sick. They may need to be reminded and reassured that cancer can strike anyone . . . and does.

To maintain self-esteem, involve patients as much as possible in the decisions that must be made. Allow them to give advice or instructions and make decisions; by doing so, they will be more likely to accept these as well.

Trust

Patients need to know that they are receiving the best care possible—that their doctors and family will aggressively pursue treatment and pain management to ensure the best possible outcome.

HELPING THE PATIENT COPE

Coping involves efforts to reduce stress in the face of adversity. Patients may put up psychological walls, known as defense mechanisms, to avoid or deny their situation. Sometimes, these reactions help cushion patients and get them through the process of gradually accepting their illness. As a result, these reactions are mainly a concern if they persist.

Patients who have a tendency to be overly watchful and who want to accumulate as much information as possible can usually feel more in control if they are assured that they will be involved in all decision making. Finding or even starting a support group with other cancer patients, especially those close in age and of the same sex, can serve to alleviate many fears, help patients share their fears and problems, and make them feel less isolated (see the next section). Teens, for example, need to talk with others their own age who have had cancer; women with breast cancer can be most benefitted by contact with other women who have had or currently have breast cancer.

Families should try to be as open about cancer and the threat it implies as possible. Try not to keep secrets from either the patient or close family and friends, and be honest with young children whose grandparent, parent, or sibling has received a diagnosis. The more that anger, anxiety, sorrow, and other negative emotions are openly expressed, the closer and more bonded the family will feel during this difficult time. Children need not be excluded from this emotional upheaval—they can understand more than many people give them credit for.

Children who receive a diagnosis of cancer can understand that they have a sickness, and they can also acknowledge that if they listen to the doctor, he can help. While we all need to vent our anger in such trying times, adolescents in particular need opportunities to express their feelings. In addition to cancer being a threat to health and welfare, cancer in teenagers may also be viewed as a threat to their emerging independence and desire to emotionally separate from authority figures. Cancer makes them dependent again. If possible, they need to feel independent and in control. Middle-aged patients, on the other hand, characteristically need support and help in coping with the needs of other family members. Middle-aged patients often feel sandwiched—responsible for caring not only for their children but for their elderly parents as well. They worry about how those dependent on them will cope while they are ill. Friends and family members can help out by providing practical help with the children or elderly parents. Friends and family can also help by offering emotional support, reminding patients of their strengths, and encouraging and guiding them to use coping strategies that have worked in the past. They can encourage patients to use relaxation techniques, help them observe thought processes and change them if they are self-defeating, offer help in practicing self-hypnotic pain control strategies, set realistic goals, and work on asserting themselves and improving communication skills. These skills are described in more detail in Chapter 12.

Again, while we tend to focus on the patient in these discussions, it is important for caregivers to care for themselves and their own needs. Relatives and friends will certainly want to know details and to offer help. Don't feel compelled to go into the many details with everyone. Find ways of avoiding the need to tell everyone everything; it may be a good idea to appoint a friend or relative to tell a circle of common friends about the status of the patient. Be specific in communicating with others about how they can help. It is acceptable to tell acquaintances or even close friends who want to visit that someone is not feeling up to visitors today. Thank them, and remember that this is a time when the needs of the patient and caregivers must come first.

Although caring for an ill member of the family takes a lot of time and effort, it's important that the family continue with their individual lives as much as possible. Not only is it important for the caregivers, but the patient will feel less of a burden if everyone can maintain their normal routine.

THE POWER OF SUPPORT GROUPS

Although not everyone will benefit, many cancer patients derive an enormous sense of relief and comfort when they join a group of other cancer patients (see discussion in Chapter 12). Meeting regularly with other people who have similar problems can dramatically reduce one's sense of isolation, loneliness, and fear. Such group settings allow patients to share their experiences and feelings, and hear those of others; they can empower patients by providing additional emotional support, companionship, and information—as well as a sense of connection and perhaps meaning. Many patients also find that support groups help them find the strength to regain their fighting spirit.

Many hospitals, physicians, and local branches of the American Cancer Society can offer referrals to local support groups.

WHEN DEPRESSION PERSISTS OR IS SEVERE

When a patient becomes so anxious or depressed that his negative moods are constant, or if excessive feelings of guilt, sadness, anxiety, worthlessness, helplessness, and hopelessness override all else and don't pass with time, then a major psychiatric illness is brewing. Professional help may be appropriate to try to cut short the spiral of negative emotions that can severely compromise the patient's quality of life and may even lead to thoughts of suicide. The power of depression over suicidal thoughts is so strong that people who are depressed are much more likely to feel suicidal than even patients in pain.

Although severe pain or other symptoms can trigger depression and thoughts of suicide, the opposite should never be assumed. That is, pain should never be viewed solely as a result of a patient's psychological state. Although there is no such thing as a "pain detector"—no blood tests or X-rays that disclose how much pain a patient experiences—a patient's own report should be the last word. Many studies show that self-reports are more reliable than the observations of nurses, physicians, and family members. As a rule, then, it should be assumed that a patient's pain is just as he says it is, even if he is depressed.

When pain and depression do occur together, they both need to be carefully assessed and treated. In most cases, relieving the pain will relieve the majority of psychiatric symptoms.

Yet, some patients do develop major depression (as opposed to reactive depression); it is more common among those in pain, who have advanced cancer, who are physically disabled, or who have previous histories of depression or major psychiatric illnesses.

Depression and Cancer

Depression can compromise health, not only by affecting sleep, appetite, and mood, but it can also induce biochemical changes in the body that researchers suspect may compromise the immune system and may even stimulate tumor growth. Some studies have suggested that cancer patients with symptoms of depression, such as feelings of helplessness and hopelessness, recover more slowly and don't live as long as those with a positive outlook. In a 1985 study at King's College Hospital in London, for example, researchers found that breast cancer patients who felt helpless and hopeless, or who just accepted their disease with stoicism, were more likely to die within ten years than women who displayed a fighting attitude. Similarly, other women with breast cancer who looked at the brighter side—who didn't attribute their discomfort to the disease advancing—not only were less psychologically stressed, exhibiting lower levels of anxiety and depression, but also were less likely to report pain. In fact, how the women viewed the meaning of the pain—whether it meant the disease had advanced or not—was a much better predictor of how intense the pain was than where the tumors were located. And although it's difficult to extrapolate from animal studies, research in which rats and other animals learn that they are helpless to escape (feelings of helplessness are a symptom of depression) shocks or other negative experiences have shown that these rats had depressed immune function and faster growth of cancer. Indeed, many studies have shown that stress not only can make pain worse but can trigger changes in the levels of a host of hormones that may suppress the immune system, and that feelings of helplessness and powerlessness increase the deleterious effects of stress.

Cancer is often associated with depression and anxiety. Women with breast cancer who have had mastectomies, for example, have a 50 percent chance of also developing depression, anxiety, and sexual problems. When they also receive chemotherapy, their rate of depression and other psychiatric problems may soar to 80 percent. Knowing this in advance should spur patients and their families to take a proactive approach and to look for help early. Like pain, depression is not good for a healthy recovery.

With psychiatric illnesses in particular, the role of the family is extremely important. One of the insidious features of depression and other psychiatric disorders is that the person who is suffering may not recognize the signs, and because they are feeling low, may not be motivated to seek help. Families need to play a vital role here (see next section).

With counseling and support, however, cancer patients can be greatly helped in changing their outlook, which not only vastly improves their quality of life but also can have a dramatic effect on their illness. A study by Stanford's Dr. David Spiegel, for example, found that breast cancer patients who have a fighting spirit, feel they have a greater sense of mastery over their lives, and have better coping strategies do significantly better after a mastectomy; their recurrence of symptoms takes longer to appear, they suffer less pain, and they live significantly longer than women who feel helpless, hopeless, and resigned to the disease. Thus, treating depression is a vital part of any comprehensive treatment for cancer pain.

Depression and Pain

People in pain and in the advanced stages of cancer have a greater chance of being depressed or of suffering from other mood disorders than those not in pain and those in earlier stages of the disease. Likewise, those who were depressed or who were in pain before their illness are at greater risk for experiencing more intense pain than the nondepressed patient. A Finnish study reports, for example, that pain thresholds are lower (meaning that patients are uncomfortable and distressed by pain more easily) in pain patients suffering from major depression than those with milder depression; and similarly, patients with mild depression had lower pain thresholds than those who showed no symptoms of depression. Patients who are depressed also report that their pain interferes with their lives more often than patients who are not depressed, despite similar intensities of pain. Spiegel's breast cancer patients, for example, who joined support groups and had lower rates of depression, not only lived longer but experienced 50 percent less pain. Researchers suspect that there are similarities in the biochemistry of chronic pain and depression. Thus, on the one hand, relieving pain can often help relieve depression and other mood disturbances, and successfully relieving depression can, on the other hand, help reduce the pain.

HOW TO HELP THE DEPRESSED OR ANXIOUS PATIENT

Families can help ease a loved one's depression or anxiety in important ways. Here are some suggestions:

- Help the patient sort out genuine losses from irrational ones, guiding the patient to acknowledge and mourn those losses. The genuine losses might include dwindling independence, loss of a positive self-image, and in some cases, the vanishing of dreams and goals. Encourage the patient to talk about these issues and, in response, try to express an understanding of those thoughts. Don't try to deny them. Statements that begin, "Don't be silly . . ." discount what the patient is feeling. On the other hand, "How does that make you feel? That must be so hard for you" are expressions of empathy and understanding.
- Support the patient in reframing feelings of helplessness by developing, in concert with the patient, small achievable goals that are realistic and practical. Help the patient maintain a sense of control by empowering him or her with choices related to care and comfort.
- Try to engage the patient in more positive thinking that involves active loving, laughing, looking on the bright side, and focusing on positive thoughts, even in the face of serious illness.
- Help the patient separate his or her identity and personality from the illness and a sick body; the patient's body may be impaired or weakened, but he or she is still the person others love and respect.
- Help the patient cope with fears of pain by reassuring him that aggressive pain management strategies are available and will be used and pursued if they are needed. To address feelings of loneliness and meaninglessness, reassure the patient that he is a highly valued and loved member of the family and community, and that he isn't alone—either physically or emotionally—you are in it together. Patients may tend to view their glass as "half empty" rather than "half full," and may need to be reminded of their blessings, although without minimizing the seriousness of their illness and concerns.

- The patient may lament what he can't do if the illness is debilitating or life threatening; he may regret what he didn't do in his life. In a loving, supportive manner, help him focus instead on what he *can* do and what he *has* achieved. For example: "I know how disappointing it is for you not to be able to go to Billy's games now, but isn't it great that you have more time to help him with his homework." Or "I hear what you're saying, Mom, but you have been a wonderful mother/friend/ neighbor/artist and that counts for a lot. I'm proud of you."
- Help the patient distinguish between realistic fears and exaggerated, distorted ones. For example, if the patient believes that he is dying when it is clear that his prognosis is good, dispute his belief with statistics, pointing out that averages mean that as many people live longer as shorter, and that a positive attitude can help. If he is truly dying and is frightened that it will be a painful, lingering, agonizing experience— challenge and dispute this in a loving but factual manner, assuring him that the pain and discomfort can be greatly relieved and controlled these days.
- When someone believes the worst, it is understandable that irrational fears will surface. Accurate, factual information is essential to reassure the patient in these instances.
- Acknowledge that sadness is a legitimate emotion and a normal response. Feeling appropriately sad, though, is different from depression, which is psychologically immobilizing and physically draining. Don't minimize a patient's (or your own) expressions of sadness, or try to change the subject. Crying together can create a strong and loving bond between you. Yet, remember to introduce thanks and joy for what the person has offered and still offers to those around him. At this time, patients may feel more despair than integrity if they see a long recovery or period of dependence ahead of them. Acknowledge that the illness is unexpected and unfortunate, but help the patient focus on small goals for today, or for the week, whatever is appropriate at the time.
- If the patient is terminal and frightened, acknowledge his or her fears; don't minimize them or brush them off with simple reassurances. Convey that you really hear what he is saying. For example: "I know what you're saying and you're right, dying is scary because you don't know what's beyond." Yet reassure him that those around him will help him live life to its fullest for as long as possible. Help him accept and mourn his losses. Focus on past accomplishments and what has been meaningful in the patient's life, and how they can strive to live each day as fully as possible until the very end.
- Don't allow the patient to feel that he has failed the family by getting ill or by not getting better. The patient also shouldn't be made to feel

that tears, grief, and acknowledgment of losses are weaknesses. Rather, courage can be emphasized—courage to face the losses and the grief, to express the sadness and the struggles associated with serious illness. Patients need to grieve these losses, so denying them may be harmful.

- Whenever possible, reassure the patient that he is not alone and not to blame.
- Don't worry about not saying "the right thing." These are difficult issues and you don't have to give any answers. The important thing for the patient is to know he is listened to and loved; you can help by providing understanding and encouragement.

Treating Depression with Medication

Your primary physician may suggest a medication to ease depressive symptoms. At Memorial Sloan-Kettering Cancer Center, patients are often started on a stimulant such as an amphetamine, followed a few days later by a tricyclic antidepressant such as amitriptyline (Elavil), imipramine (Tofranil), doxepin (Sinequan, Adapin), or nortriptyline (Pamelor, Aventyl) to prolong the short-term benefits of the amphetamine. Those benefits include improved attention, concentration, and appetite as well as an improved sense of well-being, while diminishing fatigue and weakness. Amitriptyline is particularly useful for relieving insomnia, anxiety, or agitation; while imipramine may be chosen if the patient is having slowed physical reflexes and showing fatigue. But because tricyclics carry a range of side effects, such as dry mouth, nausea, constipation, and blurred vision, a newer generation of antidepressants (such as Zoloft, Prozac, Wellbutrin, Setraline, maprotiline [Ludiomil], amoxapine [Asendin]) may be prescribed.

When both anxiety and depression are problems, some doctors prefer using an anti-anxiety medication such as alprazolam (Xanax).

Treating Anxiety with Medication

Although many patients are somewhat anxious during exams, treatments, and other procedures, a person's anxiety sometimes may become so severe that it interferes with his ability to function, comprehend, and take an active part in what's going on.

When the anxiety is linked to acute pain, a painkiller usually helps; if it's linked to trouble with breathing, then oxygen, morphine, or a mild sedative should help. When the patient is on corticosteroids, side effects may include insomnia and signs of anxiety, in which case a tranquilizer such as Oxazepam (the trade and generic name; or Serax), Lorazepam (the trade and generic name; or Ativan), diazepam (Valium), or alprazolam (Xanax) can usually help. An anti-psychotic drug such as a haloperidol (Haldol), chlorpromazine (Thorazine), or prochlorperazine (Compazine) may be useful when

tment and recovery may be
ocusing on goals and hopes
enjoying a visit with a loved
en a full recovery may no
ntial because hope restores
ness, a peaceful, pain-free
cancer patients. Other pa-
and try experimental an-
y in which a patient with
given two weeks to live.
ormously, and in 10 days'
flew his own plane. But
active or inert, his faith
athbed. His doctor tried
ication, and the tumors
two months. Then the
few days, he was back

ing fro
eful if a
Typical Dis
of the tran-
movements.
es should be
ior to being

ers, and anti-
ause they have
s of the opioids
d in Chapter 12
nseling and psy-
in easing depres-
ic; these therapies
g while enhancing
rapy which targets
generate and main-
in Chapter 12).

OF SUICIDE

uncontrolled pain to
done to hasten their
r is it uncommon for
t, if the disease gets
ave an intense need
ver their lives—and
unicated to the pa-
Nevertheless, sui-
bout potential sui-
eat.

here ever is a time
when a disease is
h so he can "die
isted suicide, see

potential threat
hat higher risk.
totally helpless,
who experience
t suicide. Those
cal mood dis-

feelings—such as hope,
in have a powerful effect
ussed in Chapter 12, how
things to themselves, can
lves or who generalize one
ny events in their lives are
ad event in perspective; and
ion and illness. One study at
looked at a possible link be-
c or optimistic—and the activ-
found to have a greater ability,
ff disease; pessimists were found
ced immune functioning. Simi-
feel as if they have more control
r than those who feel passive and
archers have studied optimism and
lplessness, and have developed con-
ir coping skills and outlook; in other
timistic and hopeful attitude.
full recovery and many healthy and

uctive years ahead of them. Although tre
ficult, families and caregivers can help by
or the day or week—a day of no pain, a day of
one, a meal of favorite foods, and so on. Wh
longer be possible, maintaining hope is still esse
meaning to life. For those facing a terminal ill
death is not only a hope, but a reality for most
tients may find it beneficial to join a clinical tria
ticancer treatments. Doctors tell of a famous stor
huge tumors and an enlarged spleen and liver was
When given an experimental drug, he improved en
time, he was released from the hospital and even
when the patient read that the drug he took was i
waned, and in two months, he was back on his de
"a double-strength, super-refined" dose of the med
receded again, after which he was symptom-free for
man read again that the drug was "worthless." In a
on his deathbed and died soon.

PAIN, DEPRESSION, AND THOUGHTS

It is not unusual for patients with advanced cancer or
state that they wish to die, to ask that something be
death, or to talk about wanting to commit suicide. No
patients with advanced disease to want assurances tha
too bad, they will have "a way out." Many patients h
to know that, if necessary, they could have control o
deaths. Such talk should be taken seriously and comm
tient's doctor, and may even warrant professional help.
cide among cancer patients is rare. For many, talking a
cide is often more a bid to regain control than a real thre

Debate in many countries is ongoing about whether th
when the wish to die is a "rational" request, especially
terminal, painful, and the patient wishes to hasten deat
with dignity." (For a fuller discussion on suicide or ass
Chapter 15.)

While actually rare among cancer patients, suicide is a
since the symptoms of cancer put these patients at a somev
What is known is that patients who believe themselves to be
who despair at their fate, who are clinically depressed, or
unrelieved pain are many times more likely to want to commi
who have histories of major depression and other psycholo

orders (such as severe panic or anxiety disorders) as well as past drug or alcohol abuse are also at greater risk for suicidal tendencies.

Families need to be aggressive and vocal about ensuring that their loved ones are not suffering uncontrolled pain by working closely with the patient and the medical team. If pain persists, the primary doctor may recommend consultation with a pain specialist or a visit to a pain clinic (see Appendix). For the depressed patient, professional counseling may help. Often discussing the option of suicide in a calm, nonjudgmental manner may be enough to determine what is really bothering the patient the most, so it can be attended to. Often such a discussion dissipates thoughts of suicide—simply because the patient is assured that her distress is being taken seriously. If the main problem is pain or fear of pain, once it is relieved, most patients will stop talking about wanting to end their lives.

Studies of cancer patients that have actually committed suicide show that about half were suffering from major depression. And since about one-quarter of all cancer patients suffer from the symptoms of depression at one time or another, and up to 75 percent of those with advanced cancer suffer from depression, cancer patients should be considered at risk for suicide. It is essential to discuss such thoughts with the patient openly. A doctor or mental health professional can help initiate this discussion if it is too difficult for the family member.

What is most important to keep in mind is the fact that pain and depression both lead many patients to thoughts of suicide. If we manage pain and depression adequately, we will dramatically reduce the number of terminally ill patients who wish for death.

COPING WITH A TERMINAL ILLNESS

Dealing with the disability of cancer is one thing; dealing with the knowledge that you are dying is another. If a patient is terminal, he or she may experience a series of emotions, sometimes in stages, as the individual comes to terms with the realization that they are going to die. These emotions, as identified by Elizabeth Kubler Ross, are similar to those associated with other losses, such as the loss of a breast, a child, a job, and so forth. These emotions are "normal" psychological reactions that help buffer the patient temporarily from a harsh reality. Patients, and their families for that matter, need time to experience this process, and while the stages listed here are typical, each person is different. Kubler Ross outlines a pattern that is typical. Not everyone will follow these particular stages in the order listed here, and not everyone will experience each stage. One does not experience a smooth transition from one stage to another; people can get "stuck" in one or another stage. The characteristics of each stage, however, are recognizable, if not to the patient, certainly to the family.

Denial and Avoidance

Upon first learning that the cancer is terminal, the patient typically denies it to himself; he refuses to accept the reality, claiming or believing that there must be some mistake. Or he will avoid the whole issue, acting as if he didn't even hear the bad news.

Anger

Upon facing the fact that he is dying, the patient may express anger—anger that life isn't fair, that someone else who is a nasty person, perhaps, is still fine but he (the patient) is going to die; anger at God for the illness and impending death.

Depression

Depression typically follows the anger stage and is characterized by feelings of loss on all levels—loss of life and dreams, loss of family, loss of health and a positive self-image, declining self-esteem, and so on. This type of "reactive" depression is not unexpected.

Bargaining

In this stage, the patient may try to bargain with God, or whatever "Maker" the patient believes in. Bargaining is just that; the patient says I'll do this if you'll do that. For example, a patient may say to herself: "If you just let me live until my daughter's wedding, I'll be a better person. I'll go to church everyday, I'll donate more to charity." Or "If I could just live until the holidays, I'll die peacefully." Interestingly, cancer patients often make it to the important date up ahead, be it a birthday, a holiday, or a wedding. In fact, studies in Israel have found that the death rate jumps just after the Jewish High Holy Days.

Acceptance

The final stage is acceptance—a relatively peaceful state in which the patient accepts that he is going to die and is psychologically and emotionally ready to prepare for it as best he can.

No two people are the same, and we each move through or get stuck in these stages in our own unique way. While some may reach acceptance rather quickly, others may remain stuck in depression. A supportive, open environment can do much to facilitate this process.

THE TABOO OF DISCUSSING DEATH

Unfortunately, some families don't talk about dying, especially with the person who is dying. In our society, it is not uncommon for people to simply deny the existence of death. The family and the patient both act as if the patient is going to get well and live forever. These attitudes end up leaving the dying patient feeling shunned and isolated, alone at a time when he needs love and support the most. He may feel frustrated and angry inside, but unable to show it. Families that deny a dying cancer patient the opportunity to talk about his dying, or what will happen to his loved ones after he dies, are denying the patient the chance to discuss issues of vital importance to him. Some patients will need to engage in such discussions to feel more at peace as they are dying.

To some of us, perhaps to most of us, however, the act of dying forces us to face our most basic fear. For some, the dying person may stop being a person and become a symbol they fear. As a result, some of us distance ourselves from the dying at a time when a parting loved one needs us more than ever. Far more of what isn't said to a dying patient has to do with the fears that the living individuals carry.

If the family cannot cope with communicating openly about the course of the disease, they should seek the help of a hospice nurse, social worker, or other mental health professional. Of course, some patients choose not to discuss these matters. Families can help by taking any leads they hear from the patient, asking questions that encourage them to elaborate, such as "What do you mean?" "I don't know [or I don't understand]. Help me understand." Some families may be comfortable about having an experienced hospice nurse or a mental health professional try to talk to the patient about dying. At a time like this, there may be a far greater disservice done because of what isn't said than what might be said, and family members should try to bring up the subject if they can. The threat of death offers a remarkable opportunity for family members to come together and share their fears, even if they have never done this before.

FAMILY BURNOUT

At the same time the patient is experiencing a wide range of distressing emotions, families and loved ones are going through their own emotional upheaval—feeling depressed, guilty about what they could have done or can't do, worried over finances, children, and jobs, concerned over the patient's illness and disability, and in some cases, overwhelmed by impending death. These concerns, combined with the physical and emotional exhaustion of caring for someone who is ill, can take a great toll.

Families should be aware that depression in spouses of cancer patients is very common, especially among wives, among those who are less satisfied with their marriages, and among those whose spouse expresses anger or report pain. Studies show that 20 to 50 percent of spouses report symptoms of depression and feelings of helplessness. Interestingly, however, a spouse's symptoms of depression do not seem linked to the patient's feelings of depression and disability.

It is important for caregivers to continue their own lives, to give themselves breathing space to do what they enjoy—to go to a movie, exercise, visit friends. If the patient declines, it may become increasingly difficult for caregivers to sustain their constant care and vigilance. (See Chapter 15 for discussions about home and hospice care.) Families may consider seeking further help from the health-care team to step up interventions with medications for pain, shortness of breath, nausea, and other distressing symptoms. And as they shift their attention from feelings of helplessness, to activities that focus on making their loved one as comfortable and as free of pain as possible, families may feel more empowered. Ensuring that the loved one has a "comfortable death" is a major victory; fretting about the past or the future takes on less importance when the focus is on the present.

Families may also find themselves experiencing *anticipatory grief*, which means experiencing symptoms of grief even before death occurs. In fact, sometimes the living may go through the grieving process so effectively that they emotionally prepare themselves before the death occurs. If family members find they are detaching themselves from their loved ones, they may wish to discuss these feelings with other family members, a hospice nurse, or a professional counselor.

TENDING TO THE SPIRIT

Whether religion is involved or not, humans throughout the ages have thought of themselves as being more than mind and body. That third dimension is often referred to as spirit. Most of this book has addressed the body and changes that may occur with cancer. We have also discussed the mind as we have tried to broaden our concept of pain to include the larger concept of suffering, which encompasses more than pain and takes into consideration the powerful interplay between the mind and the body: how depression or anxiety can exacerbate pain and further debilitate the body; how distraction and relaxation techniques can use the mind to calm the body; how a loving hand and caring concern can ease the suffering and soothe the pain.

The Spiritual Dimension of Being Human

The spiritual dimension is that characteristic of our lives that many philosophers define as the essence of being human. Whether they have led a traditionally religious life or not, patients and family members often find themselves exploring these questions from a new perspective when dealing with a life-threatening illness. When a person is facing impending death, one becomes acutely aware of the finite nature of one's life, one's vulnerability, one's temporal existence. It may be a terrifying realm that we spend our lives avoiding, a terrain that we have built walls around and have not crossed. Or it may be a source of calm, comfort, and peace—a coming "home" or a completion of a well-spent life. In considering our mortality and humanity, especially when death seems near, we may ponder issues of meaning, values, unity, and how we humans connect with that which is greater than ourselves—be it nature and its harmony, the universal mind, or God.

Many religious traditions embrace this stage of life as a reminder that we are not alone. In death, we lose our separateness and become part of a greater whole—perhaps through worship, ceremony, song, or dance. A sense of unity and oneness may free our selves, our spirit, to be truly human. This may be unfamiliar territory to some, even to those with deep religious beliefs; death offers us the opportunity to explore these questions and approach life in new ways. When the time comes, let us hope we will be a willing partner in such explorations.

CARING FOR THE WHOLE PERSON

Dr. Balfour Mount, professor of surgery, surgical oncologist, founder of the first hospital-based inpatient/outpatient hospice program in the world, and director of the palliative care unit at McGill University, talks about addressing the whole person—looking beyond the patient's physical needs and psychosocial needs. Mount suggests that we need to understand all the dimensions of an individual's "personhood" and refers to the model proposed by Eric Cassell, an internist and humanist at Cornell University Medical College and author of *The Nature of Suffering*. Cassell views human nature as having many domains—personality, character, a past, roles with others, views of life, an unconscious life, a secret life, perceived future, and a physical body. Humans also have what Cassell calls the transcendent dimension—the need to identify with what is larger than ourselves.

"Who Are We?"

Spoken or not, this is an example of the kind of question that comes up for people who find themselves seeking meaning in their life as it draws to a close. Since it is a question without a simple and obvious answer, engaging in an exploration of all it implies may have unexpected and beneficial results.

Regrettably, contemporary society emphasizes the physical—the superficial—you. Think of all the commercials that emphasize looking good. The implicit message is that "you are your body and your image." But obviously, a person's core goes beyond image.

When an illness results in some physical decline, it doesn't take too much time to begin to reject this superficial notion—the internal dialogue may go something like: "If I am my body—if that is what defines me—how come even though my body's not working so well right now, I still feel like me. . . . There must be something more." Well, perhaps what we are is a mind—that as long as we're still thinking straight and clearly, our loved ones will identify the person they have known and loved as being intact. Over time, most people will also reject this notion as being far too simple. Just think back to a time spent with a loved one who is now no longer as sharp as she once was. Perhaps she is now forgetful or unable to follow a conversation quite as well. And yet there is a sense that the person you knew and loved is still before you—changed perhaps in some ways, but at least from one perspective, in ways that are not important enough to detract from her personhood. Recognition of a human being as something more than a body and mind is what keeps us loving each other during the aging process—often loving more profoundly, even though the body and mind become less fit. It can be argued that one of the ways to establish meaning in the face of serious illness is to work at continuing to relate to the component of the person that is more than just his or her body or mind.

Caregivers who view the patient as a whole person will consider these varied domains of personhood and how the illness affects, or doesn't affect, each one. They can help the patient transcend the illness by exploring the larger picture—the sources of meaning in life and of the larger human family.

As the body deteriorates, eroding a person's mastery and control over his life, his independence, and autonomy, more and more power is given up to others. As the body changes and our abilities to smile, laugh, touch, or gesture diminish, the way the world sees us and how we relate to those closest to us change as well.

The Search for Grace

In embracing the whole person and acknowledging the reality of progressive and inevitable physical decline, the caregiver may help the person transcend the body and embrace a dimension of grace. Balfour Mount talks about giving the person an opportunity to express her unique essence, the core of her personhood, by focusing on the person's "otherness." By doing so, one can avoid depersonalizing the person whose body and face may sometimes become almost unrecognizable. There's no one right way of approaching this opportunity, and, in fact, loving intention is often enough. Just consciously focusing one's attention on all the domains of the person will go a long way. The person may have lost her roles, but she has not lost the essence of her selfhood, which makes her unique.

What can help her express that selfhood? Perhaps a discussion of the meaning of life, and what that person's creations and accomplishments have been. Or perhaps expressing to that person how grateful others are to have been her children, friend, co-worker, will awaken the dignity and integrity of one close to death. Or mentioning how things learned from her will be passed on to grandchildren, or students, will make her feel her work lives on beyond her own life. Mount suggests asking about the places, people, music, things, and ideas that the patient has loved; of keying into the person's memory to recall a life of purpose and involvement, to talk about what hopes can be shared that day.

To help the patient talk about the meaning of his life, the listener might also ask the patient questions about his childhood, turning points in his career, the most exciting and the best of times, the worst and the hardest of times, as well as lessons that he learned along the way and would want to pass on, or the best and worst things he ever did. Would he change anything about his life or past? Does he need to forgive himself or others for things that have been said or done in the past? What is the hardest thing now or the longest part of the day now? What does he think about most these days? Can he talk about what he feels about what is happening to him now? Is there unfinished business with loved ones, with God, with himself?

"To see that hope is not the way out, it's the way through," is for Mount a healing lesson. He continues: "The healing of spirit may be accompanied by an awareness of quietness, a sense of solidity, a broadness, a security or a sense of being held. . . . The most and the least we can do is to accompany them [the dying] on their journey."

15
If Death Approaches

How people die remains in the memories of those who live on.
Cicely Saunders, founder of the hospice movement

There may come a time when most patients and their families start doubting the benefits of further treatment or intervention, wondering whether it will do more harm than good. At some point, it may be necessary to accept the fact that the cancer can no longer be treated or arrested, and that a loved one is dying. If so, this is an appropriate time for the family or other loved ones to shift their focus from trying to beat the cancer, from hoping for a cure or prolongation of life, to doing what they can to enhance the quality of life for whatever precious time is left. The overriding goal becomes trying to free the patient from discomfort and pain. Called *palliative care*, the objective of this phase of treatment is to make the patient as comfortable as possible and to satisfy his physical, psychological, emotional, and spiritual needs.

DECIDING WHEN TREATMENT SHOULD BE TERMINATED

When treating patients, doctors work from the basic premise that treatments ideally should do good and preserve life while doing no harm. In almost all cases, though, medical treatment that has the potential to benefit the patient also has some potential to do harm, by way of side effects or complications. As a result, doctors must constantly balance the potential for benefit versus risk in all their treatment recommendations. Often, in patients with cancer, there comes a point when conventional medical intervention is clearly more likely to be toxic than beneficial.

Deciding when this time has come, however, can be difficult. Ideally, this decision should be made jointly by the treatment team, patient, and family. Although many doctors recognize this stage and will tell family members that they may be at that critical turning point, other doctors may not; they may continue to treat the illness, assuming that is what the patient wants. Jerry, a 65-year-old man with advanced lung cancer, for example, had a prognosis of only several weeks left to live. Perhaps not wanting to admit failure or to let the patient and family down, his doctor ordered a CAT scan, spinal tap, and daily radiation treatments. Knowing in their hearts that Jerry was very ill, and not wanting his last days to be occupied with tiring and uncomfortable treatments that seemed unlikely to help, the family initiated a dialogue with the doctor. All were able to agree that the kindest and most humane approach would be to stop all treatment, except that specifically directed at keeping Jerry comfortable.

There is often no clear-cut point at which to know when further therapy will no longer be useful. Along the way, families may be confronted with many difficult decisions about the care of their loved ones. These may include whether or not to initiate palliative (noncurative) radiotherapy or chemotherapy, blood transfusions, platelet transfusions, antibiotic therapy, intravenous feeding, and so on. Often each decision is difficult, with no accepted and clear guidelines. The potential benefits versus the potential risks of each of these treatments are different for each person and will depend on the medical details of each case, which can best be explained by the patient's doctor, sometimes at a family meeting. Although the details of each of these treatments are beyond the scope of this book, discussing the principles that underlie these decisions is important in a book on pain.

The key questions, again, are how will the proposed therapy be likely to help, and how might it hurt. Determine whether a treatment option has a chance of producing cure, in which case the patient and family may be willing to make extreme sacrifices for even a small chance at beating the cancer. Very often, however, if initial treatments have failed to produce a cure, the new treatment options will only offer, at best, a hope that the tumor will shrink, its growth will be slowed, or its symptoms will be minimized. These are the harder decisions that the patient, family, or other caregivers along with the doctor must explore together. To make the most well-informed decision or to be better prepared for discussion with physicians, many consumers pursue some independent reading or research. (See Appendix for where to look for additional sources of information.)

The primary question is: What is the good that the treatment is trying to achieve? We have already discussed the easiest scenario about which to make a decision—when the goal is to cure the cancer. But what about treatments that are intended to prolong life without the hope of cure?

At this stage of the disease, the main questions to consider are:

- What is the chance that the disease process will be slowed and life will be prolonged?
- If life is prolonged, is this likely to be for a matter of days, weeks, or months?

- How likely is it that side effects will accompany the treatment, and what will their impact be on the time that remains?

Usually, the answers to these questions are neither certain nor simple, especially when the patient is reasonably fit and getting around well. When patients become more ill and house-bound, it is easier to see how each new treatment or test takes more and more out of them, and making decisions with them about what treatments to pursue may become more clear-cut. If curing the cancer is an unrealistic goal, then the value of each treatment option is assessed, and based on how it may impact the patient's comfort and quality of life. With advanced cancer, for example, generally even simple diagnostic tests (chest X-rays, blood tests, CAT scans, etc.) are avoided unless the results are likely to change the treatment plan.

Even when the patient, loved ones, and physician all agree that conventional therapies are likely to be useless, some patients and families may want to explore experimental drugs and procedures, if they haven't already done so. If so, ask the doctor to discuss referral to a major cancer center where experimental treatments are offered. If seeking unconventional or unorthodox therapies, discuss them with the doctor and keep him informed about decisions.

When it is decided that no further anti-cancer treatments will be pursued, stay focused on how best to ensure that the loved one will remain as comfortable as possible.

THE HOSPICE CONCEPT

From its inception in England in 1967, acceptance of the hospice movement has mushroomed in this country in just the past two decades. Its goal: to promote and support a comfortable, dignified life and death during terminal illness.

The word itself—hospice—is used somewhat as a catchall term to describe either a homelike, inpatient facility staffed by palliative care experts, or community health organizations that use the same expertise to help families with dying loved ones at home. Much more than a setting where care is rendered, though, hospice is not really a place but a philosophy.

The basis of hospice is comfort care devoted to relieving pain and the physical, emotional, social, and spiritual suffering of both the patient and family unit, without an emphasis on trying to cure the cancer or prolong life. The goals of hospice care, no matter where it is based (at home or in an inpatient unit), are to help the dying and their loved ones maintain control over their lives and avoid feelings of isolation, to help promote open communication and coping strategies at the approach of death, and to provide support and information about state-of-the-art techniques that ensure that the patient remains as pain- and symptom-free as is possible.

DYING AT HOME

As a loved one moves into the terminal phase of his illness, the family or other companions will have to decide where the final days would ideally be spent. The choices include a hospital (in which case insurance companies may limit how long they will pay for chronically ill patients to remain hospitalized), a nursing home or other long-term skilled-care facility (for which "placements" may be difficult to arrange), a residential hospice (which are still relatively rare), or at home. By far the majority of patients prefer to spend their remaining days around loved ones in the comforts of their own home. It so happens that the U.S. health-care system is currently organized in a way that makes this option the easiest, and hospitalization or institutionalization care difficult to arrange and often impractical. In England, on the other hand, hospice has developed in large part as an institutional service—as a place where people go to stay during the final phase of their illness. In the United States, individuals with advanced cancer can stay at home and still receive almost all hospital services that are intended to maintain comfort. Some communities have small "backup" units in their hospitals to allow for short stays when they are needed to stabilize a terminal patient or provide familial rest.

At home, patients are in familiar surroundings where they and their caregivers can enjoy their privacy and maintain greater autonomy than that afforded in a hospital. Home care allows the family to more gradually adjust to the fact that the person is dying and usually reduces stress since their daily routine of having visitors, cooking, shopping, watching TV, and so forth, can be maintained. It avoids constant visits to a hospital room, where visitors may sit around for hours, feeling helpless and useless. Dying at home allows family members and loved ones to actively help in the care of the patient. Some experts maintain that family members who actively help with caring for patients dying at home experience less guilt and even less grieving after the death than when a family member dies in the hospital. Dying at home also means there's a far greater chance that a family member will be present at the actual moment of death.

Families that hope to keep their loved ones at home will need to be provided with certain specialized resources and support, so they are adequately prepared for various eventualities. Caring for an ill family member requires tremendous energy, attention, and loving care. It can at times be stressful, exhausting, and difficult, because the patient's condition may change rapidly and small emergencies may arise unexpectedly. Caregivers must be able to help with the patient's daily activities, including bathing, feeding, toilet care, medication, pain relief, and so on. And since most patients need full-time care, more than one caregiver is often necessary to assure that the primary caregiver is adequately rested.

Although all this may sound like a terrifying challenge, especially for someone who is not a nurse or doctor, countless people have done it and frequently have found it to be a rewarding and gratifying experience. With good support and preparation, family members or other loving caregivers are able to provide such care in most cases.

While coping with the patient's fragile emotional and physical condition, caregivers are also trying to handle their own grief, anxiety, and depression. It is very common during these times for family members to neglect themselves as they become absorbed in the job of doing all they can for the patient. They need to be reminded that, if they don't tend to their own needs, they will ultimately be letting the patient down, for the patient would never have wanted them to neglect themselves.

More and more, insurance companies, including Medicare, will provide funds to support at-home or hospice-centered care. Some will even cover part of the costs of community, hospital, or home health-care units which provide palliative care for the dying. More and more, experienced professionals are available to help families ensure that the dying process be as peaceful and as free of pain as possible.

Families who will be caring for their loved one at home need to consider and address the following issues:

- How is the disease expected to progress; what type of symptoms might occur?
- What kind of support services are available? Who will be the main medical professional with whom the family can have frequent contact, and who will respond to the patient's needs? Are there also hospice nurses or other professionals available? Mental health professionals or clergy to discuss emotional matters? Home health aides to help bathe and care for the patient? Respite workers to relieve the caregiver? How much of these services will insurance cover?
- Is there 24-hour help available by phone or available to visit the patient at home? Is there an inpatient "backup" unit available if things ever seem overwhelming?
- What kinds of equipment should be considered and when—walker, wheelchair, bed cushions, commode, pump for pain medication, hospital bed, etc.? What can be rented rather than purchased? What is covered by insurance? Are there programs sponsored by the local chap-

ter of the American Cancer Society or a community church or syn-
agogue that offer this equipment on loan if required?

- Who will help teach the family how to provide hands-on care for the
patient and answer practical, day-to-day questions—for example, how
to move or bathe the patient, how to administer or change pain medication, and so forth?
- What is likely to happen as the patient's condition worsens? Is the family member or caregiver emotionally and physically prepared to cope?
Although usually not necessary, some families may consider using a supplemental private nurse at times to help out if they can afford the service.
- Does the family wish to consider making advance arrangements with a
funeral home to come to the home when needed?

If such resources are in place, caring for a dying loved one will not seem
so overwhelming or formidable, but part of the natural cycle of loving,
living, and dying.

DYING IN A HOSPITAL OR CARE FACILITY

Many families do not have the emotional or physical stamina, or the other
necessary resources, required to care for a dying person. Many patients
have no reliable caregiver available to them at home, and some patients
don't want to die at home—they don't want to be a burden to their family,
they may not have confidence that the family can cope well, or they may
feel the family will be unable to provide the services needed. Others may
feel that, in their deteriorated condition, they do not want to be cared for
or treated by the family.

Trying to deal with these sorts of issues can be difficult for both the
patient and family. The family may feel guilty or inadequate because they
are not up to the challenge of caring for a loved one at home. A patient, on
the other hand, may fear hurting loved ones if he spurns offers of home
care. These and related problems can all be discussed with a hospital social
worker who is specially trained to help families work through such difficult
issues.

If it is decided that the patient may be better off in a hospital or long-
term care facility, find out if there are any residential hospices or palliative
care units at a nearby hospital or long-term skilled-care facility. What are
their financial requirements? Many insurance plans will help pay for such
care. Again, hospital social workers will know what the options are, including being able to identify doctors who are experienced in palliative care who
can supervise a placement.

There is no "right answer" for everyone. While home care may be ideal for some, hospitalization may be the most appropriate for others. A combination of the two is also very common, with the patient hospitalized briefly during stressful times but the primary care setting being the patient's home.

LIVING WILLS, "DO NOT RESCUCITATE," AND "NO CODE" STATUS

In recent years, legislation has increasingly acknowledged patients' rights to exert control over health-care decisions, including the right to refuse unwanted or invasive medical intervention. These rights are most commonly honored by means of living wills or "do-not-resuscitate" (DNR) orders, or both. Many states acknowledge the legality of living wills and allow patients to choose a "health proxy," a person who can make such decisions in the event that the patient cannot.

Living wills spell out the desires of the patient to accept and to refuse certain medical interventions, such as feeding tubes, respirators, or cardiac resuscitation when hopes for a cure or quality long-term survival are futile. A DNR order is also a legal document that permits doctors and health-care professionals to no longer try to resuscitate a patient in crisis. After all, resuscitating a patient is very painful and intrusive, and while it is justified when there is an optimistic prognosis, it usually is not justified in the terminally ill.

Although the public has lobbied and demanded that these rights be available to patients, most people (well or not) still do not have such paperwork in order. Most health-care and legal and ethical experts strongly urge consumers, whether ill or not, to discuss these issues as early as possible and to keep the appropriate documents both at home and in the hands of the primary doctor. Being prepared with such documentation is like wearing a seat belt—you never know when you'll need it. (See the Appendix on where to get more information on the living will and the DNR order.)

ETHICS OF PAIN CONTROL

Toward the end of life, patients may experience severe pain. In some cases, adequately treating that pain may hasten the patient's already imminent death. Many families, with the patient's prior permission, believe that being free of pain is the highest priority at this time, even if it means the patient may be sleepier or weaker as a result. Using adequate doses of painkillers in a patient who is already severely weakened by illness, however, is *not* the same as overdosing a patient and certainly has nothing to do with suicide or euthanasia. As the World Health Organization asserts: "Any hastening of death that is linked to adequate pain control measures simply means that

DIFFICULT DECISIONS

If the end is appearing to draw near, families may need to tackle some very difficult decisions: At what point should the patient no longer be strongly encouraged to take medications or to eat? Should a feeding tube or intravenous tubes be considered?

Ideally, families have discussed these difficult issues with the patient before these decisions must be made. Yet these conversations are difficult because they are about uncomfortable topics; as a result, many families put them off. To allow a terminally ill person to die peacefully, families may choose to withhold or to stop interventions such as respiratory support, chemotherapy, surgery, and assisted nutrition. The physician's team is accustomed to these situations and should be regarded as an essential source of guidance, support, and information.

In considering these decisions, you may wish to consider these generally accepted guidelines:

Follow the patient's desires. When possible, families should know ahead of time what their loved one would desire if such decisions ever have to be made.

When to simplify medications. At some point, taking medication for a chronic medical condition, like high blood pressure or mild diabetes, may be more painful or uncomfortable for the patient than it is worth. Families should be attentive to the patient's refusals to comply or cooperate with medication schedules. With the advice of their physician, families will need to assess when may be the right time to simplify medications, maintaining only those absolutely necessary to make the patient comfortable.

Is the treatment prolonging life or prolonging death? Is the proposed treatment (the use of a respirator and the feeding tube are common examples) enhancing the person's life or merely prolonging the process of dying? Will the patient's suffering be eased by the intervention or be prolonged by it?

Again, these tough decisions need not be made alone. Physicians, nurses, and other health-care providers, clergy, and hospital ethicists have experience with them and can help.

Allowing a body that is riddled with cancer to die is a far cry from suicide or murder, even if it means refusing treatments or intervention. Instead, it is an acceptance of a fact of life—that we all die, and that we have the right to choose how we die, with whatever kind of dignity and self-determination we choose.

Feeding tubes and intravenous liquids are rarely needed. As a person's body begins to shut down—that is, begins to actively die—it is common for the patient to dramatically cut down on food and drink. Sometimes the tastes or smells of even favorite foods become unpleasant; others find it too painful to have food in their mouths or can't swallow easily. Some are too nauseated to eat. Caregivers may find themselves constantly concerned about trying different ways to get the patient to take small amounts of liquids or food—perhaps by only offering liquid food, by medicating mouth sores with a local anesthetic, offering medication for nausea, offering food through a straw, offering liquids by squirting it into the patient's mouth, offering little sponge pops, or allowing the patient to suck on a water-soaked washcloth. As discussed in Chapter 11, we feed those dear to us to show our love— sometimes even when they need love more than food.

As the body stops digesting and processing food, there may come a time when the patient cannot take any nourishment or water. Should patients be given liquids through intravenous means? Most hospitals routinely take this approach, while it is not customary practice for patients being cared for at home. Many doctors feel that intravenous infusions should be avoided if at all possible in patients with advanced cancer. Although they may make the family feel better that "something is being done," many doctors assert that such intravenous nutrition may merely "feed the tumor," that the tubes are uncomfortable, and that dehydration is not an uncomfortable state for dying patients. In fact, a survey (from the University of South Florida and Villanova University) of 212 hospice physicians reported that 86 percent of the doctors felt that it was more comfortable for patients to no longer have hydration (liquids) and nutrition toward the end of life; 11 percent were unsure. Other studies have shown that providing intravenous fluids does not prolong life, and authorities agree that this practice usually only makes patients more uncomfortable. When hydration is pursued too vigorously, symptoms may get worse—a dry cough may become congested or a patient may need to get up more frequently to urinate, which may aggravate pain. It is recommended, instead, to simply keep the mouth moist with the methods already mentioned, to stave off thirst (see Chapter 11). Whether intravenous infusions are to be used is one of the many management decisions the physician, patient, and family will need to make.

SEDATING THE DYING PATIENT IS RARELY NEEDED

Studies show that a small proportion of cancer patients may need sedation in their final days to relieve their physical suffering—which may include pain, shortness of breath, nausea, and for some delirium. The sedation calms patients and permits them to rest. Using barbituates such as amobarbital (Amytal), Nebutal, or Seconal occasionally becomes necessary to relieve unendurable and uncontrollable symptoms. Families may wish to discuss their views on sedation, especially if the person has only several hours or days, and if he or she is obviously distressed and uncomfortable. If doctors have done all they can to relieve the distress, sedation may be an appropriate step.

Although some doctors report that about half their patients lose consciousness before death, and that sedating drugs may contribute to this result, they emphasize that losing consciousness is usually the result of the many impacts that advanced cancer has on the brain and body rather than just an effect of medications used to relieve pain and promote comfort.

"RATIONAL" AND ASSISTED SUICIDE

In recent years, discussions about whether physician-assisted suicide or even socially approved euthanasia should ever be permitted have become more prominent public issues. Dr. Jack Kevorkian, the retired pathologist who has helped several terminally ill patients die, brought the issue of doctor-assisted suicide to national attention in 1989 and 1990, and it's been hotly debated ever since. And in 1992, Derek Humphries' book *Final Exit* became a national bestseller with its complete instructions for how to commit a suicide without the help of a doctor.

But there is a great deal more to the argument than the either-or choices with which the debate is usually framed. Unfortunately, we now view assisted suicide, suicide, and euthanasia as one option; our loved ones left to suffer a prolonged and agonizing death as the other. But there is a large middle ground that offers a humane and scientific approach, and it is the premise of this book: patients need *not* suffer in pain and agony; modern pain management tools are available that can ease and perhaps totally eliminate the physical pain and suffering many still endure today. In tandem with psychological support and counseling to manage anxiety and depression, patients can be in the last stages of disease and be free of pain and depression—the two primary causes of suicide in patients. Today, it is unthinkable that patients may beg to die because of their pain or depression. As the former director of the National Institute on Drug Abuse has said (which we have already quoted in Chapter 1), "No patient should wish for death because of our failure to use properly our strongest weapons against pain." Once pain and depression are treated properly, the desire to hasten death diminishes, as the quality of life improves. This is a realistic goal for every cancer patient.

In the meantime, as this debate rages on, health-care providers are legally restricted from engaging in any medical practice that is specifically intended to shorten a patient's life. If thoughts of assisted suicide have been voiced by a patient, most health-care providers will listen with a sympathetic ear, but because of these legal and ethical concerns, they are unlikely to take any direct action. If this is an issue, however, it is very important to *tell the health team,* because it sends an important signal to the team that something is *very* wrong. Such a discussion may offer an opportunity to determine the underlying problems that make the continuation of life seem intolerable; only then can these problems be effectively addressed. After such a conversation, the team may pursue more aggressive management of pain and other symptoms, seek additional support for caregivers at home, recommend consultation with a social worker, clergy, pain specialist, or psychiatrist, or whatever seems to be needed. Suicidal thoughts, however, are a clear indication to the family to make absolutely certain that "do-not-resuscitate" orders have been instituted so that unnecessary suffering will not be prolonged.

In the near future, however, the climate for treating terminal illness may change. In November 1992, several prominent physicians from leading medical schools wrote in the *New England Journal of Medicine* (November 5, 1992) to urge doctors and lawyers to develop a public policy that would acknowledge the "irreversible suffering" of "competent patients who met carefully defined criteria." Those doctors, among others, have established the following criteria for so-called rational suicide or doctor-assisted suicide.

The criteria include the following questions:

- Does the patient clearly suffer from an incurable condition and is likely to experience severe and unrelenting suffering?
- Is the patient receiving appropriate medication for their suffering; are they benefitting from the best that science has to offer in relieving their suffering?
- Is the patient lucid and alert, with no psychological illness or severe emotional problems, including depression?
- Does the patient have a realistic and accurate view of the situation? Has he or she clearly and continually asked for suicide to avoid suffering? Efforts should be made to avoid having to force the patient to beg.
- Would even uninvolved outsiders view the patient's desires as understandable? Can the patient's physician agree that the situation is hopeless and the patient likely to suffer severely? Can an uninvolved second opinion concur and the three (patient and two doctors) sign a document of informed consent?

Those who endorse assisted suicide under these conditions assert that the patient should not be abandoned at the time of death, and that if an overdose is prescribed, that the physician be present at the time the patient takes the overdose. It is tragic, many assert, that terminally ill patients are so often forced to die alone because they are fearful they would place their families or caregivers in legal jeopardy if they were present.

THE WORLD HEALTH ORGANIZATION'S
GUIDELINES ON EUTHANASIA

When patients are not lucid and competent, some families wonder whether to take a more active role. Should they wait for death passively, or should they help promote a less painful, quicker death? What is humane? What is the right thing to do? These are difficult questions, perhaps the most difficult decisions anyone will have to make in their lives, and families that have discussed these issues beforehand will have an easier time. The World Health Organization's Expert Committee on these matters has drawn up the following guidelines:

- It is ethically justifiable to withhold or discontinue life-support interventions when, as desired by the patient, doctors cannot reverse the dying process and instead merely prolong it.
- Painkillers and other drugs should be used in whatever doses are needed to relieve pain and discomfort, even if that means shortening the patient's life.
- Family members can make these decisions when the patient is unconscious, incompetent, or can no longer make these decisions himself.

These issues are difficult ones, and a fuller discussion of them is beyond the scope of this book. Readers may wish to seek more information on these issues, and several books are suggested in the box on this page.

AS DEATH APPROACHES: WHAT TO EXPECT
AND HOW TO HELP

Just as every birth is dramatically different, so is every death. In listing the following symptoms, we are not suggesting that most patients will experience them. Some patients will experience only a few. Nevertheless, we list them here as a means to prepare the family or to help them cope should these symptoms occur. Some of these symptoms are discussed in more detail in other sections of the book, particularly Chapter 11.

Further Reading on Issues Related to Assisted Suicide

Death and Dignity: Making Choices and Taking Charge by Timothy E. Quill, M.D. (New York: Norton, 1993).
Final Passages: Positive Choices for the Dying and Their Loved Ones by Judith Ahronheim, M.D., and Doron Weber (New York: Simon & Schuster, 1992).
Easing the Passage by David E. Outerbridge and Alan R. Hersh, M.D. (New York: Harper Perennial, 1991).

Dehydration

Many patients become dehydrated and may experience thirst, low blood pressure, drowsiness, confusion, weakness, and perhaps even coma. Yet many doctors assert that the condition of dehydration is not uncomfortable for the patient as long as the mouth is kept moist; in fact, some conditions such as breathlessness, cough, urinary incontinence, and pain may be relieved when water intake is reduced.

Nausea

As discussed more fully in Chapter 10, anti-nausea medication is very effective. If the patient cannot swallow easily, it may be administered rectally, through a skin patch, or by injection.

Difficulty Swallowing

Do not force any liquids or foods. If swallowing is very difficult, small amounts of liquids may be given with an eye dropper or from a wet washcloth that the patient sucks. When swallowing is difficult, make sure all medications are administered in ways other than by mouth (subcutaneously, rectally, etc.).

Confusion, Restlessness, Agitation, and Delirium

If patients seem confused, restless, agitated, or delirious, the family may wish to consult with a member of the health team. Patients will need to be reassured if they become confused. Close (even constant) supervision is preferable to the use of "restraints," although these may sometimes be necessary to remind the patient to avoid pulling at dressings and other equipment. If symptoms persist, haloperidol or other anti-psychotic medications can calm a patient; benzodiazepines are helpful for the restless and agitated patient, particularly to promote sleep and rest. Drugs may be administered in the mouth through eye droppers next to the patient's cheek (when patients can no longer swallow) or through subcutaneous pumps.

Shortness of Breath

Breathlessness is a common symptom, often made worse by panic. Patients should be sat up and reassured. Allowing cool air into the room, either through an open window, with air conditioning, or with a fan can offer relief. Cool air directly into the nose can also help. Doctors may change the morphine levels (usually upward) to relieve the shortness of breath or may prescribe a benzodiazepine, such as Xanax.

Incontinence

Catheters, tubes which directly empty the bladder through the urethra, can collect urine directly into a bag. If the patient is very close to death, however, and incontinence is a new problem, catheters may be avoided. Patients may well expel so little urine that an underpad on the bed may be sufficient. Males may use an external catheter or urine bed pan; females may be given a pad in their underwear. Sometimes, patients may have stools they can't expel—a suppository, enema, or the removal with rubber-gloved hands can deal effectively with the problem.

Muscle Twitching or Jerking

These involuntary movements may be due to a variety of causes, including high doses of pain medications. Although their appearance may be disturbing, they usually are not uncomfortable for the patient. The administration of a benzodiazepine can often relieve the twitching.

Noisy, Wet Breathing

About half of cancer patients begin to breathe noisily in the last few days of life usually due to accumulations of mucus in the back of the throat. Although not particularly distressing to the patient, the noisy breathing may be hard for the family and caregivers to endure. A drug such as scopolamine (hyoscine in Britain) usually can relieve the symptom, especially if the throat has been cleared first. Changing the patient's position and reassuring him may also help. Suctioning, usually an unpleasant event, is rarely necessary.

Sweating and Feeling Hot

In addition to a fan, steroids, aceteminophen, or an NSAID can usually help if sweating is unpleasant and uncomfortable. Bed linens may need to be changed more often to ensure the patient's comfort, assuming that doing so is not too painful for the patient.

Pain

Studies show that pain usually does not suddenly escalate near death. Pain, of course, may fluctuate at any time, but usually once intense pain has been relieved, most patients can be sustained at a relatively steady level of pain medication until death. Nevertheless, patients and families should have access to extra or "escape" doses of narcotics which they can administer as needed. Even if they never need to use them, having them available (like a seat belt) will help ease anxiety for the family.

WHEN DEATH IS VERY CLOSE

Although deaths vary widely as do individuals, the following are some signs and suggestions for when death draws very close:

- Stay with the patient—if at home, a baby monitor may be used so the caregivers can hear when the patient is awake, and sit with him. Just the presence of another person helps the dying person be less apprehensive. Touching or holding the patient can do a lot to diminish feelings of fear, loneliness, and despair.
- Patients may need to be encouraged to turn frequently to prevent too much pressure on the same spot. Patients who are weak or unresponsive will need to be turned by their caregivers.
- Fingertips and toes develop a bluish hue as circulation slows down; the skin on the arms and legs may feel cool to the touch. If tolerated, keep the patient covered with a sheet or light blanket.
- The person may sleep more or may be unresponsive.
- Intermittently, the person may become very confused about where he is, who the people are around him, and why things are happening. He may become agitated and may hallucinate about people and places. Calmly explaining to the patient that the disease is doing this to him, that he's not going crazy, and that his family and loved ones are close by is reassuring.
- Although the dying person can usually continue to hear well, sometimes vision gradually fails. Keep the patient turned toward the light with people close by, near the patient's head. Even if you are uncertain whether the patient can hear you, speak as if he or she is listening; talk to the patient as if he or she can understand every word, and don't say anything that the patient shouldn't hear.
- Urine may darken, and at times, the patient may lack control of his bladder or bowel. Underpads for the bed can be purchased in drugstores and may be placed under the patient; they will absorb any wastes and can be easily replaced.
- Mucus may accumulate in the back of the throat, causing noisy breathing or even choking. Keeping the patient's head elevated on several pillows and turned to the side may help, but be prepared to either clear mucus with a washcloth or suction tube, or to do nothing.
- Keep the mouth moist with a sponge stick, which is available from

nurses, a wet washcloth (allowing the patient to suck on it), or ice chips. If it doesn't startle the patient, a straw can be used to gently place several drops of water on the patient's lips or in the mouth. Cotton swabs dipped in olive oil can be used to moisten the tongue. Do not force anything in the mouth.

- When death is very close, breathing may seem delayed or irregular; and the patient may make rattling noises in the back of the throat. If distressing, the physician may prescribe scopolamine (hyoscine in Britain).

During this time, caregivers may wish to play soothing music and have soft light in the room. Remain close to the patient, speaking reassuringly that loved ones are close by, that the patient should try to relax, and should not be afraid. Holding a hand and talking softly can be reassuring for the dying patient. Make sure the patient is not in pain, and if in doubt, administer "escape" doses of pain medication according to your doctor's instructions. It is better to err by overmedicating than by undermedicating.

GRIEF

After a loved one dies, a sense of relief that the ordeal is over may occur, which is often coupled by feelings of guilt for having that relief. Things may seem more bearable just after a death occurs, because there is so much to do and many relatives and friends are around the household. Although sometimes a very delayed response may occur, characteristically grief soon washes over the lives of survivors.

People experiencing grief may feel just about anything, from mild pangs to severe, deep upset—even of a physical nature. There is no "right" way to grieve, or "right" schedule. It is one of the most personal of events. The following reactions occur commonly, and although unpleasant or even intolerable, are relatively normal.

- Mental pain and tension
- The need to sigh
- Empty feeling in the pit of the stomach
- Frequent crying spells
- Muscular weakness and fatigue or exhaustion
- Tightness in the throat
- A choking feeling with shortness of breath
- A feeling of being "removed" from one's own body
- Waves of physical distress often lasting 20 minutes to an hour

Those who are grieving sometimes experience a sense of unreality or feel emotionally distant from others. Crying should be encouraged to relieve stress. Sometimes, those grieving are preoccupied with visions of the dead person, or are plagued by feelings of guilt—that they could have done better for the person who died, that they were somehow inadequate, even negligent or inattentive. When a person is experiencing such feelings of guilt, they may be irritable and seem angry with others, emotionally pushing them away even at a time when others come to sympathize or make a special effort to connect. Other features of grieving include restlessness, feelings of aimlessness, hostility, passiveness in actually doing anything or taking action, and an almost neurotic desire to stick to their usual routines even when all zest and vitality are sapped from them. Patients experiencing more exaggerated responses to grief may begin to take on personality traits or idiosyncrasies of the deceased—walking or talking like him, picking up a special interest of his, enshrining the deceased, and so on.

Working through these feelings has been characterized by some as "grief work." Goals of this work include:

- Freeing the living from feeling in bondage to the dead person
- Adapting to the environment without the deceased person
- Forming new relationships and moving ahead with life

However, part of the process of grief work is to express pent-up emotions that many of the bereaved try to avoid at all costs in order to minimize distress. They may stay tense and tight, as a way to prevent "breaking down," and may react with hostility to those who mention the dead person. People grieving in this way need to be helped and should be encouraged to accept the distress of active grief, which allows the one feeling "left behind" to move forward.

BEYOND NORMAL GRIEF

Not uncommonly, people get stuck in the grieving process, unable to move through it, they may:

- *Delay it* by acting as if nothing happened. They act as if they have accepted the death easily. It may be years before the person becomes preoccupied with the death and images of the dead person; it will be at that time that the grieving process must be worked through.
- *Distort their reactions* by perhaps exaggerating their activities and sense of well-being, keeping very busy and overly cheerful.
- *Develop an illness, either physical, psychological, or both* by becoming ill, sometimes even in a way that is similar to their loved one's illness, or by developing a psychosomatic illness—that is, one that can be caused or aggravated by psychological factors, such as an ulcer, asthma, or rheumatoid arthritis.

- *Persistently reject social relationships* by distancing himself from others. As the bereaving person becomes increasingly isolated from family and friends, he or she becomes overcritical or merely disinterested in others and events.
- *Experience feelings of rage or fury,* especially against specific people, such as a doctor who treated the dead person.
- *Act cold and formal* with old friends or family members. The person may go through the motions of daily living, but with a demeanor that is stilted, formal, and without warmth.
- *Social passivity* may also manifest itself, with the grieving person unable to initiate new activities or relationships because she believes that it will all be unrewarding anyway.
- *Overgenerosity* is sometimes exhibited by the grieving person, who appears not to care anymore about money or belongings and may willingly give it away, possibly hurting family and business associates in process.
- *Chronic depression and ideas of suicide* may develop as a reaction to grief. Suicide may be considered an option if anxiety, panic, or a major depression persist. Sometimes, the depressed or anxious person becomes agitated—feeling tense, restless, and worthless, unable to sleep well, and perhaps even accusing himself of all kinds of mistakes for which he should be punished. Those with obsessive traits and histories of depression are most likely to develop this agitated form of depression.

GETTING THROUGH THE GRIEVING PROCESS

The process of grieving involves the living person's freeing himself from the departed's "hold" and finding new and rewarding patterns in daily living and social interactions. The griever must work through the pain he feels in his own way. True acceptance usually involves expressing expected feelings of sadness and loss, and even unexpected feelings of hostility and guilt that may linger. Mental health professionals have specific short-term strategies (usually eight to ten sessions) for helping people work through the mourning process. By working through a process of allowing the deceased back into our lives, thoughts, and feelings, by making our loved one a "part" of, rather than "apart from" our lives, we can learn to accept our loss, how very hard that may be, and move through the process of grieving to acceptance.

CONCLUSION

Dying is a natural and inevitable part of living. To ease a loved one's passage may be one of the most profound and generous gifts we can offer. May we learn how to make that passage as easy and comfortable as humankind knows how.

> Death and love are the two wings that bear the good man to heaven.
>   —Michelangelo

Notes

Chapter 1. Cancer Pain Undermines Cancer Treatment

1. Charles Schuster, as director of the National Institute on Drug Abuse; quoted in *Newsweek*, December 19, 1988, p. 58.

2. Kathleen Foley, as quoted in *U.S. News & World Report*, June 29, 1987, p. 56.

3. World Health Organization, *Cancer Pain Relief and Palliative Care* (Geneva: World Health Organization, 1990), Technical Report Series 804.

4. Policy statement, Wisconsin Cancer Pain Initiative.

5. James R. Oleson, personal communication, 1989.

6. Charles Schuster, as director of the National Institute on Drug Abuse. Official statement made to Strategy Session held by the Wisconsin Cancer Pain Initiative at the Wingspread Conference Center, December 1986.

Appendix
Where To Find More Information

Having cancer or caring for a loved one with cancer is an enormously stressful experience. But it is not one that a person must go through alone. Resources abound, not only for families and caregivers, but even for doctors who want to obtain more information about managing cancer and pain. Help ranges from handbooks to a friendly, informed voice you can reach by phone.

In 1984, the World Health Organization determined that cancer pain was a major public health problem worldwide. Although our current knowledge and methods can readily relieve pain in more than 90 percent of cases, only about 50 percent of patients in the *developed* world enjoy such relief. In developing countries, the estimate is as low as 10 percent. One of WHO's goals is to ensure that a global program is in place by the year 2000 in which effective treatments are readily available throughout the world. In the past five years, the topic of cancer pain has been increasingly gaining recognition.

Although the information in the written materials listed in this Appendix has been incorporated into the book, consumers may still be interested in receiving some of the following resources. *Note:* Many of these organizations can also help you locate a cancer specialist or a pain specialist nearest you. The listings here are meant to serve as a resource guide only and not necessarily as an endorsement of an organization.

ON CANCER PAIN

For a referral to the closest pain control clinic, or for the closest support groups, call the Cancer Information Service (CIS) supported by the National Cancer Institute, a nationwide toll-free telephone inquiry system: (800) 4-CANCER, or write:

Office of Cancer Communications
Building 31, Room 10a-24
Bethesda, MD 20892

In Alaska, call (800) 638-6070.

In Washington, D.C., and suburbs of Maryland and Virginia, call 636-5700.

In Hawaii on Oahu, call 524-1234 (neighbor islands should call collect).

Spanish-speaking staff members are available during daytime hours in California (area codes 213, 714, 619, 805), Florida, Georgia, Illinois, Northern New Jersey, New York City, and Texas.

The Cancer Information Service can also offer free materials, including "Harrowing News/Pain Relief" and "Fact Sheet on Cancer Pain Control Activities." CIS will provide information about research studies on new treatments for cancer and cancer pain that are open to qualified patients.

For a list of accredited pain programs, contact:

Commission on Accreditation of Rehabilitative Facilities
101 N. Wilmot Road, Suite 500
Tucson, AZ 85711
(602) 748-1212

The Wisconsin Cancer Pain Initiative (WCPI) has taken a lead nationwide in promoting excellence in cancer pain relief; its activities have inspired the development of cancer pain initiatives in at least 30 other states. It offers educational materials, in print and video, as well as information about cancer pain initiatives in other states. Its publications include "Cancer Pain Can Be Relieved," "Children's Cancer Pain Can Be Relieved," "Jeff Asks About Cancer Pain" (a booklet for teens), and "The Handbook of Cancer Pain Management" (for health-care professionals).

The WCPI may be reached at:

Wisconsin Cancer Pain Initiative
1300 University Avenue, Room 3675
Madison, WI 53706
(608) 262-0978 or FAX (608) 262-1257

The Resource Center for State Cancer Pain Initiatives was established in 1992 to promote the growth and development of state cancer pain initiatives. It can be reached directly at:

The Resource Center for State Cancer Pain Initiatives
1300 University Avenue, Room 3671
Madison, WI 53706
(608) 265-4013; FAX (608) 262-1257

For information about cancer pain initiatives around the world, contact:

Cancer Control Programme
World Health Organization
1211 Geneva 27
Switzerland

WHO has as its major initiative to stamp out cancer pain worldwide. Its excellent book, *Cancer Pain Relief* (1986) is available for $6.50 in the United States, order number ISBN 92 4 156100 9 from:

WHO Publications Center USA
49 Sheridan Avenue
Albany, NY 12210

Also available from the United Nations Bookshop, New York, NY 10017.

For an unresolved cancer pain problem that perplexes a physician, the physician may contact:

Pain Management Information Center (PMIC)
401 Harris B Dates Drive
Ithaca, NY 14850
(800) 322-7642

PMIC is a national telephone consulting service available to physicians and other health-care professionals for $95 a year. It offers doctors *immediate* and expert advice about how to treat a specific patient's cancer pain.

The U.S. Department of Health and Human Services has several publications that may be obtained from:

Agency for Healthcare Policy and
    Research Publications Clearinghouse
P.O. Box 8547
Silver Springs, MD 20907
(800) 358-9295

Publications include the following:

Cancer-Related Pain Guidelines: Clinical Practical Guidelines for the Management of Cancer Pain (tentatively scheduled for late 1993 or early 1994)

Acute Pain Management in Adults' Operative Procedures, Publication Number AH CPR 92-0019

Acute Pain Management in Infants, Children and Adolescents' Operative and Medical Procedures, Publication Number AH CPR 92-0020

Acute Pain Management: Operative and Medical Procedures and Trauma, Publication Number AH CPR 92-0032

A Patient's Guide to Pain Control After Surgery, Publication Number AH CPR 92-0021

To contact the offices of Health and Human Services, write:

U.S. Department of Health and Human Services
Public Health Service
Executive Office Center
2101 E Jefferson Street

Suite 501
Rockville, MD 20852

Or call (301) 227-6662.

To obtain the free booklets "Coping with Pain at Home: A Guide for Cancer Patients and Their Families" and "How To Talk To Your Doctor About Acute Pain" write:

Du Pont Pharmaceuticals Biomedical Department
E.I. DuPont de Nemours & Co., Inc.
Wilmington, DE 19898

To obtain information in Canada about cancer and pain, write:

Health and Welfare Canada
Room 210B/HPB Building
Ottawa, Ontario
Canada
K1A OL2

This organization has written an excellent booklet on managing cancer pain.

ON PAIN IN GENERAL

National Chronic Pain Outreach Association
7979 Old Georgetown Road, Suite 100
Bethesda, MD 20814-2429
(301) 652-4948

This organization has local branches which might sponsor support groups for patients with chronic pain. They can also make referrals and offer newsletters.

For referrals to pain specialists:

American Chronic Pain Association
P.O. Box 850
Rocklin, CA 95677
(916) 632-0922

Committee on Pain Therapy
American Society of Anesthesiologists
515 Busse Highway
Park Ridge, IL 60068
(708) 825-5586

American Pain Society
5700 Old Orchard Road
Skokie, IL 60077-1022
(708) 966-5595

The American Pain Society (APS) is a nonprofit educational and scientific organization which is the national chapter of the International Association for the Study of Pain. Comprised of specialists from diverse fields, the APS is devoted to promoting education and training in the field of pain.

American Academy of Pain Medicine
5700 Old Orchard Road
Skokie, IL 60077
(708) 966-9510

The International Pain Foundation
909 NE 43rd Street, Room 306
Seattle, WA 98105-6020
(206) 547-2157

IPF is a nonprofit, charitable, educational organization which is a unit of the International Association for the Study of Pain. Its goal is to support public and professional education about pain conditions and their treatment. They offer a pamphlet for consumers titled "About Living with Chronic Pain" (1987, South Deerfield, MA: Channing L. Bete, Inc.).

ON CANCER IN GENERAL

To obtain state-of-the-art information about treatment plans, oncologists and cancer centers, clinical trials (research studies), articles from the medical literature, a directory of doctors who treat cancer, hospitals that have cancer programs, and details about specific types of cancer, one may access the National Cancer Institute's *Physicians Data Query,* or PDQ. PDQ is a computerized database that is available to anyone. Doctors and consumers may obtain a user ID, password, and instructions to access the database by calling (800) 638-8480. That number reaches information specialists (both English and Spanish-speaking) at the National Library of Medicine. They will mail out the paperwork necessary to obtain the ID and password; it will take about two weeks to get hooked up.

As an alternative, consumers may call (800) 4-CANCER to get connected to the Cancer Information Service of the National Cancer Institute. The counselors who answer the phones can help callers obtain information directly from the database. They also have a series of pamphlets available free of charge on specific issues related to cancer.

To contact the National Cancer Institute, you may also write:

National Cancer Institute
Office of Cancer Communications
Building 31, Room 10A-24
Bethesda, MD 20892

To obtain current treatment guidelines for almost any type of cancer, free of charge, dial (301) 402-5874 on the phone of a FAX machine and listen to the recorded message and its directions for obtaining information by FAX machine. For help, call (301) 496-8880.

Another way to access the medical databases (known as MEDLARS, an umbrella database comprised of about 40 specific databases, including Medline and CancerLit) is through a public library or medical library. Reference librarians will do a search for you, but usually for a fee. Call the reference desk, and ask if they can access Medline or MEDLARS. All these searches will result in a bibliography with citations and abstracts of journal articles on specific topics published in the medical literature.

The American Cancer Society, a national, nonprofit organization, has more than 3,500 offices in the United States and Puerto Rico, and it publishes several useful booklets. Write them at:

American Cancer Society
1599 Clifton Road, NE
Atlanta, Ga 30329-4251

Or call them at (404) 320-3333 or (800) ACS-2315.

Some of their booklets include the following: "Questions and Answers About Pain Control: A Guide for People with Cancer and Their Families" and "Living with Cancer." It also offers booklets for patients concerning diet and nutrition, treatments, emotional support, symptom control, and dying at home. In addition, the ACS can provide information about local support groups and educational programs. Check with a local office.

For information on some one hundred hotlines for specific diseases, call the National Health Information Center at (800) 336-4797.

For a breast cancer hotline, call Y-ME National Organization for Breast Cancer Information and Support at (800) 221-2141 or (708) 799-8228.

For information specifically about children with cancer, contact:

Candlelighters Childhood Cancer Foundation
7910 Woodmont Avenue, Suite 460
Bethesda, MD 20814

Or call: (301) 657-8401 or (800) 366-2223.

An advocacy group for cancer survivors is:

The National Coalition for Cancer Survivorship
1010 Wayne Avenue, Fifth Floor
Silver Spring, MD 20910
(301) 585-2616

Groups that provide support and information for people who have had cancer treatment are:

Post-Treatment Resource Program
Memorial Sloan-Kettering Cancer Center
410 E. 62nd Street, Room 740
New York, NY 10021
(212) 639-3292

and

The Wellness Community
2200 Colorado Avenue
Santa Monica, CA 90404
(310) 453-2200

This group has branches in cities throughout the country.

When cancer affects one's appearance, it can be devastating to one's body image and self-esteem. To help women resume normal lives after cancer, a program called Look Good . . . Feel Better has recently been developed by the charitable organization The Cosmetic, Toiletry and Fragrance Association Foundation in conjunction with the American Cancer Society and the National Cosmetology Association.

Available through the organization is free information on applying beauty techniques to restore one's appearance after treatment for cancer. Available in more than 40 states, the program may be located in local hospitals, cancer centers, community centers, or through the American Cancer Society. In some areas, free consultations are available as well as group meetings. Patient educational materials and free makeup kits are also available.

For information, call (800) 395-LOOK.

INTERDISCIPLINARY CLINICS IN THE UNITED STATES

The following is a brief list of some of the leading programs in the country that focus on pain management:

Cleveland Clinic Foundation Research Institute
Cleveland, OH
(216) 444-3900

Johns Hopkins Pain Management Service
Baltimore, MD
(301) 955-1816

Mayo Clinic's Pain Management Center
St. Mary's Hospital
Rochester, MN
(507) 255-5921

Mensana Clinic
Stevenson, MD
(410) 653-2403

New York Pain Treatment Program
Lenox Hill Hospital
New York, NY
(800) 548-3242

Pain Control & Rehabilitation Institute of Georgia
Atlanta, GA
(404) 297-1400

Pain Service
Memorial Sloan-Kettering Center
New York, NY
(212) 639-2000

Pain Clinic
Anderson Hospital and Tumor Institute
University of Texas System Cancer Center
(713) 792-6600

Pain Treatment Center
University of Rochester Medical Center
Rochester, NY
(716) 275-3524

University of Miami Comprehensive Pain & Rehabilitation Center
Southshore Hospital
Miami, FL
(305) 672-3700

University of Washington Pain Center
Seattle, WA
(206) 548-4282

NEW MIND-BODY APPROACHES

Hypnosis

American Society for Clinical Hypnosis
2200 East Devon Avenue, Suite 291
Des Plaines, IL 60018
(708) 297-3317

or

Society for Clinical and Experimental Hypnosis
129 A King's Park Drive
Liverpool, NY 13090
(315) 652-7299

This organization has a membership of 1,100 professionals.

The American Council of Hypnotist Examiners has 7,400 members and may be able to recommend a certified hypnotist close to your home. Contact them at:

The American Council of Hypnotist Examiners
1147 E. Broadway, Suite 340
Glendale, CA 91205
(818) 242-5378

Acupuncture

To obtain referrals close to your area, contact:

American Academy of Medical Acupuncture
58200 Wilshire Boulevard, Suite 500
Los Angeles, CA 90036
(213) 937-5514

or

American Association of Acupuncture and Oriental Medicine
1400 16th Street, NW, Suite 710
Washington, DC 20036
(202) 265-2276

Biofeedback

Information and referrals may be obtained from Association for Applied Psychophysiology and Feedback (formerly The Biofeedback Society of America) and the Biofeedback Certification Institute of America, both located at:

10200 W. 44th Avenue, Suite 304
Wheatridge, CO 80033
(303) 422-8436

Stress Reduction

Audiotapes on this technique are available from:

Stress Reduction Tapes
P.O. Box 547
Lexington, MA 02173

For information about five-day and eight-week training workshops, contact:

The Stress Reduction Clinic
University of Massachusetts Medical Center
Worcester, MA
(508) 856-1616

General Mind-Body Information

For general information on mind-body research, contact:

The Fetzer Institute
9292 West KL Ave.
Kalamazoo, MI 49009
(606) 375-2000

SUPPORT GROUPS

In addition to the American Cancer Society, the American Self-Help Clearinghouse can help you locate a group for specific medical programs. They may be reached at:

St. Clares-Riverside Medical Center
25 Pocono Road
Denville, NJ 07834
(210) 625-7101

COUNSELING AND PSYCHOTHERAPY

For a referral to a counselor, ask your doctor for a psychiatrist, clinical psychologist, or psychiatric social worker. National organizations that might have local branches or can offer referrals include:

American Psychiatric Association at (202) 682-6000
American Psychological Association at (202) 336-5700
National Association of Social Workers at (202) 408-8600
Center for Cognitive Therapy at (215) 898-4102

CARING FOR PATIENTS AT HOME

For information on controlling symptoms related to cancer, write:

National Hospice Organization
1901 No. Moore Street, Suite 901
Arlington, VA 22209
(703) 243-5900

For support of children with life-threatening illnesses and their families, call or write:

Children's Hospice International
1101 King Street, Suite 131
Alexandria, VA 22314
(703) 684-0330

The American Association of Retired Persons has a pamphlet called "A Path for Caregivers" (stock no. D1297). It may be obtained by writing to:

AARP Fulfillment
1909 K Street, NW
Washington, DC 20049

LIVING WILLS/RIGHT TO DIE

The following association will provide standard living-will forms and information about them. To be sure that they are valid in a particular state, check with an attorney or a hospice nurse or professional.

Society for the Right to Die
    and Concern for the Dying
250 West 57th Street
New York, NY 10107
(212) 246-6973

GRIEF

To obtain a referral or information about grief, contact:

Association for Death Education and Counseling, National Office
638 Prospect Avenue
Hartford, CT 06105
(203) 232-4825

Grief Education Institute
2422 S. Downing Street
Denver, CO 80210
(303) 777-9234

Family Services America
11700 W. Lake Park Drive
Milwaukee, WI 53224
(414) 359-2111

For a magazine called *Bereavement: A Magazine of Hope and Healing,* contact:

Bereavement Publishing
350 Gradle Drive
Carmel, IN 46032

For a free brochure, "Grief Is Not a Sign of Weakness," write:

Theos Foundation
International Headquarters
1301 Clark Building
717 Liberty Avenue
Pittsburgh, PA 15222

More Information on Medications

Table A.1. *A Basic Drug List*

Category	Parent Drug	Alternatives
Non-opioids	Aspirin	Acetaminophen Ibuprofen
Weak opioids	Codeine	Oxycodone
Strong opioids	Morphine	Hydromorphone Fentanyl Methadone Levorphanol
Adjuvant analgesics		
Anticonvulsants	Carbamazepine	Phenytoin Clonazepam Valproic acid
Major tranquilizers	Haloperidol Prochlorperazine	Chlorpromazine
Minor tranquilizers	Diazepam Hydroxyzine	Flurazepam Lorazepam
Antidepressants	Amitriptyline	Nortriptyline Imipramine Doxepin Desipramine
Corticosteroids	Dexamethasone	Prednisone

Table A.2. *Basic Adjuvant Drugs*

	Analgesic Effect	Antidepressant Effect	Anxiolytic Effect	Muscle Relaxant	Antiemetic	Anti-Confusional
Anticonvulsants						
Carbamazepine	+ [a, c]					
Phenytoin	+ [a, c]					
Psychotropic Drugs						
Prochlorperazine			+		+	
Chlorpromazine			+	(+)	+	
Haloperidol			+		+	+
Hydroxyzine	+		+		+	
Diazepam			+	+		
Amitriptyline	+ [b, c]	+	(+)			
Corticosteroids						
Prednisolone	+ [c]	(+)			+	
Dexamethasone	+ [c]	(+)			+	

[a] Often of benefit in shooting and stabbing pain.
[b] Often of benefit in superficial, burning pain.
[c] Often of use in nerve pain.
Note: Plus indicates the tendency of the medication to cause the effect.

Table A.3. *Equivalent Dosing: How the Doctor Switches Between Drugs*

Drug	Oral Dose	Ratio Between Oral and IM and Sub-q Injection	IM or Sub-q Dose
Morphine			
Repeated dose (after patient has been on medication for at least a week)	30 mg	3:1	10 mg
Single dose	60 mg	6:1	10 mg
Hydromorphone (Dilaudid)	8 mg	5:1	1.6 mg
Methadone hydrochloride (Dolophine)	20 mg	2:1	10 mg
Levorphanol (Levo-Dromoran)	2 mg	1:1	2 mg
Meperidine hydrochloride (Demerol)	300 mg	4:1	75 mg
Codeine	200 mg	1.5:1	130 mg

Note: One of the leading causes of undermedication is that errors are made in dosing when patients are switched from one method of administration to another (e.g., from receiving injections to receiving pills) or from one drug to another. This table is the same guide the doctor would probably use when planning such a change. The "conversion ratios" are approximate and may differ somewhat between patients. The ratio is given between oral medication and intramuscular (IM) or subcutaneous (sub-q) injection.

The reference dose against which other drugs are measured is 10 mg of intramuscular morphine in the treatment of severe pain.

Table A.4. *Guidelines for the Use of Opioid Analgesics in Patients with Chronic Cancer Pain (Moderate to Severe)*[a]

| | Pure (morphine-like) Agonists | | | Equianalgesic Dose[d] | Recommended Schedule[e] | Formulations[b] | Comments[f] |
Generic Name	Trade Name[b]	Route[c]					
Immediate-release morphine	MSIR Roxanol	Oral		30–60 mg[g]	2–4 hr	15 or 30 mg 2 mg/ml 4 mg/ml 20 mg/ml	1, 2
Controlled-release morphine	MS Contin Oramorph	Oral		30–60 mg[g]	12–8 hr	15, 30, 60, or 100 mg	2, 3
Morphine		IM		10 mg	2–4 hr	Various	2, 4
Morphine	RMS	Rectal		15 mg		5, 10, or 20 mg	—
Hydromorphone	Dilaudid	Oral		7.5 mg	2–4 hr	1, 2, 3, or 4 mg	5
Hydromorphone	Dilaudid	IM		1.5 mg	2–4 hr	1, 2, 4, or 10 mg/ml	5
Hydromorphone	Dilaudid	Rectal		7.5 mg	3–6 hr	3 mg	5
Meperidine	Demerol Pethedine	PO		300 mg	2–4 hr	50 or 100 mg 50 mg/5 ml	6
Meperidine	Demerol Pethedine	IM		75 mg	2–4 hr	Various	6
Diamorphine	Heroin	Oral		60 mg	—	—	7
Diamorphine	Heroin	IM		5 mg	—	—	7
Methadone	Dolophine	Oral		20 mg	4–12 hr	5, 10, or 40 mg 1, 2, or 10 mg/ml	8
Methadone	Dolophine	IM		10 mg	4–12 hr	10 mg/ml	8
Levorphanol	Levo-Dromoran	Oral		4 mg	4–8 hr	2 mg	9
Levorphanol	Levo-Dromoran	IM		2 mg	4–8 hr	2 mg/ml	9
Oxymorphone	Numorphan	IM		1 mg	3–6 hr	1 or 1.5 mg/ml	10
Oxymorphone	Numorphan	Rectal		5–10 mg	3–6 hr	5 mg	11
	Brompton cocktail	Oral		—	—	—	

(continued)

Table A.4. *Guidelines for the Use of Opioid Analgesics in Patients with Chronic Cancer Pain (Moderate to Severe)[a]* *(Continued)*

	Pure (morphine-like) Agonists					
Generic Name	Trade Name[b]	Route[c]	Equianalgesic Dose[d]	Recommended Schedule[e]	Formulations[b]	Comments[f]
Propoxyphene	Darvon	Oral	65–130 mg	4–6 hr		12
Codeine		Oral	200 mg	3–6 hr	15, 30, or 60 mg	13, 14
Codeine		IM	130 mg	Same	30 mg/ml	13, 14
Oxycodone	Roxycodone	Oral	20–30 mg	3–6 hr	5 mg	15
Hydrocodone		Oral	—	4–6 hr	1 or 20 mg/ml	13
Dihydrocodeine			—	—	—	13
Fentanyl	Sublimaze	IV	0.1 mg	Continuous	50 μg/ml	16
Fentanyl	Duragesic	TD	0.1 mg	72–48 hr	25, 50, 75, or 100 μg/hr	17
Sufentanil	Sufenta	IV	0.15 mg	—	50 μg/ml	16
Alfentanil	Alfenta	IV	0.75 mg	—	500 μg/ml	16
Partial Agonists						
Buprenorphine	Buprenex	IM	0.4 mg	4–6 hr	0.3 mg/ml	18, 19
Buprenorphine	Temgesic	SL	0.8 mg	6 hr		18, 19
Dezocine	Dalgan	IM	10 mg	3–4 hr	5–15 mg/ml	20, 21
Mixed Agonists/Antagonists						
Butorphanol	Stadol	IM	2–2.5 mg	3–4 hr	1 mg/ml	18, 21
Pentazocine	Talwin	Oral	180 mg	3–4 hr	50 mg	18, 22
Pentazocine	Talwin	IM	60 mg	3–4 hr	30 mg/ml	18
Nalbuphine	Nubain	IM	10 mg	3–6 hr	10 mg/ml	18, 21

[a] See Chapters 6 and 7 for more complete explanations.

[b] Listing is partial, comprised mostly of formulations available in the United States. **Mg** (milligrams) unless stated otherwise.

[c] For parenteral routes (i.e., those taken in ways that do not involve the digestive tract), only the most commonly used route is listed; most medications, however, can be administered intramuscularly (**IM**), subcutaneously (sub-q), or intravenously (**IV**). PO means medication by mouth. TD means transdermyl—medication absorbed through the skin. SL means sublingual—absorbed under the tongue.

[d] Equianalgesic dose refers to the dose that provides the equivalent pain relief (analgesia) as 10 mg of intramuscular morphine. Equianalgesic doses are based on values most frequently cited in the medical literature and on clinical experience, although these sometimes conflict. They are approximate and are intended to serve as guidelines only.

[e] This is a rough guideline only; physicians may deviate from these schedules as they tailor medication schedules to particular patients.

[f] Side effects and precautions for all the opioid medications include constipation, sedation, dysphoria (unpleasant moods or feelings), confusion, hallucinations, nausea, vomiting, respiratory depression (which is rare in patients who have developed a tolerance to opioids), urinary retention (difficulty urinating), and itching. How patients react to opioids differs from patient-to-patient and medication-to-medication, often even in the same patient.

[g] See Comment 3, below.

Notes

1. Usually recommended as the first drug of choice for moderate to severe cancer pain.
2. Despite a few studies that suggest a conversion ratio of 1:6 for a switch from intramuscular (**IM**) administration to one by mouth (PO), clinical experience suggests that a ratio of 1:3 with regular use is generally considered more applicable. In other words, if a patient is going from an intramuscular (or intravenous or subcutaneous) route with a dose, for example, of 10 mg, to an oral route of morphine, the physician is likely to prescribe 30 mg PO to get equivalent pain relief.
3. Controlled release means that the medication is timed release; it provides slow absorption of the medication and, consequently, doses may be farther apart. Using controlled-release formulation may result in more consistent blood levels of medication and, therefore, more consistent pain relief with fewer episodes of "breakthrough pain." Controlled-release medication is extremely useful in providing a basic level of pain relief and its infrequent dosing schedule is very convenient for the patient. Physicians will usually supplement these doses with "rescue doses" of shorter acting medications to relieve pain that "breaks through" despite the controlled-release medication being prescribed. Controlled-release medications should not be broken, crushed, or chewed.
4. Morphine is the standard against which other analgesics (pain relievers) are compared.
5. Becomes effective relatively rapidly and offers short-acting relief, so it is particularly effective for breakthrough pain.
6. Although useful for acute pain (such as from surgery), it is not recommended for chronic pain such as cancer pain.
7. Not available in United States. Has been found to be no more effective than morphine.
8. May accumulate in the body and produce sedation and perhaps respiratory depression, particularly in the elderly and in those with impaired kidney function. Should be administered initially prn (as needed) rather than a-t-c (around-the-clock).
9. See comments on methadone.
10. Not available for oral administration.
11. Named as such because it was conceived at Brompton's Hospital in the United Kingdom. Usually consists of morphine hydrochloride (15 mg), cocaine hydrochloride (15 mg), 90 percent alcohol (2 ml), syrup (4 ml), and chloroform water (15 ml). Studies show no benefits over using oral morphine; use should therefore be discouraged.

(continued)

325

Table A.4 Guidelines for the Use of Opioid Analgesics in Patients with Chronic Cancer Pain (Moderate to Severe)[a] (Continued)

12. Traditionally used for mild pain, often combined with aspirin or acetaminophen. Usually not appropriate for cancer pain because it is too weak.

13. For mild to moderate pain, traditionally administered as a combined product with aspirin or acetaminophen.

14. Although equivalent pain relief may be obtained at this dose (200 mg), unpleasant side effects are likely and so a stronger opioid is usually recommended instead.

15. For mild to moderate pain, traditionally marketed as combined product with aspirin or acetaminophen. Recently made available without aspirin or acetaminophen for mild to severe pain.

16. Not available orally. Used primarily as a component of anesthesia or in intensive-care settings.

17. Once the blood has achieved a consistent level of medication (steady state), doses last about 72 hours. From the first dose, it will take usually about 12 to 24 hours to achieve a steady state. If side effects occur and medication is removed (patch removed), adverse effects may persist for 8 to 12 hours. Extremely useful for patients who do not want to take medication frequently or who cannot swallow.

18. May cause the same side effects and the same precautions should be taken as for the "pure" opioids; also has the potential to cause withdrawal or abstinence syndrome in patients who have become physically dependent on opioids. Usually not recommended for cancer patients.

19. Sublingual (under the tongue) form not currently available in the United States. Probably has a ceiling dose for pain relief. Unlike other similar medications, may have a role in managing cancer pain.

20. Recently introduced in the United States, so clinical experience is limited.

21. Not available as an oral medication.

22. Not recommended for cancer pain.

Source: Adapted from Richard B. Patt, ed. *Cancer Pain.* Philadelphia: Lippincott, 1993. Used with permission of the author and publisher.

Table A.5. *Non-steroidal Anti-inflammatory Drugs*

Generic Name and Class[a]	Trade Name[b]	Approximate Half Life (hr)	Usual Dosing Schedule	Usual Recommended Starting Dose (mg/day)[c]	Usual Maximum Recommended Dose (mg/day)	Comments[d,e]
Para-aminophenol Derivatives						
Acetaminophen	Tylenol, Datril, Panadol	2–4	4–6 hr	2600	6000	1
Salicylates						
Acetylsalicylic acid	Aspirin, etc.	3–12	4–6 hr	2600	6000	m2
Choline magnesium trisalicylate	Trilisate	8–12	8–12 hr	1500 × 1 then 1000 q 12	4000	3
Salsalate	Disalcid	8–12	8–12 hr	1500 × 1 then 500 q 12	4000	3
Diflunisal	Dolobid, Dolobis	8–12	12 hr	1000 × 1 then 500 q 12	1500	4
Pyrazolon Derivatives						
Phenylbutazone	Butazoladin, Antadol, Phebuzine	50–100	6–3 hr	300	400	5
Oxyphenbutazone	Tandearil, Rapostan, Rheumapax, Oxalid	50–100	6–8 hr	300	400	6
Acetic Acid Derivatives						
Indomethacin	Indocin, Indocid, Indomethine	4–5	8–12 hr	75	200	7
Sulindac	Clinoril, Arthrobid	14	12 hr	300	400	8
Tolmetin	Tolectin	1	6–8 hr	600	2000	
Ketorolac	Toradol	4–7	4–6 hr	120	240	9
Suprofen		2–4	6 hr	600	800	
Fenamates						
Mefenamic acid	Ponstel, Ponstan, Ponstil, Namphen	2	6 hr	4	1000	10
Meclofenamate sodium	Meclomen	2–4	6–8 hr	150	400	11

327

Table A.5. *Non-steroidal Anti-inflammatory Drugs (Continued)*

Generic Name and Class[a]	Trade Name[b]	Approximate Half Life (hr)	Usual Dosing Schedule	Usual Recommended Starting Dose (mg/day)[c]	Usual Maximum Recommended Dose (mg/day)	Comments[d,e]
Proprionic Acid Derivatives						
Ibuprofen	Motrin, Advil, Nuprin, Rufen	3–4	4–8 hr	1200	4200	12
Naproxen	Naprosyn, Naprosine, Proxen	13	12 hr	500	1000	13
Fenoprofen	Nalfon, Fenopran, Nalgesic, Pro-gesic	2–3	6 hr	800	3200	
Ketoprofen	Orudis, Alrheumat	2–3	6–8 hr	150	300	
Flurbiprofen	Ansaid	5–6	8–12 hr	100	300	
Diclofenac	Voltaren	2	6 hr	75	200	
Oxicams						
Piroxicam	Feldene	45	24 hr	20	40	14
Pyranocarboxylic Acids						
Etodolac	Lodine	7.3	6–8 hr	800	1200	15
Naphthylalkanones						
Nabumetone	Relafen	22–30	12–24 hr	1000	2000	15

[a]This listing includes various related chemical compounds.

[b]These are predominantly U.S. trade names.

[c]Doctors usually give elderly patients, or those on multiple medications or with impaired kidneys, one-half to two-thirds the recommended starting doses. If pain goes unrelieved, the doses are usually increased as tolerated, usually on a weekly basis. Since few studies on the NSAIDs in cancer patients have actually been conducted, the dosing guidelines are from clinical experience, and may vary among patients.

[d]All of these medications (except in some cases acetaminophen) are associated with a variety of side effects; the most prominent one is gastrointestinal irritation. Other side effects include increased risk of bleeding (hemorrhage), confusion, kidney or liver problems, periods of breathing problems (bronchospasm), rash, and allergy.

[e]At high doses, doctors may wish to check stools every two weeks for blood; and conduct other tests such as liver function tests and urine analysis, every month or two.

Notes

1. Available over the counter in various preparations. Possesses weak anti-inflammatory activity and is therefore not a first drug of choice for bone pain or pain that is accompanied by inflammation. For patients at greater risk for gastrointestinal problems (such as ulcers) or bleeding complications (for example, the patient is on a blood-thinning medication), this drug is an excellent choice. Taken in large quantities, this drug can be fatal due to liver failure. When used continuously at high doses, doctors will often wish to check kidney, liver, and bone marrow function periodically.

2. Standard to which other medications in this category are compared; available over the counter in various preparations. May not be as well tolerated as other alternatives.

3. May be particularly useful in some cancer patients due to its minimal effect on thinning blood or irritating the gastrointestinal tract. Available in liquid formulation.

4. Causes less gastrointestinal irritation than aspirin.

5. Not one of the preferred medications for a first-line approach for cancer pain because of its greater risk in having an ill effect on bone marrow. If used, doctor may wish to monitor the bone marrow periodically with blood tests.

6. May cause less stomach irritation than phenylbutazone.

7. Available in sustained release (meaning that the medication may be taken less often because each dose lasts longer) and for rectal administration. Although a strong anti-inflammatory medication, its use is associated with a higher incidence of gastrointestinal irritation and central nervous system problems than some of the alternatives.

8. Seems to be associated with fewer kidney problems than other NSAIDs.

9. In low dose ranges, seems to be as effective as morphine, but like other NSAIDs, has a ceiling dose above which no further pain relief is achieved.

10. Since this medication is often associated with gastrointestinal problems after one week of use, it is usually not recommended for cancer pain.

11. This medication is associated with a relatively high incidence of gastrointestinal irritation.

12. Available over the counter in low-dose formulations; relatively economical and well tolerated for long-term use.

13. Relatively well-tolerated and rapidly absorbed.

14. Convenient once-a-day dosing is an advantage for many patients with cancer. Higher doses (more than 20 mg) are associated with increased risks of ulcers, especially in the elderly. May take 5 to 7 days to reach maximum effectiveness. When patient has liver or kidney impairment, the drug may accumulate in the body.

15. Recently released in the United States; may be administered 1 to 2 times a day.

Source: Adapted from Richard B. Patt, ed. *Cancer pain.* Philadelphia: Lippincott, 1993. Used with permission of the author and publisher.

Table A.6. Guidelines for the Use of the Antidepressants in Patients with Chronic Cancer Pain[a,b,c]

Generic Name	Trade Name[d]	Dose Range[e]	Anticho-linergic[a]	Sedative Effects	Orthostasis[a]	Comments[f,c]
Amitriptyline[g]	Elavil Endep	10–300 mg	+++	+++	++	1, 2, 3, 4
Imipramine[g]	Tofranil	20–300	+++	++	+++	1, 4
Doxepin[g]	Sinequan Adapin	30–300	+++	+++	+++	1, 5
Desipramine[g]	Norpramin Pertofrane	75–300	+	+	+	1
Nortriptyline[g]	Pamelor Aventyl	50–100	++	+	+	1, 5, 6
Trimipramine[h]	Surmontil	50–225	+++	+++	+++	—
Protriptyline	Vivactil	15–40	+++	+	++	—
Amoxapine[h]	Asendin	200–300	+	+	++	7
Fluoxetine[h]	Prozac	20–60	0	+	0	8
Second-Generation or Atypical Heterocyclics						
Trazodone[h]	Desyrel	50–600	0	+++	+++	9
Maprotiline[h]	Ludiomil	75–300	+	+++	+	—

[a]Doses and the rating of anticholinergic side effects (that is, dry mouth, urinary retention or difficulty in urinating, constipation, sweating), sedation, and orthostasis (low blood pressure upon standing up suddenly) listed here are only intended as rough guidelines. Other than dry mouth, most of the effects are uncommon with the low doses usually used for pain. Plus indicates a greater tendency to cause the side effect when compared to other medications.

330

[b]These antidepressants are most often used for managing pain associated with nerve damage, which is often felt as a burning sensation.

[c]These heterocyclic antidepressants may produce pain relief at low doses without affecting mood; these doses are usually too low to counter depression. Initial treatment is usually prescribed as a low, nighttime dose. While sleeping problems are usually resolved quickly with these doses, maximal pain relief often takes 1 to 3 weeks. Doses may be increased as tolerated, particularly when depression is also present. See Chapters 8 and 14 for more details.

[d]In the United States.

[e]The values listed reflect the range between minimum and maximum recommended doses. In general, the higher range of doses are intended to treat clinical depression, and even then, it is recommended that dosage be reduced for maintenance therapy. In general, when antidepressants are prescribed for nerve pain, they are prescribed in the low range of the dose spectrum, often initially at the lowest possible dose.

[f]As a class, these antidepressants, known as the heterocyclic antidepressants, are generally associated with the anticholinergic side effects (see note a). Infrequently, they may cause high blood pressure (hypertension), rash, bone marrow depression, vision or sexual problems, enlarged breasts sometimes with milk secretions (gynecomastia), jaundice (yellowing skin), and hair loss (alopecia). Noteworthy side effects are listed.

[g]In controlled studies, these medications have been shown to have a pain-relieving effect that is independent of the drug's antidepressant effects.

[h]For these medications, pain relief independent of antidepressant effects has not been shown reliably in controlled studies.

Notes

1. Preferred for managing nerve pain because of greater clinical experience with this drug.
2. Best studied drug of this class for relieving nerve pain, and therefore thought to be most reliable. Its use, however, must be balanced against the relatively greater potential for anticholinergic side effects (see note a).
3. Available as an intramuscular (IM) medication.
4. May be associated with weight gain.
5. Available in liquid formulation for oral use.
6. Is very similar to amitriptyline, and because of its lower incidence of side effects, many doctors favor its use.
7. Occasionally associated with side effects known as extrapyramidal side effects (sudden involuntary movements, such as jerking).
8. Unlike other heterocyclic antidepressants, this medication appears not to produce sedative effects and may even produce stimulation. Its use may be associated with weight loss.
9. A side effect that men should be aware of is that the drug occasionally causes unexpected or prolonged erections; should that occur, discontinue use and contact the physician.

Source. Adapted from Richard B. Patt, ed. *Cancer Pain.* Philadelphia: Lippincott, 1993. Used with permission of the author and publisher.

Table A.7. *Guidelines for the Use of Anticonvulsants in Patients*
with Chronic Cancer Pain[a]

General Name	Trade Name	Dose Range		Comments[b]
		Usual Starting Dose	Usual Dose Range	
Carbamazepine	Tegretol	100 mg twice a day	200 mg three times a day to 400 mg four times a day	1
Clonazepam	Klonopin Rivotril	0.5 mg twice a day	2 to 8 mg per day	2
Phenytoin	Dilantin Epanutine	300 mg per day	300 to 400 mg per day	3
Valproic acid	Depakene	125 mg three times a day	500 mg three times a day to 1000 mg three times a day	4
Divalproex	Depakote			

[a]When nerve pain is described as shooting, piercing, or intermittent, these medications are often prescribed. Also used for other types of nerve pain when antidepressants do not seem to help.

[b]All of these medications have a relatively high incidence of side effects as doses are increased. The most prominent side effects include mental cloudiness and sedation. Less common side effects are slurred speech, loss of muscle coordination (ataxia), unusual eye movements (nystagmus), confusion, dizziness, and nausea.

Notes

1. Often selected first because of clinical experience and effectiveness. Side effects such as dizziness, loss of muscle coordination, sedation, lethargy, and confusion are more common than with other related drugs listed in table. If started at low doses and increased gradually, side effects are minimized. Periodic monitoring of bone marrow function is usually recommended. See Chapter 8 for more detail.

2. Dizziness, sedation, and fatigue are relatively common. If used for a long time, withdrawal symptoms may occur if drug is stopped suddenly. May also relieve anxiety.

3. Gingival hyperplasia (an overgrowth of gum tissue) may occur but may be prevented or managed with regular oral hygiene measures (see Chapter 11). Other side effects may include acne or excessive hair growth.

4. May cause pancreatitis, nausea and vomiting, insomnia, headache, tremor, hair loss, weight gain, and rarely, impaired liver function.

Source: Adapted from Richard B. Patt, ed. *Cancer Pain.* Philadelphia: Lippincott, 1993. Used with permission of the author and publisher.

Table A.8. *Miscellaneous Drugs with Analgesic Potential*

Generic Name	Trade Name	Usual Dose Range	Comments
Oral Local Anesthetics/Sodium Channel Blockers			
Mexiletine	Mexitil	600–1200 mg/day	1
Tocainide	Tonocard	200–400 mg three times a day	2
Psychostimulants			
Dextroamphetamine	Dexedrine	5–20 mg every 6–12 hr	3
Methylphenidate	Ritalin	5–20 mg twice a day	3
Major Tranquilizers			
Methotrimeprazine	Levoprome	10–50 mg/4–8 hr	4
Phenothiazines	—	—	5
Anxiolytics/Antihistamines			
Hydroxyzine	Vistaril, Atarax	50–100 mg/4–6 hr	6
Antihistamines			7
Benzodiazepines			8
Miscellaneous			
Baclofen	Lioresal	20–120 mg/day	9
Nifedipine	Procardia	10–60 mg/day	10
Phenoxybenzamine	Dibenzyline	10–120 mg/day	11
Clonidine	Catapres		12
Tetrahydrocanna- binol	Marinol	5–10 mg	13

Notes

1. Frequently considered for management of nerve pain in patients who have not obtained relief from trials of antidepressants or anticonvulsants. Potential side effects include nausea, vomiting, constipation, heartbeat irregularity (cardiac arrhythmia), confusion, stuttering or stammering, unusual eye movements (nystagmus), and tremor.

2. Considered an option for nerve pain when patients have not obtained relief from trials of antidepressants, anticonvulsants, and mexiletine. Side effect profile similar to but more severe than that of mexiletine. In rare cases, drug has been associated with incidences of pneumonitis, hepatitis, and immunologic, allergic, and psychotic reactions.

3. Usually used as a stimulant to enhance alertness in patients who are sedated from the use of opioids. Although not specifically used as a pain reliever, this medication has been reported to relieve pain with some reliability. This effect together with its rapid antidepressant activity are beneficial side effects.

4. A phenothiazine, its pain-relieving effect may be as strong as that of morphine. Also good for treating nausea. Often causes sedation which may be useful for anxious patients with advanced illness who have not responded to more conventional pain relievers or who are unable to take opioids. May lower blood pressure. Not available orally.

5. With the exception of methotrimeprazine, these drugs do not seem to have any pain-relieving effect, but can be useful for their sedative and anti-nausea properties in treating agitation and vomiting.

6. An antihistamine that has been shown to have pain-relieving effects. Often administered with an opioid for acute pain and anxiety. Role in cancer pain is controversial.

7. With the exception of hydroxyzine, generally regarded as not having any pain-relieving effects, although sedation and anti-itching action may be useful.

8. Direct pain-relieving or coanalgesic activity has not been demonstrated. Well-established role in treatment of insomnia and anxiety. May have an indirect role in managing pain when complaints are presumed to stem in large part from anxiety or sleep deprivation. Should not be used as a substitute for analgesics.

Table A.8. *Miscellaneous Drugs with Analgesic Potential (Continued)*

9. This antispasmodic agent has not been studied in cancer patients but may be useful as an adjuvant (in addition to other medications) for nerve pain.

10. A calcium channel blocker, this medication has not been studied in patients with cancer pain. May be useful for certain types of headache. May cause low blood pressure upon standing suddenly or swelling in the extremities.

11. Although different from nifedipine, its action and side effects are similar.

12. A medication usually used to treat high blood pressure; may be useful in managing opioid (and nicotine) withdrawal. Experimental intraspinal use now being researched.

13. The active compound in marijuana. Ability to relieve pain is controversial. Use may be associated with mind-altering effects which some patients find undesirable. Sometimes prescribed to counter nausea and vomiting and, more recently, as an appetite stimulant.

Source: Adapted from Richard B. Patt, ed. *Cancer Pain.* Philadelphia: Lippincott, 1993. Used with permission of the author and publisher.

Table A.9. *Comparison of Selected Corticosteroids*[a]

Generic Name	Approximate Duration	Equivalent Dose	Relative Anti-inflammatory Action
Short Duration	12 hr		
Cortisone		25	0.8
Hydrocortisone		20	1
Intermediate Duration	12–36 hr		
Prednisone		5	4
Prednisolone		5	4
Methylprednisolone		4	5
Triamcinalone		4	5
Long Duration	48 hr		
Paramethasone		2	10
Dexamethasone		0.75	25
Betamethasone		0.6	25

[a]Based on oral administration. Steroidal anti-inflammatories (as opposed to the non-steroidal anti-inflammatories, the NSAIDs) may relieve pain by reducing inflammation and swelling. May also reduce nausea as well as boost mood and appetite.

Source: Adapted from Richard B. Patt, ed. *Cancer Pain.* Philadelphia: Lippincott, 1993. Used with permission of the author and publisher.

Glossary

absolute alcohol   A chemical substance commonly used in semipermanent nerve blocks. It is intended to relieve certain pains for a period of months but may injure nerves indiscriminately and so this and phenol, a chemical substance also often used for this purpose, are used with caution to avoid complications and unwanted results. See **nerve block; neurolytic drugs.**

acute pain   Pain stemming directly from an injury. This pain is usually sharp and easily identified by its source. Many of its features contrast with those of chronic pain. See **chronic pain.**

addiction   Psychological craving for a drug; the need to obtain and use a drug for nonmedical reasons overwhelms and controls the addict's life, despite the risk of harm. Extremely rare in the cancer patient, but still feared by patient and doctor alike. Distinct from **tolerance** and **physical dependence.**

adjuvant medications   Medications prescribed to enhance the pain-relieving effects of painkillers or to relieve the side effects of medications. Also known as **co-analgesics.**

alopecia   A condition in which one's hair falls out. Sometimes associated with chemotherapy or radiation therapy.

analgesics   Medications that relieve pain.

anesthesia dolorosa   A painful numbness occurring in a small proportion of patients after a destructive (neurolytic) nerve block, especially after a **peripheral nerve block.**

anorexia   A condition in which one has a reduced appetite.

anti-emetic   Any drug that helps relieve vomiting and nausea.

asthenia   A condition in which the patient experiences overall weakness.

a-t-c   A prescription to take a medication at scheduled intervals, "around-the-clock," not as needed (prn).

b.i.d.   An abbreviation used with prescriptions, meaning to take a drug twice a day.

biopsy   A procedure to remove a small bit of tissue from a growth to have it analyzed and to determine whether the growth is harmless or cancerous. Depending on the tumor's location, surgery may be involved or the procedure may be performed in a doctor's office with only a needle. General anesthesia may be necessary or just a local anesthetic.

bolus An "escape" or "rescue" dose. An extra dose of medication to take as needed (prn) to relieve pain that breaks through despite medication that is given at regularly scheduled intervals.

bradycardia A condition in which the heart beats slowly, under 60 beats per minute. Opposite of **tachycardia.**

cachexia A condition in which the patient experiences significant weight loss and weakness.

cancer Any of 100 different diseases in which a mass of abnormal tissue grows uncontrollably with the potential to spread throughout the body.

catheter A tiny tube. In cancer patients, it is used to administer intraspinal morphine easily to the patient. The tube is left in place, usually in the back.

ceiling dose A dose beyond which a drug will do no further good. Aspirin and acetamenophin, for example, have ceiling, or maximum, doses; morphine and other opioids do not.

central nerve block An injection within the spinal canal, between two of the spinal bones. May be an **epidural** or **spinal injection.**

chemotherapy A therapy for cancer in which drugs (including hormones) are administered intravenously or less often orally.

chronic pain A pain that has persisted for four months or longer. Rather than being sharp and easy to locate, it tends to be dull and achy and often cannot be pinpointed. Treating this kind of pain often requires a combination of medical and psychological approaches.

cingulotomy A relatively safe, promising form of neurosurgery for pain when excessive depression or anxiety persists or when drug use is excessive.

co-analgesic See **adjuvant.**

cryoablation A type of semipermanent nerve block in which the needle tip is frozen to relieve pain. Such blocks are used less often than blocks with **absolute alcohol** or **phenol.**

debulking Refers to surgery that reduces the size of a tumor, as opposed to removing the entire tumor. It may render certain tumors more responsive to chemotherapy or radiation.

deep brain stimulation (thalamic stimulation) A procedure in which a tiny electrode is placed in the brain to relieve pain; it is still considered experimental.

dependence Also called physical dependence, a common and natural result of the body growing used to a medication, particularly an opioid such as morphine. If the drug were suddenly stopped, the patient would undergo physical problems associated with withdrawal (also

A permanent catheter with one end that leaves the
|omen to be connected to an external pump, which
|ation.

of pain An explanation of how electrical stimulation
|s block the sensation of pain.

| used with prescriptions, meaning to take a medication

|ation for intramuscular, meaning to take a medication
|jection in muscle tissue.

id therapy A technique, which may be **epidural** (or **in-**
l or **subarachnoid**), in which morphine (or another opioid)
| directly near their receptors in the spine. Only tiny amounts
|ded, and usually pain relief is potent, but with few side ef-
|An invasive but efficient means of delivering medication.

(or **subarachnoid** or **spinal**) **morphine** A procedure in which
|pain-relieving medication is mixed with the spinal fluid; since
|s procedure brings the medication close to the drug receptors in
| spine, even less morphine is needed than with epidural mor-
|ine.

a A condition in which there is not enough blood getting to cell
|tissue, often producing pain.

|he abbreviation for intravenous, meaning to take medication or nu-
|trition through a tube (catheter) or by injection in the vein.

anesthetic nerve block A procedure to temporarily relieve pain in
which a medication that causes numbing is injected near a nerve or
in the painful area. Novocaine is the most well-known medication
used for this purpose, but longer acting drugs, such as lidocaine and
bupivicaine, are now more commonly used.

umbar puncture A procedure in which a needle is introduced between
two bones of the spine to remove a small amount of spinal fluid for
diagnostic purposes or to inject medication for anesthesia.

malignancy A growth of abnormal cells that has been determined to be
cancerous; unless treated, the growth will continue to grow at the
expense of healthy cells.

meningitis A serious infection near the spine that occasionally occurs with
intraspinal opioid therapy. It can usually be treated with hospitalization and intravenous antibiotics; surgery, however, may sometimes
be necessary.

metastasis The process by which cancer cells spread from the original site
of the tumor to other areas of the body; cancer growths that have
spread from their original site are called **metastases.**

called abstinence '
of the drug '

destructive b'
manent .
just puttii
destroyed. .

diaphoresis   A con
ing.

diagnostic nerve block
formed specifically
locate which nerves

diuretic   A medication that .
help breathing difficult.

drug receptors   Places on the
phine receptors are mostly .
cord. Like a lock and key,
type of drug.

dura   The sac that contains the spinal

dysphagia   Difficulty in swallowing.

dysphoria   A mental state in which the ;
pleasant sense of not feeling like ones

dyspnea   Difficulty in breathing.

epidural abscess   An infection near the spine t
intraspinal opioid therapy.

epidural injection   An injection within the spina.
sac (dura) that contains the spinal cord and
(cerebrospinal fluid or CSF). Temporary or lt
tions of this type are commonly used for laboi
pain. Steroid injections may be used for back pain
tered epidurally. Alcohol and phenol are injected o.
in the epidural area. See **epidural morphine**.

epidural morphine   One type of intraspinal opioid therapy. M.
another opioid) is administered into the epidural space, u.
continuous basis through a **catheter**.

equianalgesic doses   The necessary doses of different drugs to p.
equivalent painkilling effect.

escape dose   Also called a rescue dose. See **bolus**.

external pump   The type of pump used to give morphine intravenously
subcutaneously, or intraspinally; the device can be hooked to a temporary or implanted catheter for home use. Usually portable and battery driven; family can operate but requires supervision by a nurse
or doctor.

externalized catheter
skin of the abc
delivers medic

gate control theory
can sometim

h.s.   Abbreviation
at bedtime

IM   An abbrevi
through i

intraspinal opi
trathec:
is given
are ne
fects.

intrathecal
the
thi
th
p

ischem

IV   T

loca

mg The abbreviation for milligrams, meaning one-thousandth of a gram. A unit of measurement for many medical prescriptions.

microgram One-millionth of a gram; abbreviated μg.

ml The abbreviation for milliliter, a liquid unit, meaning one-thousandth of a liter.

morphine An opioid medication; the first drug of choice for severe cancer pain.

myelogram A diagnostic X-ray procedure involving an injection of X-ray dye into the spinal fluid.

myelopathy An injury to the nerves in the spinal cord.

narcotic medications A group of drugs used for severe cancer pain. Morphine is the most common of these for severe cancer pain. See **opioids.**

neoplasms Abnormal growths comprised of cells that are different from normal cells. Neoplasms (meaning "new growths") may be harmless (benign) or cancerous (malignant).

nerve block A procedure involving an injection near a nerve to produce numbness and relieve pain. There are many different types of nerve blocks. See **local anesthetic nerve block.**

neuroablation See **nerve block; neurolytic drugs.**

neurolytic drugs Chemical substances used in semipermanent nerve blocks. Since these substances may injure nerves indiscriminately, they must be used carefully to avoid paralysis. A commonly used substance for this procedure is alcohol or phenol.

neuropathic pain Pain that stems from a damaged nerve; it is usually burning, tingling, numbing, or itching in character.

neuropathy Damage to nerves.

nociception The process of pain transmission; usually related to a pain receptor.

nociceptor A nerve receptor that responds to a painful injury.

oncology The study or science of cancer; a person who specializes in the study of cancer is an **oncologist.**

opiate See **opioid; narcotic medications.**

opioid Narcotic painkiller, the most common of which is morphine; the drug of choice for severe or chronic pain. A person taking these drugs often develops physiological conditions known as **physical dependence** and **tolerance** which have nothing to do with **addiction** and can be easily treated.

pain threshold The point at which a sensation or stimulus is perceived to be painful. Pain thresholds differ among individuals and even in the same individual over time.

pain tolerance   How much pain a person is willing or able to endure. Pain tolerance may be lowered by factors such as fatigue, anxiety, fear, depression, boredom, mental isolation, and anger, and raised by sleep, rest, symptom relief, sympathy, understanding, medications, and diversions.

palliative care   Medical care that focuses on the comfort of the patient when a cure is not a realistic goal.

p.c.   An abbreviation used with prescriptions, meaning to take a medication after meals.

PCA   An abbreviation for patient-controlled analgesia. With this form of care, the patient may control the timing of medication; it may refer to an oral medication or a pump system in which the doctor has pre-programmed the amount and frequency of doses of pain-killer.

percutaneous cordotomy   Similar to a nerve block, but usually performed by a neurosurgeon. A needle is advanced between two of the spinal bones and directly into the spinal cord where a small hole is burnt. A very effective method for relieving pain on one side of the body below the mid-chest.

peripheral nerve block   An injection to relieve pain that involves a nerve in the periphery, meaning one of the nerves that is not part of the spinal cord.

permanent catheter   A more durable spinal catheter implanted under the skin for long-term use. With this method, there is less chance of infection and less chance that the tube will become dislodged.

"permanent" nerve block   A term used to describe injections of neurolytic substances because these substances injure nerves involved in the transmission of pain. There are no truly permanent nerve blocks, because even after they are destroyed, most nerves will grow back, usually within three to six months.

phenol   See **absolute alcohol.**

physical dependence   An expected physical condition which results from the continued use of some medications, such as opioids. If medication were suddenly stopped, flu-like symptoms (withdrawal) would occur. Distinct from **addiction** and **tolerance.**

pituitary ablation   A procedure in which a few drops of alcohol are introduced into the pituitary gland to relieve bone pain, especially from breast or prostate cancer. This procedure is performed only in a few cancer pain centers.

PO   An abbreviation used with prescriptions, meaning to take a medication by mouth.

pr   An abbreviation used with prescriptions, meaning to take a medication, usually a suppository, through the rectum.

prn   An abbreviation used with prescriptions, meaning to take medication "as needed" as opposed to scheduled intervals (around-the-clock or **a-t-c**). Discouraged as the sole means to treat pain, especially when it is constant (chronic) pain.

prognosis   The doctor's determination of what the outcome of an illness will be. This is an inexact "science" in diseases of cancer.

prognostic (predictive) nerve block   A temporary or local anesthetic block that is performed specifically to predict the results of a more permanent block. Determining how much of the pain is relieved, whether there are side effects, and if the patient prefers the numbness that comes with the procedure, all help the patient and doctor decide whether or not a more permanent nerve block is recommended as a means of relieving pain.

pruritis   A condition marked by excessive itching.

pseudo-addiction   A drug-seeking behavior that is often construed as a psychological craving for a medication, usually an opioid such as morphine, but in fact is the result of undermedication and the desire for pain relief.

psychosurgery   Procedures in which brain pathways are disrupted so that pain is not felt by the patient, though it still exists—in other words, the perception of pain is changed. It has been almost abandoned because of the frequency of undesirable personality changes. See **cingulotomy.**

q.i.d.   An abbreviation used with prescriptions, meaning to take a medication four times a day (in a 24-hour period).

q3h   An abbreviation used with prescriptions, meaning to take a medication every 3 hours.

q4h   An abbreviation used with prescriptions, meaning to take a medication every 4 hours.

radiation therapy   A therapy for cancer that uses a type of X-ray to kill or shrink tumors. Such therapy is prescribed by a medical specialist, usually a radiation oncologist.

rescue dose   Also known as an escape dose. See **bolus.**

sequential drug trial   Treatment with a series of different analgesics, undertaken to determine the best medicine for a particular person. Should be conducted prior to trying more invasive treatments.

singultus   A condition marked by excessive hiccoughing. May occur with brain tumors and stomach or chest tumors.

spinal cord stimulation   A procedure in which an electrode is surgically placed in the epidural space to relieve pain; used mostly for pain due to causes other than cancer.

spinal injection A procedure in which a needle is advanced through the epidural space into the sac containing the spinal cord and its surrounding fluid. Local anesthetics are often administered in this manner, primarily for cesarean section and for other (not just minor) surgery. Morphine, or another opioid, may be administered here to provide pain relief in special circumstances but requires the placement of a catheter (a tiny tube) for long-term relief. (See also **intrathecal morphine.**) In special cases, a qualified doctor (an anesthesiologist) may use an injection of alcohol or phenol in the spine to destroy selected nerves for long-term relief. See also **absolute alcohol.**

spinal morphine See **intrathecal morphine.**

spinal port Instead of exiting from the skin of the abdomen, the other end of this catheter is attached to a silicone bubble left under the skin. A pump is then attached to the port through a tiny needle that is changed weekly.

spinal pump An implanted pump—Infusaid™, Synchromed™, or Medtronic™ pump—that may be computerized and inserted under the skin to give morphine through a permanent catheter. The device only needs to be refilled every 1 to 2 months and can be adjusted with a special laptop computer. It is very costly and cannot be reused, and so is only recommended for special cases.

spinal tap A diagnostic procedure in which a needle is introduced between two bones of the spine to remove a small amount of spinal fluid.

stat A medical abbreviation meaning immediately.

subarachnoid morphine See **intrathecal morphine.**

subcutaneous Abbreviated SQ or sub-q, meaning just below the surface of the skin. It usually refers to a way to take a medication—that is, through a needle positioned under the surface of the skin.

tachycardia A condition in which the heart beats rapidly; usually applied to rates faster than 100 beats per minute. Opposite of **bradycardia.**

t.i.d. An abbreviation used with prescriptions, meaning to take a medication 3 times a day.

temporary catheter Not everyone receives adequate relief from intraspinal morphine, so a temporary tube or catheter is usually taped to the back for a trial period before a more permanent one is inserted. If someone is very sick, the temporary catheter can be left in indefinitely, although there is some risk of infection.

temporary nerve block A local anesthetic that is injected to make a nerve or nerves inactive to pain. The effect of the medication is temporary, although sometimes long lasting pain relief can result after one or several temporary blocks. Sometimes a steroid is added to reduce inflammation around a nerve that is irritated.

TENS unit (transcutaneous electrical stimulation) A simple, portable device the size of a beeper which delivers gentle shocks to the skin to relieve pain. It is not effective for severe pain.

therapeutic nerve block A nerve block that is not just diagnostic or prognostic, but that may relieve pain for some time.

thermoablation A type of nerve block in which the needle tip is heated to relieve pain. Such blocks are used less often than those with alcohol or phenol. See **cryoablation**.

thrompocytopenia A condition that may occur with cancer or after radiation treatment or chemotherapy in which spontaneous bleeding or greater than normal bleeding may affect the patient because of low platelet count.

titration An adjustment to a dose of a medication for a particular patient at a particular time.

tolerance A condition in which a patient will need larger doses of a drug over time to receive the same relief. It is an expected effect of using opioids and is unrelated to addiction. Distinct from **physical dependence** and **addiction**.

transcutaneous electrical stimulation See **TENS unit**.

Selected Bibliography

For the General Consumer

American Cancer Society and National Cancer Institute. *Questions and Answers About Pain Control: A Guide for People with Cancer and Their Families.* New York: American Cancer Society, 1992.

Cancer Pain: A Monograph on the Management of Cancer Pain. A Report of the Expert Advisory Committee on the Management of Severe Chronic Pain in Cancer Patients. Canada: Minister of Supply and Services, 1987. (Cat. No. H42-2/5-1984E.)

Melzack, Ronald. "The Tragedy of Needless Pain," *Scientific American,* Vol. 262, No. 2, February 1990, pp. 27–33.

National Public Radio. *Pain and Medicine.* Cassette tape, #ME-890503, 1989.

Public Health Service, National Institutes of Health. *Relieving Pain.* Washington, D.C.: U.S. Department of Health and Human Services, 1988.

Swedlow, Mark, and Vittorio Ventrafridda, eds. *Cancer Pain.* Lancaster, England: MTP Press Ltd., 1987.

Twycross, Robert, and Sylvia Lack. *Oral Morphine: Information for Patients, Families and Friends.* Beaconsfield, Bucks, England: Beaconsfield Publishers, Ltd., 1987. (Revised edition, 1991.)

Walsh, T. Declan. *Common Misunderstandings About the Use of Morphine for Chronic Pain in Advanced Cancer.* New York: American Cancer Society, 1985. (Reprinted from *Ca-A Cancer Journal for Clinicians,* Vol. 35, No. 3, 1985.)

World Health Organization. *Cancer Pain Relief.* Geneva: World Health Organization, 1986.

World Health Organization. *Cancer Pain Relief and Palliative Care.* Geneva: World Health Organization, 1990. Technical Report Series 804.

Yasko, Joyce M., and Patricia Greene. *Coping with Problems Related to Cancer and Cancer Treatment.* New York: American Cancer Society, 1987.

For the Technical Reader

Abram, Stephen E., ed. *Cancer Pain.* Boston: Kluwer, 1989.

Aronoff, Gerald M., and Wayne O. Evans. *Handbook on the Rational Use of Medication for Pain.* New York: Delacorte, 1987.

Cassell, Eric. *The Nature of Suffering.* New York: Oxford University Press, 1991.

Enck, Robert E. *The Management of Terminally Ill Patients*. Baltimore: Johns Hopkins University Press, 1993.

Foley, Kathleen M., J. J. Bonica, V. Ventafridda, and M. V. Callaway, eds. *Advances in Pain Research and Therapy, Volume 16: Proceedings of the Second International Congress on Cancer Pain*. New York: Raven Press, 1990.

Foley, Kathleen M., course director. *Management of Cancer Pain: Syllabus of the Postgraduate Course, Memorial Sloan-Kettering Cancer Center*, November 14–16, 1985. New York: Memorial Sloan-Kettering Cancer Center, 1985.

Janssen Pharmaceutica. *Pain Management Refined: New Approaches*. Faculty Review Meeting, May 20, 1992.

Kanner, Ronald. *Diagnosis and Management of Pain in Patients with Cancer*. Basel, Switzerland: S. Karger AG, 1988.

Patt, Richard B., ed. *Cancer Pain*. Philadelphia, Pa.: Lippincott, 1993.

Queen's Medical Center Cancer Institute. *Cancer Pain Can Be Relieved*. Pain Management Conference, March 6, 1992.

Ventafridda, Vittorio. "Continuing Care: A Major Issue in Cancer Pain Management," *Pain*, Vol. 36, 1989, pp. 137–143.

For Part I

Breura, Eduardo. "Continuing Challenges in the Management of Cancer Pain," *Oncology* (Special Supplement), August 1989.

Brigden, Malcolm, and Jeffrey B. Barnett. "A Practical Approach to Improving Pain Control in Cancer Patients," *Western Journal of Medicine*, Vol. 146, No. 5, May 1987, pp. 580–584.

"Cancer Pain and the War on Drugs." Special issue of *American Journal of Hospice & Palliative Care*, Vol. 8, No. 6, November/December 1991.

Cleeland, Charles S. "Barriers to the Management of Cancer Pain," *Oncology* (Special Supplement), April 1987, pp. 19–25.

Cleeland, Charles S. "The Impact of Pain on the Patient with Cancer," *Cancer*, Vol. 54, No. 11, December 1, 1984, pp. 2635–2641.

Daut, Randall L., and Charles S. Cleeland. "The Prevalence and Severity of Pain in Cancer," *Cancer*, Vol. 50, No. 9, November 1, 1982, pp. 1913–1918.

Deschamps, Michele, Pierre R. Band, and Andrew J. Coldman. "Assessment of Adult Cancer Pain: Shortcomings of Current Methods," *Pain*, Vol. 32, 1988, pp. 133–139.

Enck, Robert E. "Understanding Tolerance, Physical Dependence and Addiction in the Use of Opioid Analgesics," *American Journal of Hospice & Palliative Care*, January/February 1991, pp. 9–11.

Ferrer-Brechner, Theresa. "Treating Cancer Pain as a Disease." In C. Benedettei et al., eds., *Advances in Pain Research and Therapy*, Volume 7. New York: Raven Press, 1984, pp. 575–591.

Fishman, Baruch, et al. "The Memorial Pain Assessment Card," *Cancer*, Vol. 60, 1987, pp. 1151–1158.

Foley, Kathleen M. "The Cancer Pain Patient," *Journal of Pain and Symptom Management*, Vol. 3, No. 1, Winter 1988, pp. S16–S19.

Hill, C. Stratton, Jr., "A Call to Action to Improve Relief of Cancer Pain." In C. Stratton Hill, Jr. and W. S. Fields, eds., *Advances in Pain Research and Therapy, Volume 22.* New York: Raven Press, 1989, pp. 353–361.

Hill, C. Stratton, Jr., "Opinion: Narcotics and Cancer Pain Control," *Ca-A Cancer Journal for Clinicians* (A Journal of the American Cancer Society), Vol. 38, No. 6, November/December 1988, pp. 322–326.

Hill, C. Stratton, Jr., "Relationship among Cultural, Educational, and Regulatory Agency Influences on Optimum Cancer Pain Treatment," *Journal of Pain and Symptom Management,* Vol. 5, No. 1 (Supplement), February 1990, pp. 537–545.

Posner, Robert B. "Physician-Patient Communication," *American Journal of Medicine,* Vol. 77 (Supplement), September 10, 1984, pp. 59–64.

Liebeskind, John C. "Pain *Can* Kill," *Pain,* Vol. 44, 1991, pp. 3–4.

For Part II

American Pain Society. *Principles of Analgesic Use in the Treatment of Acute Pain and Cancer Pain,* 3rd ed. Skokie, Ill.: American Pain Society, 1992.

Berry, Joni I. "The Use of Analgesics: In Patients with Pain from Terminal Disease," *American Journal of Hospice Care,* September/October 1988, pp. 26–42.

Enck, Robert E. "Complications in Pain Management," *American Journal of Hospice & Palliative Care,* November/December 1990.

"Management of Cancer Pain," Special Issue of *Cancer* (A Journal of the American Cancer Society), Vol. 63, No. 11, June 11, 1989.

Patt, Richard B. "Control of Pain Associated with Advanced Malignancy." In G. M. Aronoff, ed., *Evaluation and Treatment of Chronic Pain,* 2nd ed. Baltimore: Williams and Wilkins, 1992, pp. 213–339.

Patt, Richard B. "Interventional Analgesia: Epidural and Subarachnoid Therapy," *American Journal of Hospice Care,* Vol. 6, 1989, pp. 11–14.

Patt, Richard B. "Nonpharmacologic Measures for Controlling Oncologic Pain," *American Journal of Hospice & Palliative Care,* Vol. 7, 1990, pp. 30–37.

Patt, Richard B. "PCA: Prescribing Analgesia for Home Management of Severe Pain," *Geriatrics,* Vol. 47, 1992, pp. 69–84.

Patt, Richard B. "Pain Therapy." In E. A. M. Frost, ed., *Clinical Anesthesia in Neurosurgery,* 2nd ed. Boston: Butterworth, 1990.

Patt, Richard B., and J. Loughner. "Management of Pain in the Cancer Patient." In S. Rosenthal, J. R. Carignan, B. D. Smith, eds., *Medical Care of the Cancer Patient,* 2nd ed. Philadelphia: Saunders, 1992, pp. 255–264.

Patt, Richard B., and Subhash Jain. "Recent Advances in the Management of Oncologic Pain," *Current Problems in Cancer,* Vol. XIII, No. 3, May/June 1989.

Payne, Richard. "Novel Routes of Opioid Administration in the Management of Cancer Pain," *Oncology* (Special Supplement), April 1987, pp. 10–17.

Portenoy, Russell K. "Drug Therapy for Cancer Pain," *American Journal of Hospice & Palliative Care,* November/December 1990, pp. 10–19.

Portenoy, Russell K. "Management of Pain in Patients with Advanced Cancer," *Resident & Staff Physician*, April 1987, pp. 59–66.

Portenoy, Russell K. "Practical Aspects of Pain Control in the Patient with Cancer," *Ca-A Cancer Journal for Clinicians* (A Journal of the American Cancer Society), Vol. 38, No. 6., November/December 1988, pp. 327–352.

Portenoy, Russell K., and Steven D. Waldman. "Recent Advances in the Management of Cancer Pain: Pharmacologic Approaches," *Pain Management*, May/June 1991, pp. 10–24.

Twycross, Robert, and Sylvia Lack. *Oral Morphine in Advanced Cancer*, Beaconsfield, Bucks, England: Beaconsfield Publishers Ltd., 1984.

Waldman, S. D., and Richard B. Patt. "Guide to the Clinical Use of Controlled-Release Morphine and Transdermal Fentanyl," *Pain Digest*, Vol. 2, 1992, pp. 200–206.

Walsh, T. Declan. *Common Misunderstandings About the Use of Morphine for Chronic Pain in Advanced Cancer*. New York: American Cancer Society, 1985. (Reprinted from *Ca-A Cancer Journal for Clinicians*, Vol. 35., No. 3, 1985.)

Walsh, T. Declan. "Symptom Control in Patients with Advanced Cancer," *American Journal of Hospice & Palliative Care*, November/December 1990.

Yasko, Joyce M., and Patricia Greene. *Coping with Problems Related to Cancer and Cancer Treatment*. New York: American Cancer Society, 1987.

For Part III

Acute Pain Management Guideline Panel. *Acute Pain Management: Operative or Medical Procedures and Trauma. Clinical Practice Guideline*. AHCPR Pub No. 92-0032. Rockville, Md.: Agency for Health Care Policy and Research, Public Health Service, U.S. Department of Health and Human Services, February 1992.

Anderson, Patricia. *Affairs in Order: A Complete Resource Guide to Death and Dying*. New York: Macmillan, 1991.

Bailey, Lucanne M. "The Role of Music Therapy." In *Management of Cancer Pain: Syllabus of the Postgraduate Course, Memorial Sloan-Kettering Cancer Center*. November 14–16, 1985. New York: Memorial Sloan Kettering Cancer Center: 1985.

Barkwell, Diana P. "Ascribed Meaning: A Critical Factor in Coping and Pain Attenuation in Patients with Cancer-Related Pain," *Journal of Palliative Care*, Vol. 7, No. 3, 1991.

Borysenko, Joan. "Behavioral Considerations in the Development and Management of Cancer," *Resident & Staff Physician*, Vol. 33, No. 1, January 1987.

Cleeland, Charles. "Psychological Aspects of Pain Due to Cancer," *Cancer Pain*. Boston: Kluwer, 1988.

Coyle, Nessa, Jean Adelhardt, Kathleen Foley, and Russell Portenoy. "Character of Terminal Illness in the Advanced Cancer Patient: Pain and Other Symptoms During the Last Four Weeks of Life," *Journal of Pain and Symptom Control*, Vol. 5, No. 2, April 1990, pp. 83–93.

Davidson, Paul. "Facilitating Coping with Cancer Pain," *Palliative Medicine*, Vol. 2, 1988, pp. 107–114.

Droughton, Mary Lynn. "Head and Neck Carcinomas," *Journal of Palliative Care*, Vol. 6, No. 4, 1990, pp. 43–46.

Enck, Robert E. "Delirium: Diagnosis and Management," *American Journal of Hospice & Palliative Care*, January/February 1988, pp. 17–19.

Enck, Robert E. "The Management of Large Fungating Tumors (Malignant Ulceration)," *American Journal of Hospice & Palliative Care*, May/June 1990, pp. 11–12.

Gaylin, Willard. " 'Doctors Must Not Kill,' " *Journal of the American Medical Association*, Vol. 259, No. 14, April 8, 1988, pp. 2139–2140.

Goleman, Daniel, and Joel Gurin, eds. *Mind/Body Medicine: How To Use Your Mind for Better Health*. Yonkers, N.Y.: Consumer Reports Books, 1993.

Jay, Susan M., Charles H. Elliott, Ernest Katz, and Stuart E. Siegel. "Cognitive-Behavioral and Pharmacologic Interventions for Children's Distress During Painful Medical Procedures," *Journal of Consulting and Clinical Psychology*, Vol. 55, No. 6, 1987, pp. 860–865.

Krant, Melvin. "The Adult with Cancer: In Preparation for Death," *Resident and Staff Physician*, May 1982, pp. 89–93.

Lloyd, Chris, and Laura Coggles. "Contribution of Occupational Therapy to Pain Management in Cancer Patients with Metastatic Breast Disease," *American Journal of Hospice Care*, November/December 1988, pp. 36–38.

Lundberg, George D. " 'It's Over, Debbie' and the Euthanasia Debate," *Journal of the American Medical Association*, Vol. 259, No. 14, April 8, 1988, pp. 2142–2143.

Martin, Edward W. "Confusion in the Terminally Ill: Recognition and Management," *American Journal of Hospice & Palliative Care*, May/June 1990, pp. 20–24.

Miser, Angela W. "Assessment and Treatment of Pain in Children with Cancer," *Anesthesia Progress*, Vol. 34, 1987, pp. 113–127.

Patt, Richard B. "Non-Pharmacologic Measures for Controlling Oncologic Pain," *American Journal of Hospice & Palliative Care*, November/December 1990.

Pronsati, Michelle P. "PTs Provide Human Link in Cancer Treatment," *PT Advance for Physical Therapists*, Vol. 1, No. 4, May 7, 1990.

Ritchie, Karen. "Guilt and the Cancer Patient," *Cancer Bulletin*, Vol. 43, No. 5, 1991, pp. 430–432.

Roy, David J. "Need They Sleep Before They Die?" *Journal of Palliative Care*, Vol. 6, No. 3, 1990, pp. 3–4.

Rhymes, Jill. "Hospice Care in America," *Journal of the American Medical Association*, Vol. 264, No. 3, July 18, 1990, pp. 369–372.

Sankar, Andrea. *Dying at Home: A Family Guide for Caregiving*. Baltimore: Johns Hopkins University Press, 1991.

Schwartz, Lauren, Mark Slater, Gary Birchler, and J. Hampton Atkinson. "Depression in Spouses of Chronic Pain Patients: The Role of Patient Pain and Anger, and Marital Satisfaction," *Pain*, Vol. 44, 1991, pp. 61–67.

Siegal, Tali. "Muscle Cramps in the Cancer Patient: Causes and Treatment," *Journal of Pain and Symptom Control*, Vol. 6, No. 2, February 1991, pp. 84–91.

Tennant, Forest J., Jr., "Management of Patients Dependent upon Prescription Opioids," *Resident and Staff Physician*, April 1986, pp. 41–47.

Thorpe, Deborah M. "Sleep Disturbances in the Cancer Patient," *The Cancer Bulletin*, Vol. 43, No. 5, 1991, pp. 393–396.

Vachon, Mary L. S. "Counselling and Psychotherapy in Palliative/Hospice Care: A Review," *Palliative Medicine*, Vol. 2, 1988, pp. 36–50.

Varni, James W. "Acute and Chronic Pain in Adults and Children with Cancer," *Journal of Consulting and Clinical Psychology*, Vol. 54, No. 5, 1986, pp. 601–607.

Vaux, Kenneth L., "Debbie's Dying: Mercy Killing and the Good Death," *Journal of the American Medical Association*, Vol. 259, No. 14. April 8, 1988, pp. 2140–2141.

Wall, Patrick D., and Mervyn Jones. *Defeating Pain*, New York: Plenum Press: 1991.

Index